My Garden of Flowers
What the Professionals are Saying

"*My Garden of Flowers* is a unique book documenting the career of a remarkable first-generation neonatologist. Dr Kaur has captured the history of neonatology together with the trials and triumphs of her NICU patients. Beautifully illustrated, with wonderful testimonials and poetry, this is a fantastic resource for families and healthcare providers."
— *Avroy Fanaroff, MD, Emeritus Eliza Henry Barnes Professor of Neonatology, Rainbow Babies & Children's Hospital, Emeritus Professor of Pediatrics, Case Western Reserve University School of Medicine, Cleveland, Ohio*

"Beautifully written and illustrated, *My Garden of Flowers* recounts the NICU experiences of parents whose infants received care from Dr. Manjeet Kaur. The parents' stories are uplifting, and I encourage all care providers who work in the NICU to read them."
— *Richard A. Polin, MD, Director, Division of Neonatology, New York Presbyterian Hospital, Professor of Pediatrics, Columbia University, New York*

"Dr. Kaur's amazing and rich history of caring for vulnerable neonates is truly a legacy, as this book illustrates. Filled with vivid and tender stories, photos, and images, one sees her garden of the precious lives of her NICU graduates and their families. This is an essential resource for both providers and parents. The heartwarming stories from former NICU families indeed provide an emotional connection to help other parents overcome obstacles and gain strength."
— *Mope Akintorin, MD, Chair, Division of Neonatology, Cook County Health and Hospital, Chicago, Illinois*

"*My Garden of Flowers* is a true labor of love with its touching accounts of the journeys of the tiny babies and their families in the NICU and beyond. Dr Kaur's passion and lifelong dedication is exquisitely captured on every page — especially in the poems composed for and dedicated to her tiny patients. This book provides NICU families an instant support system that identifies with every roller-coaster moment they experience. The simple diagrams and explanations of common medical problems and terminology is an invaluable reference for parents navigating the complex and often prolonged NICU stay. *My Garden*

of Flowers is inspirational not just for families but also for the medical staff; it serves as a reminder of why we do what we do every day. We are blessed to see miracles daily, and the true superheroes are these babies and their families!"

— *Monika Bhola, MD, Associate Professor of Pediatrics, Rainbow Babies and Children's Hospital, University Hospital Cleveland Medical Center, Cleveland, Ohio*

"One rarely finds a book that offers such hope, miracles, and love. *My Garden of Flowers* shows us how precious life is, and makes the parents' emotional difficulties while on the NICU journey a little easier. I loved reading what the families were feeling; their real-life examples take us on the journey with them. Also great are the illustrations and medical terms that families may expect to encounter in the NICU. I recommend this book to anyone who has been touched by the hope for survival, the miracle of life, and the love for each other and a neonate."

— *Margi Bowers, MSN, MHA, RN, NE-BC, Nurse Manager NICU, Penn Medicine, Lancaster General Health Women & Babies Hospital*

"This very moving book brought tears to my eyes. It's a must read for all parents with premature babies. Well written and easy to understand, it lets us follow a deeply committed neonatologist as she chronicles the development of the neonatal ICU, and shows us how the care for very premature infants has evolved. The commitment of the staff who work in these units inspires confidence and provides realistic reassurance to the parents who find themselves in this difficult time. It warmed my heart to read about the reunions and the achievements of the neonatal grads. Many will draw strength from this chronicle."

— *Nikki H. Chawla, MD, Pediatrician, Seminole, Oklahoma*

"Doctor Kaur is not only clearly skilled in caring for the sickest of newborn babies but is also extremely adept at telling the poignant and touching stories of those fragile children for whom she has provided that care. This book is a jewel and an essential tool for families who are facing a NICU admission. It offers hope and support during the most stressful event in their lives, provides a wealth of information, and is an incredible resource for an often unexpected and occasionally terrifying journey through the bewildering experience of having a critically ill newborn. I applaud Doctor Kaur's skill, faith, insights, and hope, which she instills in those whom she touches, both in her life and through her words."

— *Brent D. Wright, MD-PhD, Ob-Gyn, Mendocino Coast District Hospital, Fort Bragg, California*

"A devoted and loving neonatologist shares the treasury of photos, newspaper clips, and personal stories of patient successes collected during her thirty years of leadership. *My Garden of Flowers* is for families of children about to enter, already in, or graduated from a NICU. Dr. Kaur's long-term contact with families allows us a hopeful view into the future for many of these children— among them a successful cellist and a noted sports figure. The doctor's own moving poetry is dispersed throughout. The book also provides a practical orientation to the procedures used to care for common disorders of high-risk neonates. There are helpful diagrams, growth tables, nutritional information, a list of support groups, and a glossary. In all, this is a stimulating and inspirational treatise by a physician in love with her rewarding career."

  — *Jeanette R. Pleasure, MD, neonatologist; Former Clinical Professor at UC Davis*

"Dr. Kaur reminds us of how miracles occur through the power of community, dedication, and love. *My Garden of Flowers* provides comfort and inspiration for healthcare providers and the families of preterm infants."

  — *Jochen Profit, MD, MPH Assoc. Professor of Pediatrics and Neonatology, Stanford University, Lucile Packard Children's Hospital*

"The collection of family stories in *My Garden of Flowers* can provide parents comfort and support in the NICU and in life beyond it. At CHEO, we're also proud that Dr. Kaur's training here inspired her to pursue a career in neonatology— improving the lives of all the families in this book and many, many more."

  — *JoAnn Harrold, Director MD, Division of Neonatology, Children's Hospital of Eastern Ontario, Ottawa, Canada*

What the Parents are Saying

"As the mother of a micro-preemie, I was profoundly touched by *My Garden of Flowers.* It will provide great hope and reassurance to new NICU families. I founded Hand to Hold to ensure that NICU families know they're not alone on their journey. Through her book, Dr. Kaur shares the same message. There is great comfort in knowing others have endured, overcome, and thrived after such traumatic birth experiences. Dr Kaur has been and will continue to be a blessing to all who've been in her care as well as to those who now find ease and hope in her book."

  — *Kelli Kelley, NICU Graduate Mom, Founder and Executive Director, Hand to Hold*

"It's uplifting to read about Dr. Kaur and the NICU staff helping the families of preemies. The stories of what families face when they have a medically needy infant are real; and the stories of people like us who have feared it, lived it, and made it through are amazing! *My Garden of Flowers* is well written and offers great tools and a medical glossary to help understand the medical terminology you hear when your little miracle comes into this world with complications you never expected. If I'd had this book when I had my premature 29-week-gestation triplets, I'd have been better prepared and more knowledgeable and able to help in those critical days we faced after their birth."
— *Bev Doughty, NICU Graduate Mom*

"*My Garden of Flowers* offers a firsthand look into the development of the Lancaster General NICU unit and the lives touched by the compassionate and innovative care found there. Our daughter was born premature, and we are forever grateful for Dr. Kaur's expertise and vision to bring a NICU to Lancaster, and for her tender heart and friendship. Reading this book, one cannot escape the truth that Dr. Kaur viewed all the babies in her care as beautiful gifts from God who deserve the best care and chance at life. Dr. Kaur is not only an accomplished physician but also a beautiful person who loves her patients and their families, and it shows clearly throughout the book. Many authors delve into what to expect during a normal pregnancy and delivery, but Dr. Kaur brings guidance and hope to those who find themselves on a different path. Parents will find *My Garden of Flowers* an invaluable tool to help navigate an unexpected journey."
— *Kimberly Eltman, NICU Graduate Mom*

"*My Garden of Flowers* is wondrous. Dr. Kaur pours out her heart and soul, gracing us with her inspired poetry and medical expertise in what will surely become "The NICU Family Bible." How I wish we'd had such a book to cling to twenty years ago when our twin boys, Quinn and Dylan, were born severely premature!"
— *Kerry Loughlin, NICU Graduate Mom*

My Garden

of

Flowers

Miracles in the
Neonatal Intensive Care Unit

What Every NICU Family Needs to Know

Manjeet Kaur, MD

DCH, FAAP, FRCPC

INSPIRANTE
PUBLISHING LLC
LITITZ, PENNSYLVANIA

Inspirante Publishing LLC
InspirantePublishing@gmail.com

https://mygardenofflowers.wordpress.com

Book Design:	Mike Lovell
Editor:	Mike Lovell
Artwork:	Larissa Hise Henoch, LHH Design Inc. based on original drawings by Manjeet Kaur
Permissions:	Family stories and photographs are used with permission of the families; newspaper articles and photographs are used with permission of LNP Media Group; Shert's wedding photo is used with permission of Brittani Elizabeth Photography; Growth Charts are used with permission of Dr. Tanis Fenton of the Cumming School of Medicine, University of Calgary.

Important notice for parents and practitioners

The information provided throughout this book is intended as guidelines only, and should not be substituted in any way for recommendations by your physician or medical team.

There are continuing new developments in the field of neonatology. Best practices may vary from time to time, and readers should always confirm that they evaluate the information, methods and products relevant to each particular situation.

Readers are advised to check the most current information provided by manufacturers of equipment, pharmaceuticals, and nutritional supplements about their products, methods and procedures for their administration and use.

The publisher, author, editors, and other contributors assume no liability in any way for any injury or damage arising from the use of products, methods and practices described throughout this work.

Publisher's Cataloging-in-Publication Data

Names:	Kaur, Manjeet, 1949- author.	Lovell, Mike (Editor).
Title:	My garden of flowers : miracles in the neonatal intensive care unit : what every NICU family needs to know / Manjeet Kaur MD ; editor, Mike Lovell.
Description:	First edition.	Lititz, PA : Inspirante Publishing LLC, [2019]	Includes bibliographical references and index.
Identifiers:	ISBN: 978-1-7326462-0-9	LCCN: 2018954836	ebook ISBN: 978-1-7326462-1-6
Subjects:	LCSH: Neonatal intensive care.	Neonatal intensive care--Psychological aspects--Personal narratives.	Neonatal intensive care--Nursing.	Newborn infants--Family relationships-- Personal narratives.	Newborn infants--Care.	Breastfeeding--Complications.	Neonatal emergencies--Personal narratives.	Newborn infants--Handbooks, manuals, etc.	Newborn infants--Diseases--Treatment--Handbooks, manuals, etc.	Parents of children with disabilities--Counseling of.	Parents of children with disabilities--Handbooks, manuals, etc.	Infants--Nutrition.	Children--Death--Psychological aspects--Personal narratives.	Parental grief--Counseling of.	BISAC: MEDICAL / Nursing / Critical & Intensive Care.	MEDICAL / Perinatology & Neonatology.	MEDICAL / Physician & Patient.
Classification:	LCC: RJ253.5 .K38 2019	DDC: 618.92/01--dc23 First Edition

Cover Photo: Dr. Kaur holding Quinn and Dylan; born in 1997 at 25 weeks gestation. Their story is on page 148.

PRINTED IN THE UNITED STATES OF AMERICA

2 4 6 8 9 7 5 3 1

Dedication

Above all, to the Almighty for His innumerable blessings.

~

To the numerous buds of life that have been entrusted to our care and have bloomed into a wonderful Garden of Flowers—little miracles—"my godchildren," and remembering those who were called to leave the garden and join the angels.

~

To my NICU family

Our wonderful staff, nurses, and colleagues—a great team! Your dedication and friendship have made it an incredible place to work in over the past three decades.

~

To my mentors

The late Dr. Brock MacMurray, formerly Chief of Neonatology, Children's Hospital of Eastern Ontario, Ottawa, Canada. "A dedicated neonatologist who taught and inspired me in my love for the field of neonatology."
Dr. Jeanette Pleasure, formerly Chief of Neonatology, Medical College of Pennsylvania in Philadelphia. "A caring physician who always provided gentle guidance."

~

To my family

To my parents

My late father, Mr. Kartar Singh, one of the most knowledgeable persons that I have ever known, and whose approval I can feel from the heaven above.

My mother, my friend, Mrs. Parkash Kaur, whose unfaltering love and blessings have been my support always.

Our Biji, Mrs. Iqbal Kaur, for her love and dedication for all time.

My children—all physicians now themselves

Harsimran Singh my firstborn, whose professionalism and work ethic, love, and strength shine bright, always bringing me renewed energy.

Arunjot Singh my diligent and smart comedian, whose kind caring ways, compassion, support, and anonymous sweet gestures always bring me smiles and a unique fulfillment.

Jasmeet Singh my lovely bright daughter, now a wonderful mother herself, has brought me a new dimension of love, that of the loving daughter that I had longed for.

Aditi Singh my pretty, brilliant, daughter who has been a sweet addition to the family, and whose love and tender, winsome ways bring me great joy.

My grandchildren—the light of my life bring me a unique happiness

Cutie Kabir, my honeybunch, and "favorite buddy" for all time.

Adorable Pareesa—my frolicsome li'l chum, my Goo Goo!

All my dear family, godchildren, and friends—throughout my life I have cherished your love and support.

My sisters and brother, Drs. Neelam, Kirti, and Davinder, and their families, godchildren Melanie and Monica, my three special friends in USA, India, and Canada ironically with the same first name—Madhu, and so many others who have enriched the journey of my life.

My husband, Surender—you are my cheerleader, my inspiration, and my dearest friend. You give me the fortitude to face the world.

Contents

Part IV Discharge—Homeward Bound

Contd/-

Appendices

Foreword

*P*rior to Dr. Kaur coming to Lancaster in 1984, the role of the pediatricians in caring for the sick newborn was to stabilize and transport the baby to one of several larger facilities that were forty to seventy miles away. This not only separated a mother from her baby, but also added risk to the infant during the transport. As pediatricians, we were often pushed to our limits clinically in order to avoid these problems.

By agreeing to singlehandedly set up a NICU in Lancaster, Dr. Kaur took on a challenge that few others would have attempted. During those first few years she often worked for twenty-four hours or more at a time to stabilize a sick infant—there was no one else who could do what she did.

Her dedication to setting up a NICU in Lancaster never wavered. Although it took some years of self-sacrifice to make it happen, under her leadership our NICU became a reality that is now widely recognized for the quality of its care. This would never have happened without her vision and determination.

Since those founding years, Dr. Kaur and I have worked together on many occasions, and she has become a trusted colleague on whom I can always rely for advice and guidance in the care of our tiny patients.

Despite the workload, Dr. Kaur never stopped treating each infant and each family with love and compassion. She developed deep relationships with these families that have been long-lasting and meaningful. Few situations in life place us in a more vulnerable situation than watching our newborn struggle to live. Dr. Kaur was always there to administer excellent care to the infant and to provide reassurance and empathy to the family.

The NICU that Dr. Kaur created has been of inestimable value to the Lancaster community, and her book—My Garden of Flowers–Miracles in the Neonatal Intensive Care Unit—is a testament to her legacy. In 2002 the Lancaster General Hospital recognized Dr. Kaur's achievements and honored her by naming the neonatology division at the Women's and Babies Hospital the "Manjeet Kaur MD Division of Neonatology."

The vignettes of some of her tiny patients that are included in this book testify to the impact she had on the families she cared for. And, what greater celebration of life than to see these babies who had such a tough start now living their lives as accomplished adults—many of them now with families of their own. The families who have shared the stories of having their babies in the NICU deserve our thanks for their frank honesty and open-hearted sharing of their intimate experiences.

This book provides an invaluable resource for families to demystify what happens in the NICU, and to help them prepare to cope with caring for their child.

Firstly, it provides essential information in simple terms about what happens in the NICU and the various medical conditions that are commonly encountered there.

But, perhaps more importantly, it addresses the emotional reality of Neonatal Intensive Care. The compelling messages from the Family Stories are that "You are not alone," and reassurance for parents that "These tiny, critically ill infants will typically grow to adulthood and lead normal healthy lives."

This book brings hope and support for families who suddenly find themselves with a baby needing intensive care. It has practical advice, and the charts, checklists and homeward bound section will be a real resource to help parents caring for their new little "NICU grad" once they come home from the NICU.

In 2015 Manjeet Kaur retired from clinical medicine but has continued her contribution to the practice of neonatology through an active teaching program at the Women's and Babies Hospital. In 2016 the Lancaster General Health Foundation initiated the Dr. Manjeet Kaur NICU Scholarship Fund to honor the vital contributions that Dr. Kaur has made at Women & Babies Hospital and in our community. The scholarship will provide an annual award to assist with further training and education related to neonatal care.

Preparing this book has been an ambitious undertaking, and Dr. Kaur is to be thanked for her work in making this further contribution to support the families that she so cares for, and the tiny babies that she so loves.

Steve Tifft, MD

January, 2018

Sincere Thanks

To the wonderful families who opened their hearts, sharing their experiences of hope and fear in the stories while in the Neonatal Intensive Care Unit and beyond:

Beisker family

de Lorraine family

Deatrick family

Doughty family

Eltman family

Gerhart family

Getzloff family

Grove-Workman family

Harriger family

Herr family

Huntley family

Hussar family

Hynes family

Loughlin family

Mahajan family

Medina family

Miller family

Mummau family

Oree family

Patterson family

Sauder family

Sharpe family

Sheid family

Sherts family

Sturla-Womack family

...

To my NICU family—our wonderful staff, nurses, and colleagues
> Thank you for sharing your precious memories. This book holds only some of the stories shared, and I am sure each of us have many more.

...

For sharing your experiences and heartfelt memories
> Mary Ann Wolpert, NICU Staff Nurse CLIV, and Carolanne B. Hauck—Chaplain

...

> Christine Hansson, RN—Clinical Educator (Lactation Support)

> Anand B. Mahajan, MD, and Joel Seacrest, MD (Medical Review)

> Arunjot Singh, MD, MPH (Medical Review and invaluable suggestions)

> Charity Grove, RN (Resources for NICU Families)

...

To Amy Colm—for your patience and expertise, as we worked through so many iterations during the preparation of the materials for this book.

...

To Larissa Hise Henoch—for your skill in taking my original diagrams and charts and transforming them into professional artwork that adds so much to this book.

...

To Mike Lovell, my editor at LifeReloaded Specialty Publishing, for traveling this journey with me with gentle patience, support, and numerous suggestions, as we brought this memoir to reality.

...

To my husband—Dr. Surender Singh, for his insight, inspiration, and vital suggestions through the long process, as we brought my dream to life over the past two years.

...

An Invocation

May my mind be like the lotus, O'Lord,
Remaining pure and serene amidst the murky marshes.
May my heart sing in dedication, salutations to thee,
Resounding in sweetness as the nightingale's melody.
May my hands always rise to give what is but thine,
The infinite gifts of thy bequest, a greater joy tis hard to find.
May my lips bespeak but kind, tranquil words—a notion,
Of sweetness, of care, of love and devotion.
May the tiny lamp that I kindle at your feet today,
Light my way, to thine glorious kingdom one day!

—Manjeet Kaur

Introduction

If you are reading this book, then you are most likely a parent or member of a family that has suddenly found itself with a baby who has been admitted to a Neonatal Intensive Care Unit (NICU). Or perhaps you are already some time into your pregnancy, and you have just received the news that your baby is likely to be born prematurely and may need intensive care.

Whatever brings you here, most people have little or no awareness of the NICU. The discovery that you are about to be thrown into this unexpected ocean of technology, surrounded by beeps and alarms, can be frightening, unnerving, and downright scary.

The stories in this book—stories of the tiny, sick babies who have now blossomed into wonderful adults leading normal and fulfilling lives—will give you hope and reassurance. Other parents have been where you are, and have heard the same upsetting news. Caring for little "NICU grads," as we call them, is challenging and there are often bumps in the road.

These stories, told in the parents' own words, share their fears and uncertainties and are a testimony to their courage, the fierce determination of these sick little infants to survive, and the power of faith in the Divine.

There is always apprehension when we are faced with the unknown. This book will also give you information to make you aware of the **common medical issues** that occur in the newborn and to understand what happens when a baby is born and admitted to intensive care. Once discharged, there are a lot of special considerations for **caring for your new baby at home**, and the book includes practical guidance in the form of **information, checklists, and charts**. The chapter on **coping tips** is drawn from the experience of parents who have walked this path. The appendices include a comprehensive **glossary** to demystify the medical jargon and an **index** that will help you find information as you need it.

For a couple, the discovery of having a baby is an exciting and blessed experience—a time of dreaming and great expectations. In today's world, a birth is supposed to be perfect. It's a world where we believe in zero tolerance at work and in day-to-day behavior; a world where we aim to control all aspects of our lives, and where with every morn attempt to plan our days on daily planners or e-scripts. For years, we plan that birth for the right time and the right schedule to fit our jobs and our homes. And then, for some, BOOM—the shock of the unexpected—everything goes haywire:

"Honey, my water broke!"

"Know that you are not alone!

"But you're only twenty-five weeks! We haven't even started decorating the nursery; we haven't picked names," and so on. The truth is, we only have so much control before we bow to the inevitable, the plan from above. Everything is running on track and going well for a term birth, and suddenly something snaps, and the baby ends up in the intensive care unit. Though prenatal care helps, there are situations in which things don't work perfectly, and we may not always find a cause for prematurity or a difficult birth. There are situations in which, finding no reason, we say, "It's just destiny!"

The mother's first thoughts often are *Why me? What did I do wrong?* "There are so many people who don't take much care, who even do drugs. I didn't touch alcohol or drugs! I took my vitamins just like the doc said" is an oft-repeated lament of moms. Then, gradually, comes acceptance and realization that you were not to blame for your child's needing intensive care. It's called "life," and this has happened to many families before for no known reason.

Part I is a reminiscence of my experiences over the past three decades, starting with the founding of the NICU. It feels wonderful to travel down memory lane and relive those precious moments, some fluid and some poignant, especially while narrating memoirs related to our little miracles. I hope you enjoy reading them as much as I did penning them.

The Family Stories section in **Part II** has narratives from twenty-five families whose babies have been cared for in the NICU. Each story tells of their NICU experiences and of their joys and upheavals as they incorporated these tiny NICU graduates into their homes and daily family life. These stories were written by the parents and families themselves, and have been included with minor edits. These are the heartfelt sagas of anguish and despair, of hope, courage and achievement—each of the little ones is a special hero of the NICU family.

These family stories illustrate how nurturing and close relationships and support can make those heartrending, labor-intensive times into memorable and precious experiences for both families and staff. For those who suddenly find themselves facing the challenge of a NICU admission, *know that you are not alone!* Families before you have gone down the same road and are able to talk positively about their experiences—so will you.

Knowledge brings empowerment, courage, and determination. The ocean of information available on the Internet today can be overwhelming. **Part III** describes in simple terms, some of the **common problems encountered in the NICU**, including resuscitation and discharge planning. You may face other problems that have not been touched on, as they're beyond the scope of what can be covered in this book. You can also expect to find that opinions vary among caretakers. Management is evidence-based, but may differ in various situations.

There is a lot that can be done ahead of time to make things easier when the baby comes home. The chapter *Homeward Bound* presents planning checklists and other resources to assist families for dealing with this stressful and emotional time. These support systems will be a useful aid to get you prepared, and to know what to expect.

The coping tips in **Supporting You!**, are derived from experiences of prior NICU families, and are a wonderful example of parents helping parents.

As Henry Wadsworth Longfellow states so beautifully in "A Psalm of Life":

> *Lives of great men all remind us*
> *We can make our lives sublime,*
> *And, departing, leave behind us*
> *Footprints on the sands of time;*
> *Footprints, that perhaps another,*
> *Sailing o'er life's solemn main,*
> *A forlorn and shipwrecked brother,*
> *Seeing, shall take heart again.*

This section also includes a directory of many resources that are dedicated to assisting and supporting parents throughout the stages of infancy and early childhood.

The stories and support resources that are shared in this book give an insight into the challenges of a premature, or a difficult birth and the role of the NICU and its staff in providing neonatal intensive care.

Each NICU baby is a tiny miracle—a story of courage; of climbing mountains, even while skidding down those steep slopes only to ascend again—always victorious, as per potential, no matter how tough the load! Small rejoicings for tiny steps forward on that oft-spoken-about roller coaster are cherished moments. "Hope and faith," as some parents have written, are what kept them strong amidst all adversity. Often, after the baby goes home, we hear, "I made so many friends there. I'll always remember this time passionately but not negatively."

We in the NICU hope parents will believe that, even though it may be hard to accept at the time!

I have received calls, as have other staff members, on birthdays, at the births of siblings, school events, graduations, and weddings. Time is a great healer, and the pain that parents experienced in their early days turns to joy as their little bud blossoms to become a beautiful youngster. I consider every call a compliment of the highest category, one that makes all the difficulties, the trials and tribulations of those long on-call nights, worthwhile.

And—if you are reading them while your baby is in the NICU—it is my sincere hope that these stories of rough roads and valor will inspire confidence and give you courage as you face the challenges on the road that lies ahead.

Disclaimer: The stories of our little miracles in **Part II** depict events as their families perceived them, so any medical interpretations in their narratives are parental views only.

The medical data provided throughout this book are guidelines only and should not be substituted in any way for recommendations by your physician or medical team.

A Prayer

May only goodness enter this door,
May love and comfort light this floor.
In the midst of clamor, may peace pervade,
And the tumultuous woes of our babes abate,
While noisy beeping, whistles, and bells,
A novel birth of tiny footsteps foretell.
Monitors, vent, lines, a prescription,
Every effort to obtain a benediction.
May all who enter feel the encircling flow
Of love, labor, and dedication aglow.
We pray, oh Lord, and we implore
Bless our NICU
With healing, hope, and grace evermore.

—Manjeet Kaur

PART I

The Building
of a
NICU

Memoirs of a Neonatologist

Love

Let love be an infinite gift,
That rejoices in giving.
A giving that resonates with joy …
Therein lies the gift of giving!
—Manjeet Kaur

I have always felt a special love for children. When I was about seven or eight years old, I would sit in a revolving chair in my grandfather's medical clinic in Delhi pretending to be a doctor. I saw how his patients loved him.

"I want to be a children's doctor," I would say—I had not yet learned the word "physician." I was one of the lucky ones who hone in on their vocation early in life.

≋

If I could pinpoint a moment that is etched in my mind when I knew that Neonatology was to be my life's career choice, it would be when I performed my first intubation during the first week of the Neonatal Intensive Care Unit (NICU) rotation of my Pediatrics Residency (training) at CHEO (Children's Hospital of Eastern Ontario) in Ottawa, Canada. We suddenly heard the monitor alarms go off during our daily morning rounds in the NICU. I even remember the name of the tiny baby from almost forty years ago. "Charity just extubated!" called the nurse who had run to assess the cause of the alarm.

"Who wants to intubate?" asked Dr. Brock Mac-Murray, the Chief of Neonatology, and who was soon to become my mentor. I quickly volunteered, enthusiastic to learn a new procedure. We did nasotracheal intubations at CHEO back then, a procedure in which the endotracheal tube (ETT) is passed through the nose and then gently guided through the pharynx (throat) into the windpipe with the help of a curved Magill forceps. I performed the procedure with my heart racing as the nurses and residents looked on. The baby pinked up as Dr. MacMurray listened to the chest for tube placement and gave a thumbs-up

I can do this! I thought. What a fine, challenging and rewarding job!

≋

I never forgot the encouragement from my mentor, and throughout the next six weeks I thoroughly enjoyed a rotation that many residents dreaded. When we relocated to Philadelphia it was easy for me to pick Neonatology as the specialty that I wanted to pursue throughout my medical career—a calling I was to learn would not only be a profession but also a dedication.

≋

These memoirs are the story of that career as it unfolded over the next three decades. I hope that you enjoy reading them as much as I have enjoyed writing them.
Manjeet Kaur

≋≋

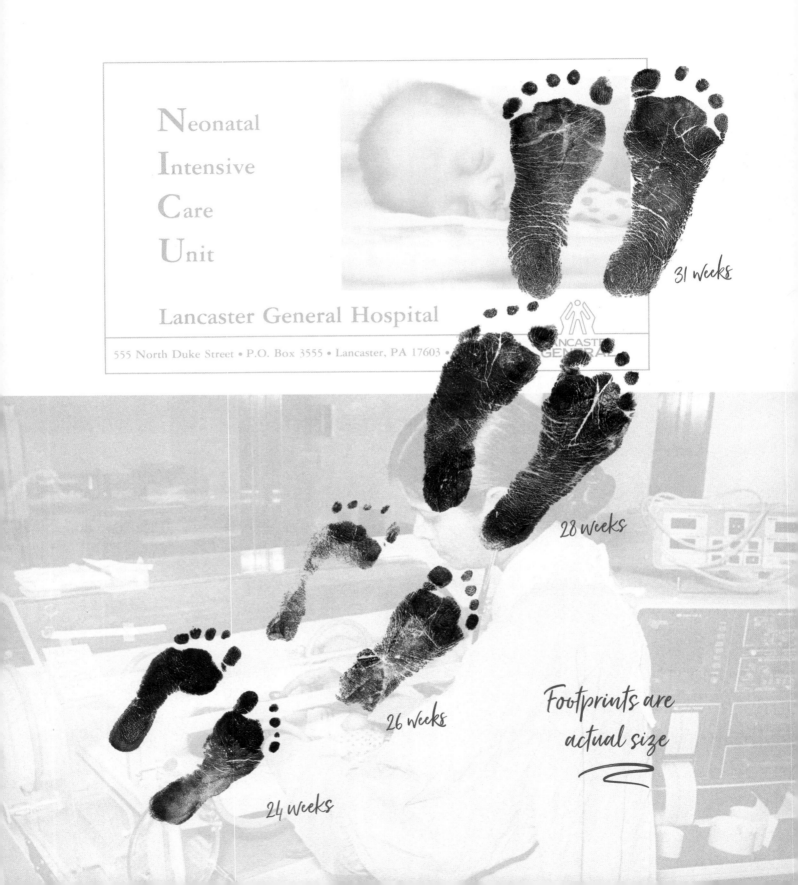

Neonatal Intensive Care Unit

Lancaster General Hospital

555 North Duke Street • P.O. Box 3555 • Lancaster, PA 17603 •

31 weeks

28 weeks

26 weeks

24 weeks

Footprints are actual size

Establishing the
NICU
at Lancaster General Hospital

As I look back, time stands still and the years fade away. It's the summer of 1984. I had completed my fellowship in Neonatology and stayed on as a faculty member at the Medical College of Pennsylvania (now Drexel) in Philadelphia, when my husband, a cardiologist and also an attending,[1] opted to go into private practice.

When an opportunity came up in Lancaster, Pennsylvania, our friends were highly encouraging, suggesting that it would be a good place to practice. Coming from New Delhi, where I attended Maulana Azad Medical College, then Canada, where I completed my pediatric residency at Ottawa Children's Hospital, and on to the United States—I had already experienced quite a cultural and emotional roller coaster.

I was used to the peace and beauty of the countryside, having studied at a boarding school in the Himalayan ranges in Mussoorie and then in a small town, Ferozepur in Punjab, Northern India, and I loved the natural beauty of Lancaster, which was then considered Amish country. My husband, who had grown up in urban New Delhi, was initially not so sure about settling in a small town.

> " I connected with Lancaster at first sight. The delightful blossoms of this lovely countryside beckoned me almost as Avonlea had enticed Anne in *Anne of Green Gables.*

---

1   An attending is a staff physician who has completed his/her training and is now practicing medicine and often teaching medical students and fellows in their specialty. Usually an attending has titles such as assistant, associate, or professor.

I connected with Lancaster at first sight. The delightful blossoms of this lovely countryside beckoned me almost as Avonlea had enticed Anne in *Anne of Green Gables*. The greenery of the farms, orchards, and rolling hills; the graceful boughs of the willows; the pure loveliness of the cherry blossoms, creeks, and covered bridges—complete with horse-drawn buggies—were very endearing. It appeared a picturesque place, "a home away from home," I called it, as it reminded me of my school town in India, which I had loved.

My first meeting with Paul Wedel, the President, and Nevin Cooley, the Vice President of Lancaster General Hospital[2] (LGH) came after I had already spoken to pediatric groups called MBMA (now Lancaster Pediatric Associates) and BHPT (now called Roseville Pediatrics). Though supportive, there was a lot of ambivalence regarding the initiation of Neonatology at LGH. As an obstetrician put it, "We have Hershey Medical Center only twenty-five minutes away. We don't have the numbers needed to support a NICU."

However, I received a very warm welcome when I joined LGH in May 1984. Most of the staff were very excited, but like anything new, there was certainly some resistance to change.

Dr. William Boben, then the Chief of Pediatrics, traveled with me for meetings at other hospitals in the area: St. Joseph's, Ephrata, and Columbia Community, where we presented our plans for the establishment of a new Neonatal Intensive Care Unit at Lancaster General. Though the initiation had been somewhat dubious, the poignant reception by the area hospitals as we presented the plans was very encouraging. Advertising was mainly via newspapers and television back then, and we started in a rather non-ostentatious manner. The practice of neonatal intensive care was still in its infancy back in 1984,

2   Now Penn Medicine Lancaster General Health

INTELLIGENCER JOURNAL, Lancaster, Pa., Monday, May 14, 1984 —5

Pediatrics Specialist Joins Staff at LGH

Lancaster General Hospital announces the appointment of Manjeet Kaur, M.D., to the Department of Pediatrics, Division of Neonatology.

Before coming to Lancaster, Dr. Kaur was assistant professor of pediatrics and consultant neonatologist at Montgomery Hospital, Norristown.

Dr. Kaur is certified by the American Board of Pediatrics, a fellow of the Royal College of Physicians and Surgeons of Canada and holds memberships in the Philadelphia Perinatal Society and the American Medical Women's Association.

Dr. Kaur-is the wife of Surender Singh, M.D.

and it was still unfamiliar to most people. We spent the first three to four months reviewing literature, creating protocols, and developing brochures and teaching programs for the staff. After reviewing equip-

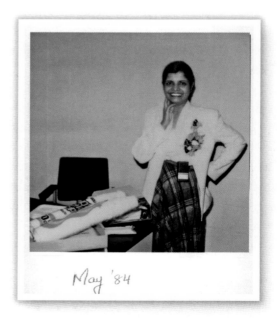

May '84

ment costs from literature and from my colleagues at the Medical College of Pennsylvania, I presented the hospital president with a budget of about $110,000. This was in 1984, and it seems unimaginable today to even consider that such a paltry sum could be the initial cost for establishing a NICU.

I promised the administration that I would oversee the unit and provide coverage until we found an additional neonatologist. This was certainly a very ambitious commitment, as my boys, Simran and Arun, were only seven and one and a half years old at the time. It's difficult to imagine now, when we're making our call schedules and trying to accommodate our days off, that back then I was on call 24/7. On occasions that I had to go out of town I would ask a pediatrician to cover for a day. If I had a baby on a respirator, I just stayed.

Of course, other than work with my NICU babies, all the rest of my time and life was my family and children. My husband was always very supportive, and our mother lived with us, which made it easier. "Work is worship," I told my seven-year-old son; just as my dad had often quoted during my childhood years. Simran's rigorous work ethic and empathetic acceptance have thus been qualities since those formative years, as I wrote in a personal reference for his college application. My younger son, Arun, was too young to understand and needed even more cuddles when I was home.

We recruited from amongst the nurses working in the regular "Newborn Nursery" and the "Preemie Nursery," where babies requiring any additional assistance were admitted. They were ready, and more than willing, to undergo further training to meet the requirements of the higher level of treatment that is provided in a NICU to enable babies to stay in Lancaster with their moms.

The staff was fabulous! I received flowers and small gifts, which remain precious memories of this day. There was an aura of excitement, as well as a lot of "ifs" and "buts," as expected; I recall the head nurse coming to my office, pen and notebook in hand, saying, "Just tell me what you need and we'll get it." Coming from Philadelphia, where I was "just" one of the attendings, this was indeed remarkable.

The enthusiasm and support of the staff made this challenge a fun and very rewarding endeavor. It was almost like setting up a house, including the décor. They were passionate about keeping babies who were previously sent to Hershey in Lancaster. Vicky, Judy, Brenda, Lynn, Tracy, Brenda, Kim, Karen, Nancy, Marion, Sherry, Betsey, Cindy, and Pat were just a few of the nurses. Miriam, our ward clerk, was very much a part of our NICU team, keeping everyone in line with the support of our administrators, Josephine and Joan.

New ventilators, monitors, and intravenous and other supportive equipment were ordered. The ebullience of the nursing staff was infectious as they embraced the change, and the now archaic monitors were replaced with state-of-the-art technology of the eighties.

" I received a very warm welcome when I joined LGH in May 1984. Most of the staff were very excited, but like anything new, there was certainly some resistance to change.

> " ... we would only keep babies that were at least thirty-two weeks gestation in Lancaster.

The Sunday News ran a feature article profiling our new unit at LGH, which included a description of some of the common problems of the newborn and the equipment that was being installed to provide treatment for these sick infants. Most of all, the article highlighted the value of this new medical service to the community, quoting Dr. Boben:

"It is one of the most difficult and heart-rending decisions for physicians and family members when a mother delivers an infant with difficulties and you have to fire this infant off to Hershey or Harrisburg or Philadelphia. ... This is not a profit-making venture for LGH; to tear a child away is very difficult ... That's why we set this up—as a service."

"New NICU Will Keep Families Together" was the headline in the Lancaster newspaper.

The times were different then. To borrow from Charles Dickens, "It was the best of times," but it wasn't the worst, though there were difficult times. It was the best of times in that one could make plans, execute them more easily, and make things happen. It was a difficult time in that we were starting from scratch, with little ancillary assistance and no such thing as computers and Internet access, which was still way into the future; however, it was a challenge and a privilege that few people get in a lifetime.

We'd planned to start out with ten NICU beds with four radiant warmers (acute care open beds

with heat source) and six incubators (or isolettes). We had decided that initially we would only keep babies that were at least thirty-two-weeks gestation in Lancaster; any smaller babies would be stabilized and transferred to Hershey, a level-3 NICU.[3]

Once the equipment was ordered, we organized seminars to train our staff. I'd been on faculty at the Medical College of Pennsylvania (MCP) before I came to Lancaster, and had left with a lot of goodwill and great friends. I was able to tap into those resources and recruit Linda, a nurse educator then at MCP, to come and participate in a two-day seminar, and we were able to cover all the basic topics between her training and the conferences that I ran.

Our staff members were like sponges, noting all the information, and asking questions while maintaining their humor. One incident stands out. The usual concluding sentence after the nurse

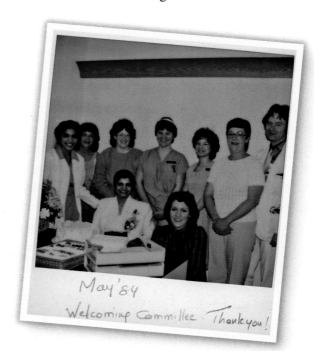

May '84
Welcoming Committee. Thank you!

---

3   Problems of prematurity are inversely proportional to the gestation. At less than thirty-two weeks, babies have increasing lung and general immaturity and are therefore more prone to experience the problems of prematurity.

At LGH: New Neonatal Intensive Care Unit will keep families together

In the room next door, friends and relatives are cheering the birth of a little boy or girl. There's Grandma with a stuffed teddy bear; an aunt with some roses; a proud new father handing out cigars.

But in this room, the parents are somber. 'They hold hands. They cry. They're frightened. They can't cuddle their newborn; because their baby has been whisked to a hospital miles away. They pray that their baby survives.

The usual celebration of the birth of a child can be usurped by the birth of a baby with severe medical problems.

"It is one of the most difficult and heart-rending decisions for physicians and family members when a mother delivers an infant with difficulties and you have to fire this infant off to Hershey or Harrisburg or Philadelphia," said Dr. William Boben, chief of pediatrics for Lancaster General Hospital.

But now Lancaster will have a new medical service to help ease some of the anguish the parents of these infants experience. After two years of planning, Lancaster General Hospital will open its four-bed (isolette) neonatal intensive care unit (NICU) the first week of September.

"We have in this county a sufficient number of deliveries to merit such a unit sixty to 80 babies are transferred out of the county each year. The volume was .there," said Boben, "but much more important than that was the human element here."

"Suddenly, unplanned, you have a sick infant at Hershey and the parents are here in Lancaster, That was the chief reason behind the process to get this into the county."

Then, as fate would have it, neonatologist Dr. Manjeet·Kaur moved to Lancaster with her husband, LGH cardiologist Dr. Surender Singh. Dr. Kaur was ready to take on the responsibility as head of the unit.

She comes to Lancaster with eight years of training in New Delhi, India. She also did a pediatric residency for three years at Children's Hospital of Eastern Ontario, Ottawa, Canada, and a fellowship in neonatology from The Medical College of Pennsylvania in Philadelphia.

Dr. Kaur was a member of the . physician team which helped a premature, 15-ounce baby in Philadelphia survive and thrive.

That little one is now two years old and developmentally normal.

Lancaster General also has the county's first pediatric_neurologist, Dr. Robert Vanucci, on its staff. He, with Drs. Kaur and Boben, will spearhead the NICU program with referring pediatricians.

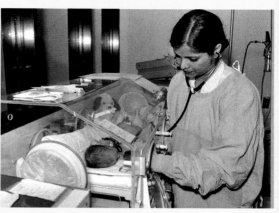

Sunday News Photo By Jack LPonard
Neonatologist Dr. Manjeet Kaur will head the new neonata1 intensive care unit at the Lancaster General Hospital. scheduled to open in early September.

Premature and/or full-term babies can require intensive care if they suffer respiratory, feeding, jaundice, hemorrhage or other severe medical problems.

An advanced, compact system for continuous monitoring of oxygen delivery in critical care situations is an integral piece of equipment in the unit. "Oxygen requirements for these babies is very critical," Dr. Kaur explained. "This sophisticated equipment lets us monitor the babies' oxygen."

Too much oxygen can cause blindness, Dr. Boben explained, and too little can cause brain damage. Thus, trained personnel, as well as up-to-date equipment is vital.

When a neonate's vital signs start to change, the medical staff needs to know it immediately. The NICU, therefore, also features also features a Neo-Trak 506 vital signs monitoring system which provides ECG, respiration, blood pressure and two-temperature monitoring.

And, there are other concerns the health-provider must consider in the treatment of these sick infants. "These little tiny babies are very defenseless," Dr. Kaur said. "And we have to treat them as soon as we see infection. We also have to prevent infection; that is why they are in isolation."

Most of the babies in the NICU will be fed intravenously

"Special solutions can keep them going for months," Dr. Kaur related. She emphasized the importance of having carefully trained personnel to implement an intravenous feeding. "A little amount of fluid which may just be a drop in the bucket to an adult can flood a tiny infant. You have to watch every cc (¼ teaspoon) being given to these babies.

In addition, an IV technique must be "right on

the money," said Dr. Boben. "It's one thing to get a needle, into an adult; but to get it into a tiny, tiny baby, everything must be just right or you will have a child with a sore arm or infection. It takes a lot of specialized nursing and physician care. It really becomes art."

Total jaundice management will also be available in the LGH NICU. "These babies can have horrendous problems with jaundice because their enzymes are immature," explained Dr . Kaur.

Premature babies are also prone to have brain hemorrhages "We monitor them with ultrasound using a little transducer which can be brought right into the nursery and put on the soft spot of the head," she said.

The body systems that can go awry in a premature (or even a full-term birth are many. And, although the LGH NICU can handle the bulk of those health disorders, there are some medical cases which will still need to be referred to hospitals outside of Lancaster.

"WE do not plan to do heart surgery on these babies," said Dr. Boben. "Or, if an infant is born with his intestines out of the body we wouldn't do that surgery here either."

So far, the equipment alone for the LGH neonatal intensive care unit has cost approximately $100,000. But, Dr. Boben said, "This .is not a profit-making venture for LGH. As perinatal events have- become more relaxed and personalized (birthing rooms, fathers at deliveries), to tear a child away is very difficult I've never yet met a mother who'd rather send her child off info the night to a distant hospital somewhere. That's why we set this up as a service."

educator finished an instruction would be "You take this action and then you hover."

One of the nurses, Vicky, was asked a question; she told me afterward that she answered correctly adding, "and then you hover." The whole class burst out laughing. Vicky herself laughed so much that her glasses fell off and broke. That was one of the highlights of those early days, and long afterward the story about Vicky's glasses remained a humorous memory.

The administration was extremely supportive, and has always continued to be so. There was a lot less formality and bureaucracy back then, even in an institution of the standard of LGH, and the nurse manager and I were at liberty to plan the running of the NICU. We had our equipment organized, had protocols in place, and after the nursing orientation we were on our way.

When needed, I attended deliveries and C-sections for the family physicians and pediatricians, and I truly think that the physicians were glad of that respite so they didn't have to leave their busy practices. The obstetricians were also happy they didn't have to wait for the family physician or pediatrician to come in as I was in the hospital and more easily available.

The first cesarean section I attended was with Brenda, an RN (registered nurse) who was pregnant and almost full-term herself. Of course, as Murphy's Law would have it, we had an LGA (large for gestational age) infant who had bilateral spontaneous pneumothoraces (air around the lungs). As Brenda tried to reach for tubes in her tackle box on the floor, we determined to make simplistic changes—along with guidelines and charts there would be additional space and tables assigned specifically for infant resuscitation. Interestingly, I attended a delivery sixteen years later of a baby with a similar last name and, on inquiring about a possible connection, was told that my first C-section baby was an uncle of this infant, was on a boxing team, and had been "student of the week" that month in the Lancaster newspaper. I received a newspaper clipping in the mail of this young man in his boxing attire the following week. Such is the close-knit community in Lancaster County.

September 1984 was the official inauguration of the Lancaster General Neonatal Intensive Care Unit. we had a ribbon-cutting ceremony attended by the staff and administrators and, most importantly, prayers by the chaplain.

"Back in 1984 ... when we needed to administer oxygen and no respiratory masks were available, the oxygen tubing would be stuck in a paper cup and the cup then placed over the infant's nose and mouth.

" The staff, though apprehensive, was very excited
—their theoretical learning was about to be tested.

Back in 1984 we made do with very little in the nursery. When we needed to administer oxygen and no respiratory masks were available, the oxygen tubing would be stuck in a paper cup and the cup then placed over the infant's nose and mouth. Although it was a primitive oxygen mask, it certainly worked well.

At times, being the single neonatologist in town was indeed a daunting task. I remember being called in the middle of the night, not only for deliveries but also for starting intravenous lines (IVs) on infants who weren't taking feeds or who were on antibiotics.

The first procedure that I determined to teach our staff was how to start IVs, so back to our great resource of The Medical College of Pennsylvania. The nurses were sent in pairs for a week for NICU orientation and to learn IV skills in babies, which was subsequently reinforced in Lancaster. This took another three to four months to accomplish, after which we felt more comfortable keeping sicker babies.

The very first baby we kept on a respirator after the inauguration of our NICU was little Lauren, a thirty-two-week-gestation infant with respiratory distress syndrome (immature lungs), which would have been one of the simpler admissions at a bigger center. Her story is included in this book. The staff, though apprehensive, was very excited—their theoretical learning was about to be tested. Lauren was Dr. Tifft's patient from what was then called the BHPT

Pediatrics. Lauren's parents were informed and were offered the choice of transferring her to Hershey Medical Center (HMC) or keeping her at LGH.

"This is our first vent baby at LGH, but I would trust Dr. Kaur if I had my own baby in here," said Dr. Tifft, and added a few other good words. I remember how comforting that was, almost as much as when my mentor, Dr. MacMurray, had spoken words of encouragement just before my Fellow of the Royal College of Physicians, Canada (FRCPC) board's practical in Canada, not so many years earlier.

That first intubation was quite a celebratory and dramatic event in our NICU. It seemed like at

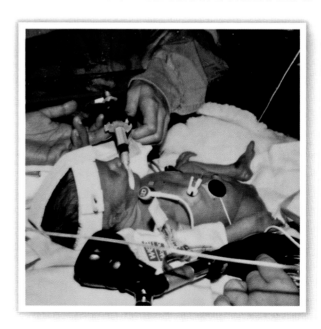

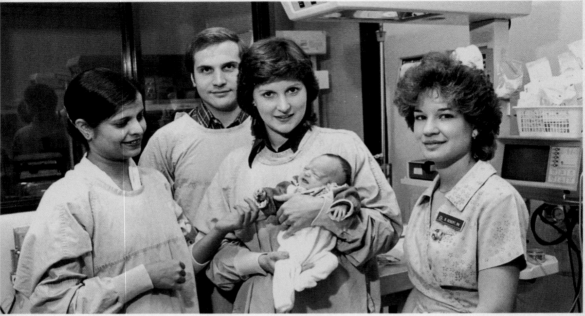

Intelligencer Journal photo by Richard Reinhold

The parents of six-week-old Lauren Sturla, born prematurely last month, prepare to take their daughter home Friday from Lancaster General Hospital— just in time for her first Christmas. Jeff and Ann Sturla, center, are seen off by Dr. Manjeet Kaur, left, head of the hospital's neonatal intensive care unit, and nurse Betsy Gebert.

Baby's Discharge is 1st For ICU

By Chris Noonan
Intelligencer Journal Staff

Six-week-old Lauren Sturla is going home for her first Christmas—but if all had gone according to plan, she wouldn't even be here yet.

Lauren was born two months premature on Nov. 12. And as is not uncommon with such infants, she had a lot of problems.

Before this September, Lauren would have been transferred to hospitals in Hersey or Philadelphia for special care. No more.

Staffers at Lancaster General Hospital's new neonatal intensive care unit monitored and oversaw her development for 39 days until she was strong enough to go home with her parents Friday.

The unit is the only one of its kind in the county. Before it was formed, 60 to 80 babies were transferred out of the county each year.

"The idea is, babies can be cared for in the county and parents don't have to travel," explained Anita Gogno, public relations director for LGH.

Lauren is the first child for Jeff and Ann Sturla. both 26, of 107 Donna Drive, Terre Hill. When Mrs. Sturla's placenta ruptured, doctors decided that the baby would have fewer problems if it were delivered prematurely.

But Lauren's lungs were underdeveloped and she needed oxygen. She was one of the first babies in the unit to go on a respirator.

She weighed four pounds, six ounces, but dropped to 3.9 pounds because she wasn't feeding correctly.

The baby's digestive system was underdeveloped. She couldn't breastfeed or handle formula, so she was fed intravenously.

But Lauren 's veins were so small and tender that they broke when nurses tried to put needles into them. "So they shaved both sides of her head to find a vein," said her mother. "They told me the veins in your head are as good to use as the ones in your arms and legs."

The sight scared Mrs. Sturla.

"We were very worried in the beginning," she said. "As soon as she was born the doctor told me to give her a kiss. I guess for 72 hours it was touch and go because of her being so early. She was hooked up to everything they could book her up to."

Mrs. Sturla visited her daughter every morning, then she and her husband would return to the hospital each night for a second visit.

Now Lauren weighs a healthy 4.13 pounds and is eating well. Her parents still have to watch over her carefully. They've learned infant CPR and will listen for warning beeps from a heart monitor the baby will wear on her chest for the next three months.

"She'll lead a normal life," her mother said. "And we can almost handle her as if she were born when she was term due."

least a dozen staff members, including nurses and respiratory therapists, were there during that procedure. "It went well!" I thought, after we placed the endotracheal tube and makeshift sandbags for support, not having very simple pieces like the angel frames that we have today. The staff was great—everyone pitching in as a team, providing long hours of care and poised to run for equipment as needed. With our first respirator in place, the staff was a bit nervous. We didn't have our own call room then, so our NICU manager had arranged the delivery of a sofa-cum-bed to my office for those times when I was unable to go home for hours or, on occasion, for days at a time.

Lauren improved over the next three days and was soon ready to go home. All had gone extremely well; the morale of the staff was pretty high and this called for another celebration! The media was there to cover the event, and the article in the *Intelligencer Journal* highlighted that the baby would need to have been transferred out of the county had this birth occurred two months earlier, before the NICU was established at LGH.

Though most pediatricians supported our endeavors, my biggest champions and supporters were Dr. Stephen Tifft, a great pediatrician, and Dr. Hilary Becker, a pediatrician who had some neonatology experience. I'll always be grateful to both of them. They not only covered for me for an occasional night here and there when I needed a break but also provided moral support

Simple things were addressed too. In those days, triple dye was applied to the cord of the infant after delivery, which worked well as an antiseptic but was unsightly with the violet stain and delayed cord separation. I had a meeting with the obstetricians and presented data and other options, just as we later did for meconium-stained babies. The maternity team always embraced changes if they were evidence-based, and especially if accompanied by appropriate presentations.

Thus began what was for me three decades of strong bonding with little angels from Lancaster—now our NICU Grads, whom I personally like to refer to as my godchildren: the diverse tiny buds who have blossomed into my wonderful Garden of Flowers.

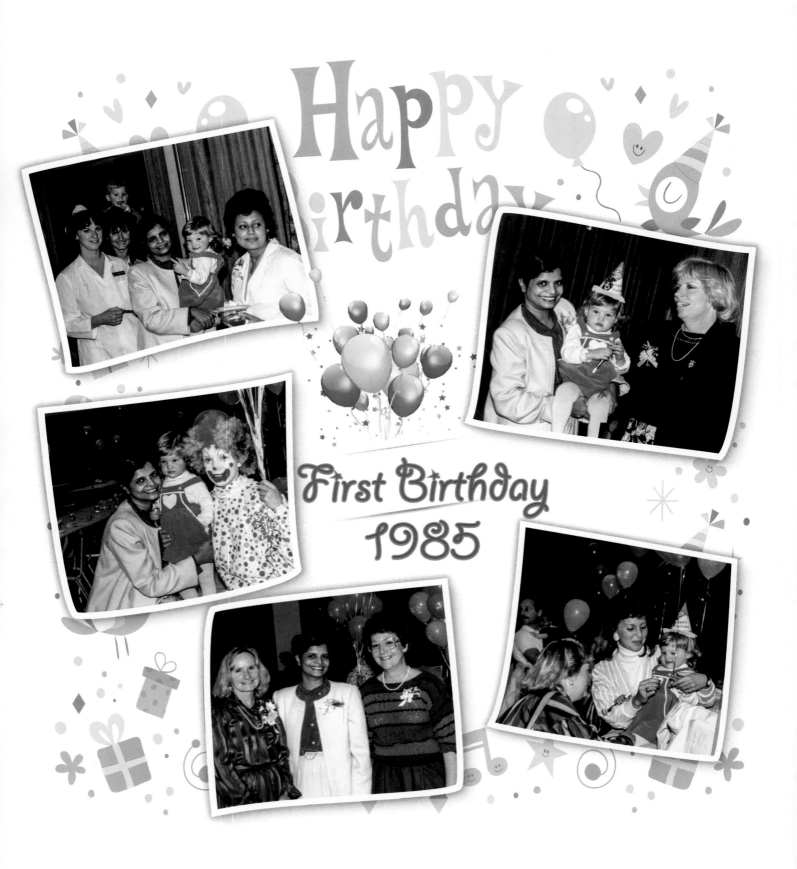

Happy Birthday

First Birthday
1985

Serving the Community

Lancaster General Hospital was founded as a non-sectarian hospital in 1893. Since its founding, it has provided an expanding range of medical, health, and education services to a community that is demographically and ethnically diverse. Lancaster is known for its sizable Amish and Mennonite population, and it includes both urban and rural communities. Since its inception in 1984 the NICU at Lancaster General Hospital made a vital contribution to the community health programs as new developments in medical technology were introduced to ensure that the sick newborn babies received the very best of care. The NICU also expanded the quality of its support to give the best family experience while the babies were in the hospital, and to ensure that the parents received the best possible support when they brought their little NICU grad home.

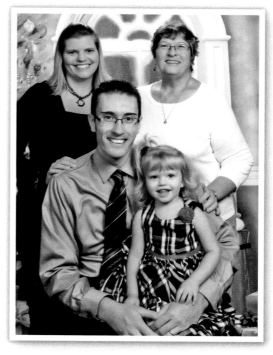

With support from our president we expanded our service to the community and I obtained privileges at St. Joseph Hospital (now called Lancaster Regional Hospital) so I could go there for deliveries and transport the sicker newborns to LGH. The staff of St. Joseph's nursery were a lot of fun to work with, and over the years some of them transferred to work with us in the NICU at LGH.

One of these babies from St. Joseph's was Bobby, a term LGA (large for gestational age) infant with meconium aspiration, perinatal distress, and seizures, possibly caused in part by the difficult delivery of this large baby. We started him on Phenobarbital and Dilantin, drugs we still use, and the pungent, odorous paraldehyde drip that we used back then, before his seizures could be controlled. With the constant care of our great staff, along with the Lord's blessings, all went well; the lad is now a thirty-year-old professor who lives in Florida with a family of his own.

> " The NICU also expanded the quality of its support to give the best family experience while the babies were in the hospital.

> "Prenatal ultrasounds were unknown or rare in the 1980s ... we never knew what we were going to get.

Over the years we have cared for babies from single mothers, babies born to mothers who did not know that they were pregnant, and babies with a wide variety of conditions such as diaphragmatic hernias, gastroschisis, encehaloceles and meningomyeloceles, sacrococcygeal teratomas, and various syndromes. Being amidst the Amish population meant more cases of dwarfism and genetic disorders, which are more prevalent within their community due to consanguinity or inbreeding.

Prenatal ultrasounds were unknown or rare in the 1980s, and every delivery could be a surgical challenge as well—*we never knew what we were going to get.* In those first two years, I certainly saw a lot of pathology that would be channeled to a center with surgical capability today.

Various community support events were held such as public educative conferences, birth fairs, and student awareness. I remember a public rhetoric at a church addressing the "Mothers of Twins Club" regarding problems of multiple gestation and support systems.

High school students were welcomed from area schools seeing the problems of teenage pregnancy and drug issues in their students, and students from Lancaster Country Day School came every year for several years as part of their field trip while completing a psychology course. We spoke about teenage pregnancy issues and the long-term effects of drug and alcohol abuse on babies—important wake-up calls for young teenagers.

The annual Birth Fair provided information and gave parents the opportunity to ask questions of the pediatric and neonatal specialists. The media recognized these services to the community, and always gave promotional coverage of these events.

Of course, we were always ready to respond when needed. I recall the wedding of one of our RNs. It was a lovely morning, and I was preparing to go to the ceremony when I got a call about a baby in distress, who turned out to have a diaphragmatic hernia (herniation of some abdominal contents into the chest). Being the only neonatologist in town, I rushed to the hospital and we got busy with respiratory support, stabilizing the infant before transferring him. At that time, surgical cases were transferred to the Hershey Medical Center (HMC) or Children's Hospital of Philadelphia (CHOP).

LANCASTER, PA, NEW ERA—TUESDAY, JUNE 4 1985

Pediatricians to Talk to Moms at Birth Fair

By NAOMI YOCOM
New Era Staff Writer

MOTHERS-TO-BE are always full of baby questions on everything from diet to diapers. "Should I breast-feed?"

Suppose the baby comes early ...? "What if my doctor isn't in when I call — who do I talk to?" "How do I take a brand new baby's temperature?" • "What should I do about colic?"

To respond to this mountain of question marks, Saturday's YWCA Birth Fair will offer a panel discussion on child care with pediatricians Drs. Clark McSparren, Margaret Knox and Hillary Becker, family practitioner Dr. Peter Altimare and neonatologist (specialist in the care of high-risk newborns) Dr. Manjeet Kaur. Registered nurse Joanna Boyer of Lancaster General Hospital will be the moderator.

Questions like, If I have a problem breast-feeding, do I go to my child's pediatrician or to my obstetrician?"

The pediatricians generally agreed that problems should be handled by whoever is best able to handle them, and all said they would encourage the woman to continue breast-feeding.

The question about breast feeding had a different shading when asked of Dr. Manjeet Kaur. neonatologist at Lancaster General Hospital. The babies she deals with may desperately need breast milk.

If this is the case. but the baby is too small to be put to the breast, Mrs. Kaur will encourage the mother to pump her breast so the milk can be frozen for the baby. Mrs. Kaur said, reassuringly. that only 6 or 7 percent or all babies are premature (defined as under 5 pounds, 8 ounces or less than 37 weeks gestation), and only 1 or 2 percent are extremely high risk. Women are more likely to give birth prematurely if they are carrying multiple babies, are under 16 or over 35, suffering from poor nutrition (often these women are from poor socio-economic backgrounds), have given birth prematurely in the past or have medical problems such as diabetes, said Mrs. Kaur.

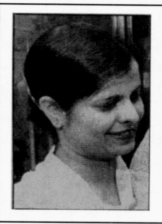

"Education and good prenatal care can help prevent some premature births. There are things that can be done during pregnancy."
-Dr. Manjeet Kaur

Also, if a mother drinks alcohol, takes drugs or smokes cigarettes she is risking premature birth.

Education and good prenatal care can help prevent some premature births, Mrs. Kaur said.

"There are thing that can be done during pregnancy." It is important to know what is normal and what ls not and what to do if there may be trouble. This is just one of the goals of the Birth Fair, which will run from 8:30 a.m. to 1:30 p.m. at the YWCA, 110 N. Lime street.

There is no admission charge.

Another story imprinted indelibly in my mind is of a courageous Amish mother of five children. She had recently been diagnosed with metastatic breast cancer while twenty-six weeks pregnant, and she presented with jaundice due to liver metastasis among other symptoms. The baby would be better off being delivered via cesarean section so the mother could begin chemotherapy. Little Miriam looked literally green at delivery; she was very sick, and needed every medical modality we had available. Mom did

survive long enough to hold and care for her baby in the NICU. I'll never forget that stoic strength of faith exhibited by the baby's father, calm and accepting, even as he had a dying wife and possibly baby as well. I'm always amazed at this profound faith and strength of the Amish, which I've witnessed time and again over the years. That day I saw living proof of that trust.

After his wife passed, the father came back to see us, bringing the little one and his other children, all

> "I'm always amazed at this profound faith and strength of the Amish.

neatly dressed in white blouses, black pinafores, and bonnets. I remember bringing them some chocolates and feeling overwhelmed with emotion at such valiant acceptance. The extended-family support of the Amish folk is phenomenal, and brings them great strength.

I had a wonderful continuity with the families over the first two years, since I was the only neonatologist at the time. This is likely one of the reasons why I'm still so connected with babies from the early days, having cared for them every day during their stay in the NICU.

The people of Lancaster County have a wonderful community spirit. We had many volunteers—always ready to do whatever was needed to keep our babies comfortable. One delightful eighty-year-old lady came to meet me. "I want to knit hats for your babies, Dr. Kaur," she said. "**I knit all day except when I am in the church or the bathtub.**" We talked about designs, not placing strings or ribbons to prevent a choking hazard. True to her word, from that day on, Mrs. Beal provided us with stacks of hats for many years.

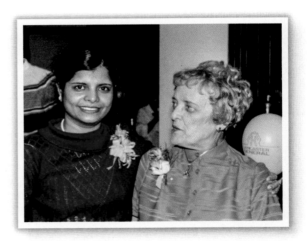

Two years on, another neonatologist joined us—one with a great love for Mickey Mouse. I've never met anyone so enamored of Mickey—ever! At his job interview he wore a Mickey tie, a Mickey watch, and to my surprise, when he took his wallet out to show me a photograph of his daughter, it was—you guessed it—a Mickey wallet! What a sweet love for a pediatrician. Dr. John Jirka turned out to be a dedicated neonatologist with a great sense of humor.

Now we could keep smaller babies in the NICU, and between LGH and St. Joseph Hospital we covered over 2,500 deliveries a year.

Like any other busy unit, we continued to have challenging cases. A call I remember vividly was one for transport of an extremely preterm infant born in a toilet bowl in a bar. Not knowing what to expect, after intubation we brought back the baby, who stayed with us for weeks. Mom, a single mother, bonded with the NICU staff and made wonderful friends in the NICU. She kept in touch with her NICU family, and I still have a painting of a little boy that Mom had made and gifted me—a precious memento!

Our NICU was certainly well supported by the administration. **Pulse oximetry** was first introduced for babies in the mid-eighties. Looking back, it's hard to imagine how we ever survived without that common, non-invasive modality for monitoring oxygenation! At that time we were obtaining capillary blood gases, which do not give a very accurate oxygen status, to monitor the babies' respiratory status. We had only just learned of this new technology when we had preterm twins delivered. We met with the administrators and expressed our request, and they promptly located the needed equipment and had it flown to us. That certainly saved the babies many sticks!

This was still the pre-surfactant era. We did have several babies with chronic lung disease and long-term vents, and we sent at least four babies home on ventilators after a tracheostomy in those early years. One of a set of twins had been sent home on a ventilator. He remained on the vent for almost eighteen months, and when we went to visit him at home he was crawling along with the long, extended

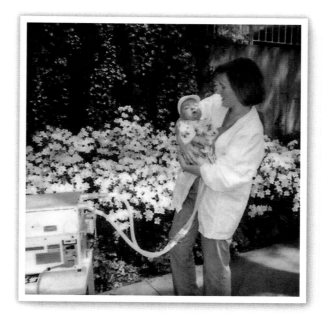

coil connected to his tracheostomy. Andrew is a fine young married man today. I remember nurses with a respiratory therapist taking little Zach for a walk with a trach and vent as he had never been out of the NICU in the first nine months of life. Another baby I remember was on a respirator for over a year. We celebrated his first birthday in the NICU, and actually cut a birthday cake for him outside the NICU.

In 1988 and 1990 we were joined by two other neonatologists, Dr. Lebischak and Dr. Mahajan. Dr. Lebischak, a bright doctor and fun-loving friend, worked at LGH for almost sixteen years before relocating to Florida. Dr. Mahajan is a caring, intelligent, and knowledgeable physician who became a good friend and was still working in the NICU in 2017. He and his wife had triplets who were in the NICU and are now great, college-going youngsters.

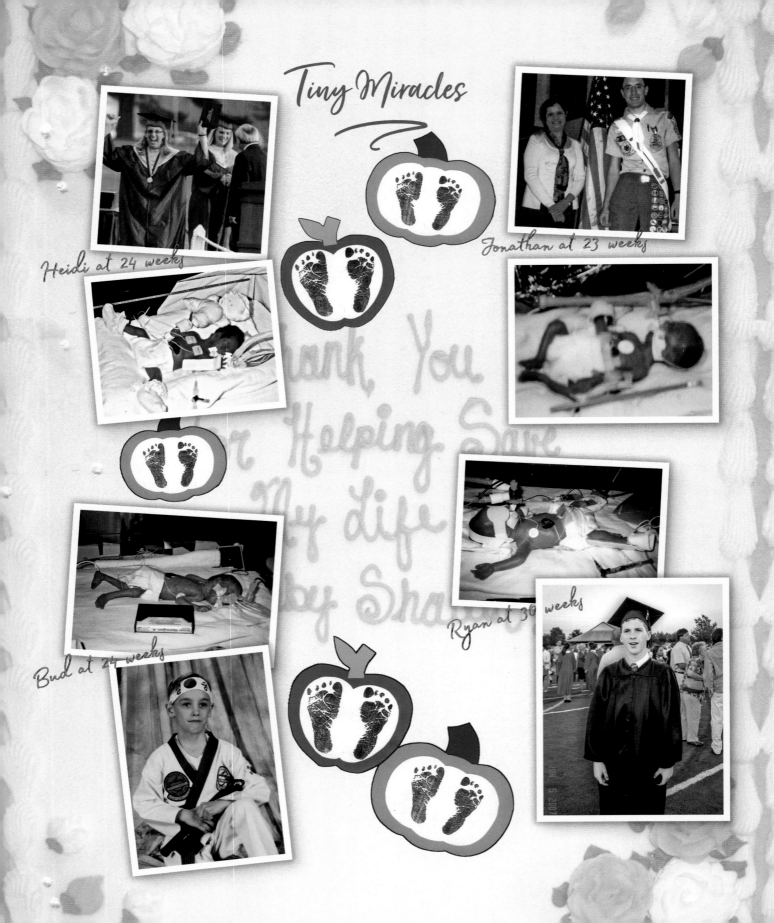

Tiny Miracles

Heidi at 24 weeks

Jonathan at 23 weeks

Bud at 24 weeks

Ryan at 30 weeks

Miracles in the NICU

People often speak of the miracles that happen in the NICU—I have truly seen the Divine Hand at work many times over the years. Situations that seemed beyond hope, and tiny, brave warriors who survived against all the odds.

We had toiled all night with a very sick infant who was born via emergency cesarean section, had very poor Apgar scores, pulmonary hypertension, and was extremely difficult to ventilate. The cord pH of this little boy was so low (representing fetal compromise) that we were unsure of his survival, and we definitely didn't expect an intact survival without neuro-developmental issues.

He ended up requiring ECMO (extracorporeal membrane oxygenation),[4] was sent out by helicopter for this specialized treatment, and then came back to us. Mom said that she named him Drew Justin, as he drew a lot of attention and was born just in time. This little one has grown up to be a cute, normal, little boy. For many years, the grateful young mom brought her sweet bundle of joy to visit her NICU family.

⁂

A term infant, delivered via a repeat C-section, presented with respiratory distress and was transferred to the NICU. The baby's oxygen requirement kept going up, and we ended up intubating her and placing her on vent support. Her need for respiratory support, however, continued to escalate over the next few days. She became hard to oxygenate despite maximal respiratory support due to persistent pulmonary hypertension (PPHN).[5] A decision was made to send her out for (ECMO), and she was transported by helicopter to a hospital in Washington, DC. They found on a scan that she had a cerebellar (brain) bleed, and the protocol at that facility determined that she didn't qualify for ECMO. They would just take her off the vent and let her go; therefore, my partner brought her back to LGH.

This little cherub had multiple pneumothoraces (lung air leaks) during the hospital course, and at one time had eight tubes in place to drain recurrent air-collection pockets around her lungs. I remember coding her and placing chest tubes. We continued to care for her as best as we could, using high ventilator support until she was finally well enough to be discharged. I have delightful photos of her at follow-up, at our NICU reunions, and ones her mom sent. Today, she is a normal adult and is working in the medical field. Amazing, isn't it?!

⁂

---

4   ECMO: a procedure in which the sick lungs are bypassed and the blood is re-oxygenated outside the body in equipment somewhat like a heart-lung machine.

5   PPHN: persistent pulmonary hypertension is a condition where oxygenated blood is diverted back from the lungs due to a narrowing of blood vessels in the lungs.

"Little Bud" was a twenty-four-week-gestation infant born with fused eyelids—a consequence of extreme prematurity. Though lots of babies who are born at that stage of immaturity survive today, in the early 1980s fused eyelids was considered to be a criterion of non-survivability. Initially thought to be non-viable, Bud had a strong heart rate and was resuscitated. He was a strong one, made it through numerous hurdles, and went home with his delightful family after a NICU stay of about three months.

His mom kept strong connections, sent photos and notes, and came for visits both at work and at home. He has certainly become an extended family for me. Every Halloween, my children had to wait for Bud's visit with his mom and two sisters before they were allowed to go trick-or-treating in case we missed Bud. One time he came to my house after earning a black belt in karate to show me how he could break a block of wood, and again after his graduation, since I had not been able to attend the ceremony—"Before he went to his girlfriend's home," his mom told me.

Of course, he was always in attendance at our various NICU reunions, and later, an ambassador at one of our hospital administrative retreats. Invariably he brought me flowers and would say, "My mom says to always greet a lady with flowers." How absolutely endearing!

> "'My mom says to always greet a lady with flowers.' How absolutely endearing!

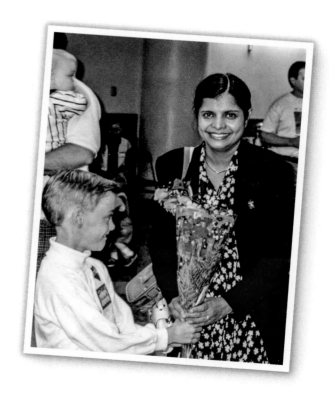

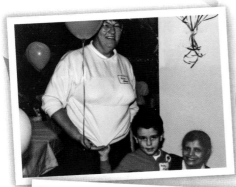

Early Days Celebrations

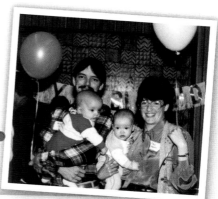

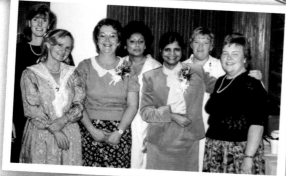

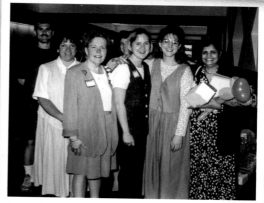

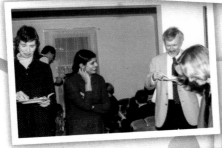

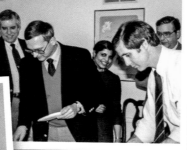

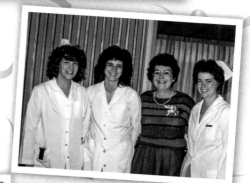

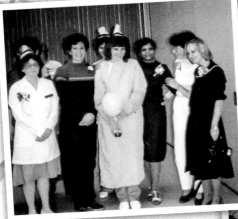

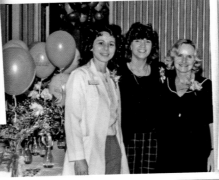

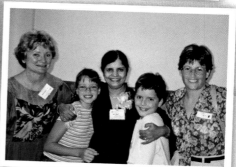

Could one ask for a better and more rewarding job?

Such stories are hard—no, impossible—to forget. True miracles: these sick children with a poor prognosis (expected outcome) and who are now doing so well. My philosophy has always been to be perfectly honest with the parents and tell them all the problems that can occur. Being prepared for the worst possibilities is far better than living in a spurious paradise. The nurses would often tell the parents, "The doctor is telling you 'as it is' and not through rose-tinted glasses." But the tenacity and resilience of those tiny newborn bundles have never failed to amaze me. The longer I've been in the profession, the more hesitant I've become to give a firm prognosis.

> "Could one ask for a better and more rewarding job?

The local newspapers have always been great supporters. Over the years they would seek out opportunities such as the birth of a tiny baby, or triplets or quads to run a feature article about the NICU which families really loved.

It's interesting how one connects with families who are undergoing the most serious problems and with some of the sickest infants. Often, to lighten the moments, we would speak to the families as we waited for events to unfold, and even nicknamed their little ones. I remember one whose mother always dressed her infant in especially long booties, resembling Dick Whittington's cat in the story of *Puss in Boots*. I called her my "Little Puss in Boots." Many years later, I received a card from the mother of a lovely eight-year-old girl, signed, "Your Puss in Boots." When we had a preterm baby born with the first snowfall, I called her "My Little Snowflake," and later we got cards that said, "from Snowflakes."

It's amazing how these little fun anecdotes become so meaningful and are so often remembered. I think parents and staff hold on to the precious lighter notes associated with those very difficult moments. Some other nicknames I remember nostalgically are "Little Mac" (who later got promoted to a "Big Mac"); "Spring Shine," obviously born on a warm spring day; "Good Golly Miss Molly," whom parents chose to call Molly; "Jane Austen's Emma," after the classic novel when the name Emma was being discussed. Each time these sweet names would bring a smile amidst the serious business of the NICU.

Sadly, not all stories are positive ones, and amidst the wonders, there were many days and long nights when tiny lungs were too immature even for pumped breaths, and hearts too tired to beat. We've fought our share of losing battles, our share of situations where nothing could be done, and others in which our current state-of-the-art technology just wasn't enough or the baby was just too early and didn't meet the limit of viability, a bud that didn't unfurl. Much

as we would like to be strong, we often cry with these families, holding their hands when there is nothing more that we can do. As clinicians, we try our best and then leave our precious bundles in His hands.

Our wonderful chaplains are always available to support the parents if they so desire. Nowadays, with protocols and support teams, a lot of support systems come into play so that assistance can be continued beyond maternal discharge as needed.

After sitting by the bedside comforting a grieving family, I would go to my office, look at my wall of photos of tiny babies now little ballerinas, soccer players, kids hanging upside down on a swing. What a comfort that was to see those faces smiling back at me.

Suddenly the secretary interrupts. "A doctor is on the line from Community hospital; he wants to talk to you regarding transport of a 30-week-gestation infant." A sense of urgency fills the air as details are obtained, the transport accepted, and some instructions are given—a pitter-patter of feet collecting equipment while informing the respiratory therapist,

transport nurses, and arranging for an ambulance. The ambulance leaves, for the transport—then back to the NICU routine ... humming of the respirators, beeping alarms, and incessant rings of the phone. A mother waits to discuss the status of her infant. The secretary calls, "It's 11:30 doctor—the pharmacy is calling for parental nutrition scripts for Baby Herr and Baby Collins." Yes! Of course let us get that done before we get busy with our new little one from Community—some semblance of routine—**the NICU routine**.

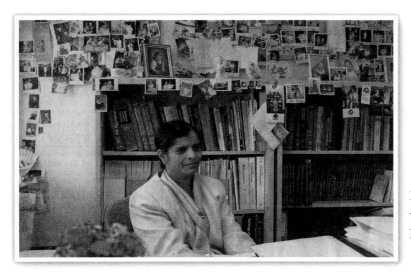

Dr. Kaur's office is decorated with pictures of the children who have been cared for by the NICU.
—Sunday News, Lancaster PA
December 7, 1997

An Art Divine

Healing is an art, an art divine,
A blessing, a sanction to seek at that shrine!
A rhapsody of love—on the clarinet of time.
Amidst turmoil and chaos at a tumultuous pace,
A promise to comfort, possibly cure, a pledge to bring solace.
Aspiring to administer a soothing therapy with grace!
                                          —Manjeet Kaur

The Divine Art of Healing

Pythagoras said, "The most divine art is that of healing. And, if the healing art is most divine, it must occupy itself with the soul as well as the body, for no creature can be sound as long as the higher part in it is sickly."

This story is of a tiny preemie born at the limit of viability at twenty-three-and-a-half-weeks gestation. Mom was in labor and in no condition to be transferred from St. Joseph Hospital, so the LGH NICU transport team was called. As I lived closest, I arrived before the rest of the team and received this twenty-three-and-a-half-week-gestation infant.

The nurses at St. Joseph, though very caring and competent, weren't experienced in dealing with extreme prematurity. Luckily, all went well; the infant was resuscitated, and transported to LGH. I distinctly remember that moment in the hallway when we spoke to the mom on a gurney on her way to her room. As I explained the odds and the risks of a micro preemie, she smiled and said, "I have faith, Dr. Kaur. He has strong protoplasm. He will be fine."

For me, it was certainly one of those moments when I felt the hand of the Divine.

> "As I explained the odds and the risks of a micro preemie, she smiled and said, 'I have faith, Dr. Kaur. He has strong protoplasm. He will be fine.'

Today, this same little one whose photograph I have with a pencil next to him, which was close to his body length, is now a handsome, courteous, six-foot-tall young man who came to the door to greet and escort me as I went to attend his Eagle Scout ceremony in a church. At his special request, I recently danced with him at his wedding and had the honor of being seated with his parents. It brought tears to my eyes as I reminisced about his birth and his NICU course.

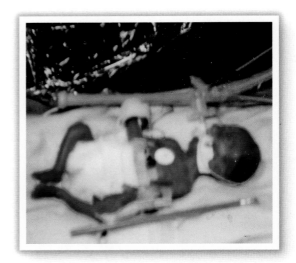

Sometimes one has to wonder if it's the faith or our efforts that make the difference. My conclusion is probably both. To me that was a moment of faith, a moment of grace.

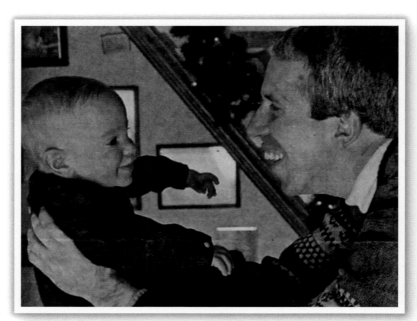

Jonathan Sherts, who weighed only 1 pound, 7 ounces at birth, has some fun with his dad, Jeff.
Sunday News Photos/Jack Leonard.

'This baby is going to make it'

And, he did

By Peggy Schmidt
Sunday News Staff Writer

Pam and Jeff Sherts, were expecting their second child on or about Feb. 2-Ground Hog Day-1990, but their son, Jonathan made his debut Oct. 12, 1989—Columbus Day—at only 23 to 24 weeks of gestation. When Pam went into labor, there was little hope the baby would survive.

But there was a heartbeat. There was a neonatologist at hand. There was the determination of Jonathan's mother that "This baby is going to make it."

And despite overwhelming odds, Jonathan did make it. He was delivered—all 1 pound, 7 ounces of him-at St. Joseph Hospital and Health Care center, with Dr. Manjeet Kaur, neonatologist, in attendance. Jonathan was quickly transported to Lancaster General Hospital, where he remained in the Neonatal Intensive Care Unit (NICU) until Jan. 20, when the nation was observing Martin Luther King's birthday.

Examination indicated Pam was in labor and her physician, Dr. Laurence W. France, offered little hope for the baby's survival. "I was prepared to

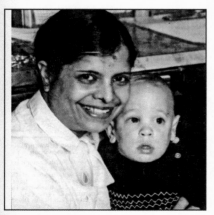

Dr. Manjeet Kaur says, for his 'corrected age,' Jonathan is doing well.

give birth to a dead fetus," Pam said, "but they put the monitor on Jonathan's head and picked up a heartbeat!"

Jonathan's eyes were still fused shut when he was born and did not open for another two weeks. His Apgar scores (a means of testing babies' vital functions) were low; the initial score was 2, although within 10 minutes a second and third test showed scores of 7 and 9, which are in the normal range.

The baby's lungs were not developed, which is typical of premature babies, and he was supported by a respirator for 40 days. He was jaundiced and needed phototherapy. He was on antibiotics and IV feedings as well. Those feedings, Dr. Kaur said, were "very specially made. We sort of custom-make each one."

Jonathan also had a heart murmur, but required no surgery; the murmur corrected itself. In addition he developed an inguinal hernia, "which is very common in premature babies, and especially boys," Dr. Kaur said. "It had to be repaired and, unfortunately, we do not have a pediatric surgeon at LGH. We had to send him out to Children's Hospital of Philadelphia."

Taking Jonathan out of LGH for surgery in Philadelphia was difficult for the Sherts family. "That was the hardest taking him out of (LGH)," said Pam. "I had built up such trust in those people."

Vickie Reay, who—along with Sandy Ness, Beth Yeingst and Suzanne Lefever—served as Jonathan's nurse in the NICU, said, "Jonathan was the most pleasant child to take care of and, in fact, he did do so well compared to other premature kids we had.

Jonathan's homecoming was a sure

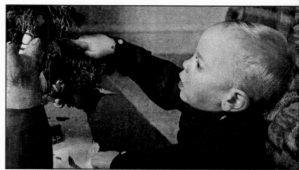

Sunday News Photos/Jack Leonard

Jonathan Sherts, who weighed only 1 pound, 7 ounces at birth

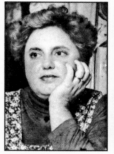
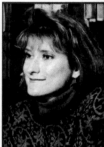

Pam Sherts, left, and nurse Vickie Reay recall Jonathan's first days.

sign of his good progress, something Pam, Jeff and their son, Steven, 6, had been praying for months.

Still, the day he came home was a difficult time for his mother. "I was scared to death," Pam said. "His life support was taken away, and I was petrified." She said she continually asked herself, "Am I going to remember what to do?"

"The first two nights were the worst, but then I gained confidence. (I thought) 'I can do this. We're going to be fine.'"

Pam and Jeff said that they have a debt of gratitude to many people. "The things that got us through," Pam said, "are the love, support and prayers of the whole community of East Petersburg, our church, Hempfield Church of the Brethren, and our families. They have been wonderful Believe it or not, our church sent meals, one a day, for an entire year.

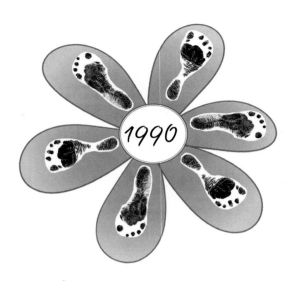

The second was an acceptance for training of Neonatal Nurse Practitioners (NNPs) as care providers for LGH.

In some states around the country, NNPs were being trained and found to be a great asset to the neonatologists. This was certainly a new concept, and when I approached the administration, some initially deemed it unacceptable. The cons given were, one—that nurses would find it hard to accept orders from other nurses even if they'd received additional training. Another—that parents wouldn't accept NNPs as care providers for their babies. I remember collecting data and making a slide presentation regarding the acceptability, role, and training needed for NNPs. I presented this to the NICU administrators and the staff, and, after much discussion, we finally got approval.

We selected three of our nurses as candidates who were sent to Washington, DC, for the NNP teaching program followed by an internship with us for six months before going on to take an exam. I affectionately called them platypi. Just as a platypus has features of both a bird and a mammal, so they were both nurses and "docs," I teased. At the time I was writing this narrative, Steve and Julie, who interned with us at LGH, are still working in our unit. This became a very successful project. We've had some of the finest NNPs, and both nurses and parents have given very positive feedback.

*T*he wheels of time moved on—a new decade—a new beginning.

The year 1990 brought two major advances in the field of neonatology.

One was the approval of the much-awaited Surfactant, a phospholipid given as a liquid through an endotracheal tube (breathing tube) into the lungs to help the underdeveloped lungs of a preterm infant. Our babies would now breathe more easily—this was indeed a breakthrough in the field of neonatology!

"The year 1990 brought two major advances in the field of neonatology. One was the approval of Surfactant … The second was an acceptance … of Neonatal Nurse Practitioners as care providers for LGH.

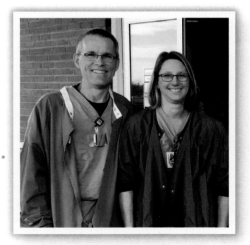

NNPs, Steve Hart and Julie Leach

LANCASTER, PA, NEW ERA

THURSDAY, MARCH 11, 1993

'Super Babies!' exclaims physician tending quads

by Jane Holahan — New Era Staff Writer

She's a tiny thing, no bigger than a woman's forearm.

Lying on her stomach in the warmer bed, with intravenous tubes stuck in her arms and a bili mask—what one nurse refers to as a little pair of sunglasses—shielding her eyes from the lamps above, she sleeps peacefully, her breathing steady and even.

Sylvia Esh, the smallest of the quadruplets born to Emma and Amos Esh Wednesday at Lancaster General Hospital, may be a bit frail, but she's doing "better than anyone expected."

And so are her three sisters.

"So far they've been extremely stable. They're taking no supplemental oxygen and their lungs are mature. We don't anticipate any problems, though it's a little early to tell. But so far things look good," says neonatologist Dr. Manjeet Kaur, who is in charge of the babies' care.

Born eight weeks prematurely the girls are now in the neonatal unit at LGH, where they will probably stay for several weeks. Since they are only a day old, Kaur is hesitant to make too many predictions, but she called Wednesday's delivery "a once in a lifetime thing. I was on the top of the world yesterday."

All four girls have lost a few ounces since their birth, which Kaur says is perfectly normal. And she says one of the girls has had a brief episode in which she stopped breathing for a moment, but that, too, is relatively normal.

It will probably be about two months before the girls can go home, and they may have to be

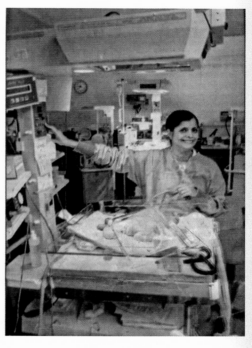

New Era Photo/Richard Hertzler

Dr. Manjeet Kaur, above, oversees one of the 11 premature babies in the neonatal center at Lancaster General Hospital. Two of the quadruplets born Wednesday can be seen in the background.

hooked up to monitors.

"We've got to worry about jaundice, infections—they're on antibiotics now—and nutrition," Kaur explains.

Another milestone in our NICU was the birth of **quadruplets (quads) in 1993**. These were surprisingly natural quads born to an Amish couple who already had three other children. Seven children under four!! All of us waited excitedly for this once-in-a-lifetime opportunity to care for quads. Born at thirty-two-weeks gestation, however, they were super babies, requiring minimal support. Mom and Dad had maintained a calm demeanor amidst all the chaos and excitement—a wonderful tribute to the Amish.

There was a lot of support, but one can only imagine raising four babies along with another three children under four.

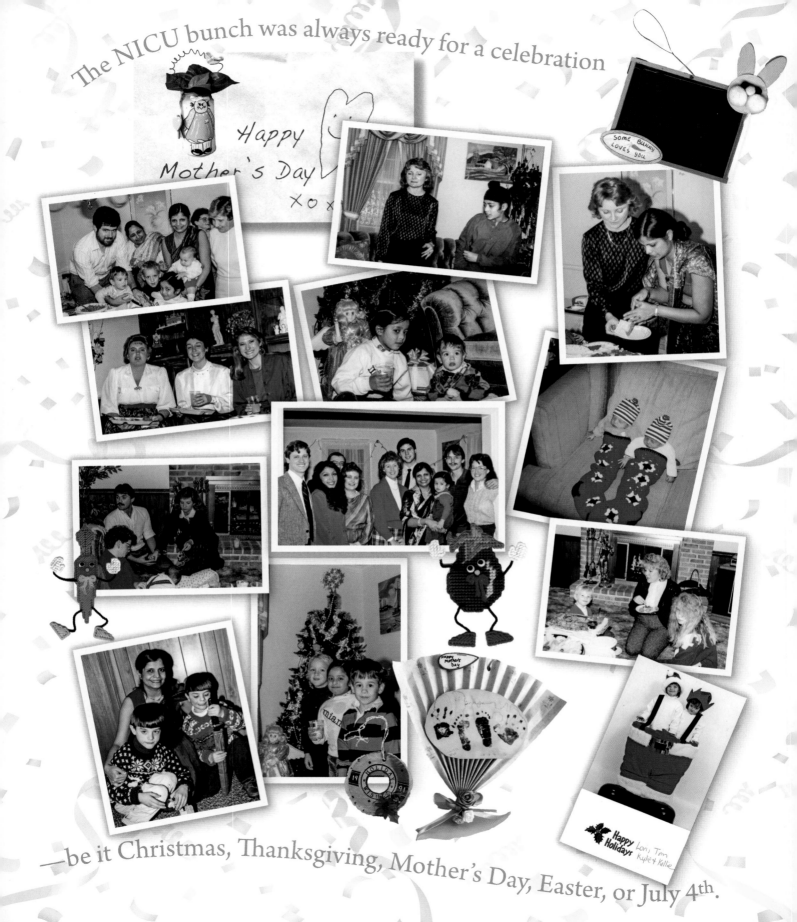

The NICU bunch was always ready for a celebration

—be it Christmas, Thanksgiving, Mother's Day, Easter, or July 4th.

Our NICU Family

Every few years we had reunions of our "NICU graduates," and we always arranged for someone to take photos. Once we started, families would often line up and we felt like Santa Claus. These are some of my dearest memories—seeing our little ones growing up and capturing those precious moments.

The nursing staff has always been one of the key pillars of our successes and an integral part of our NICU family. We have shared stories about our homes and children, and they have always been wonderful resources, both professionally and otherwise. Early on, we had Christmas parties at one of our homes almost every year. Besides the NICU staff, we invariably invited the parents of some of our graduates with their children, and together we would sing carols and hang Christmas ornaments—wonderful memories!

> "The NICU bunch was always ready for a celebration—be it Christmas, Thanksgiving, Mother's Day, Easter, or July 4th. Invariably our talented nurses made little parental gifts with infant footprints and messages of comfort.

A lot of the families of the NICU Grads have remained connected with the LGH NICU family over the years. They would come to visit, often bringing photos, and sometimes mailing us updates. I would often get a call on the child's birthday, always amazed that Mom wished to remember someone connected with such a difficult time. Christmas was always a happy time when we got tons of cards from moms giving us an update about their families and how their little NICU Grads were doing.

The NICU bunch was always ready for a celebration—be it Christmas, Thanksgiving, Mother's Day, Easter, or July 4th. Invariably our talented staff made little parental gifts with infant footprints and messages of comfort.

We always had fun on April first (April Fool's Day) too. I remember one time, in cahoots with Dr. Kegel, a fine Obstetrician at St. Joseph's Hospital, enacting a preterm birth with a nurse actually on a bed, calling out to the Nursery to come immediately for a twenty-five-week gestation birth (of course we made sure nothing urgent was happening at the time). He passed a wrapped resuscitation doll to the nurses who were too frazzled even then to realize what was happening till they opened the little bundle. Everyone chimed—"April Fool!"

The work longevity of the nursing staff in the NICU is a bona fide proof of the quality of our NICU family. We have several NICU nurses from back in the eighties and nineties still working with us, and a couple of nurses who left for family reasons came back after several years. They literally did come back to their NICU family.

We are indeed blessed to have such a dedicated staff!

A personal celebratory event that stands out in memory was my surprise fiftieth birthday party. My colleagues and staff orchestrated it, and most of our NICU staff members attended. My family was invited to the restaurant as well. Surprise! Surprise! Not only my husband and children but also my mother was there at this midday luncheon. Of course, there were a lot of "over the hill" fun jokes and gifts, one of which was a bike—so I could keep myself moving, I guess. What a great gesture, and what fun!

Such occasions remain etched in my mind, recalling the generosity and closeness of my amazing NICU family.

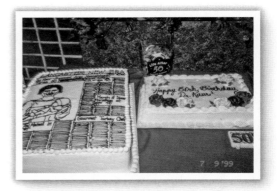

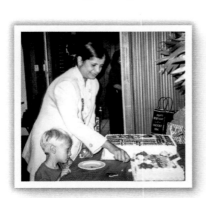

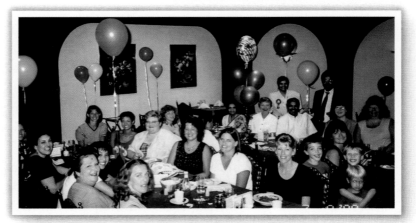

Life's Treasures

Life's greatest treasures lie not in accumulation of wealth, diamonds and pearls
But amassing great deeds:
not deeds of achievement!
nor ones acclaiming greatness!
But shimmering links of smiles, of love and happiness that glow and swirl,
The images of faces you lit up in life,
In times of duress, in times of strife.
Of the pearls of tears from pained eyes that you stole,
More precious than emeralds, more treasured than gold.
Count these treasures till your coffers fill,
The happiness in your heart, your gift … an everlasting rill!
—Manjeet Kaur

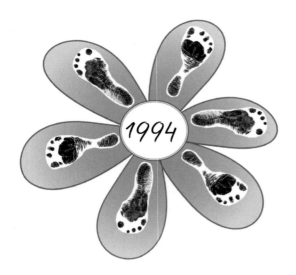

1994

It was 1994—could it be a decade since the inception of our NICU?

We had grown into a fully fledged NICU, now caring for over 350 babies each year, amongst them many micro preemies—singletons, as well as twins and triplets.

The Lancaster newspaper printed a great article reprising our first ten years and featuring Bud Getzloff who had been born at twenty-four weeks weighing one pound, nine ounces.

Cody Sheid was featured in the paper for the 10th NICU Anniversary—a little one born at twenty-six weeks weighing one pound three ounces. I attended his prestigious Eagle Scout ceremony and was filled with pride as this little hero was decorated with medals. Little Cody is now a handsome and affable young man who works at a bank.

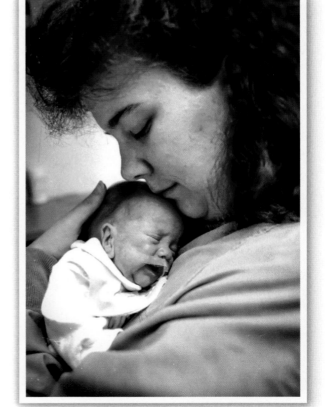

NICU puts the accent on care

By Lisa Christopher
Sunday News Staff Writer

When Rita Getzloff gave birth to a baby three months prematurely in July 1987, she didn't know whether it was a boy or a girl. All she knew was the baby was in distress.

"The way we found out the baby was a boy was the doctor came over to us and said 'I'm sorry. He didn't make it.' "

The baby, Getzloff said had no heartbeat. The medical staff tried cardiopulmonary resuscitation but to no avail. For some reason, though, when they pulled an air tube out of the baby's throat his heart started beating on its own.

"He was alive and they told us to just take things one day at a time. That's what we did," Getzloff said.

Today. William Leonard, "Bud" to his friends, who weighed 1 pound, 9 ounces at birth is a first-grader at Sacred Heart Parish School where his favorite topics are recess and lunch he said. This year, he's going to be a green Power Ranger for Halloween.

Bud is just one of the miraculous stories that has come out of the Lancaster General Hospital Neonatal Intensive Care Unit. This year, the unit celebrates its 10th anniversary.

'The staff here is an extended family to us " Getzloff said. "We spent three months with the people here. They gave us more than just medical help. They gave us moral support."

"They keep in touch. It's amazing how they remember me,' said Dr. Manjeet Kaur, chief of neonatology since the department's inception.

Kaur's office walls are lined with bright smiling little faces of the babies she's nurtured at the unit.

There's Adam. Jonathan. Bobby. Jake. Ethan. Amber and dozens more.

"Amber had eight chest tubes in her at one point. Here she is at discharge," Kaur said pointing to one of the photos. We never thought we'd see that day. We thought she'd die."

Kaur is one of three doctors assigned to the unit. But when it opened, Kaur was the only doctor. At the time, she was the mother of a 1-year-old and a 7-year-old and assigned to 24- hour-a-day, on-call duty.

At that time, the unit accepted children 32 weeks and older. Nowadays the unit can handle babies as small as 23 weeks into development. The survival rate of the unit is 55 to 60 percent. The unit can handle 18 babies at one time. Most babies spend about three months in the unit.

"Statistically, we do have losses, but it is always hard to take," Kaur said. "When I get depressed, I come into my office and see all these pictures of these faces of the babies who were once so sick and now are thriving."

Before the LGH unit opened premature babies or infants in need of specialized care ere sent to Hershey Medical Center. Having a neonatal unit in the county saves precious time in the first moments of life and enables immediate medical assistance for a baby in distress.

After 10 years on the unit, Kaur has one wish for its future.

"I would like to see us be able to do pediatric surgery here so babies won't have to be transferred to Hershey or Children's Hospital in Philadelphia," Kaur said.

Kaur said parents and medical staff bond to one another during the baby's stay in the hospital.

"You get attached to the kids here because you are together a very long time through the bard times," Kaur said.

"I think being a mother has made me a better doctor," Kaur said. 'I feel for the parents. I sit and cry with them sometimes, and while I can't get too emotional, I think the parents are comforted by the fact that their doctor feels what they are going through.

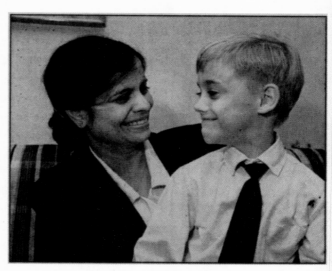

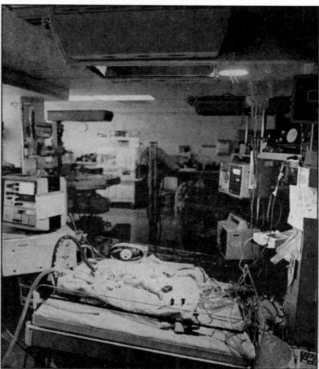

Sunday News Photos/Jeff Ruppenthal

Dr. Manjeet Kaur (top photo) talks with former patient Bud Getzloff. Cody Scheid, above, the son of Keri and David Scheid, Holtwood, is a current patient. He was born 14 weeks premature.

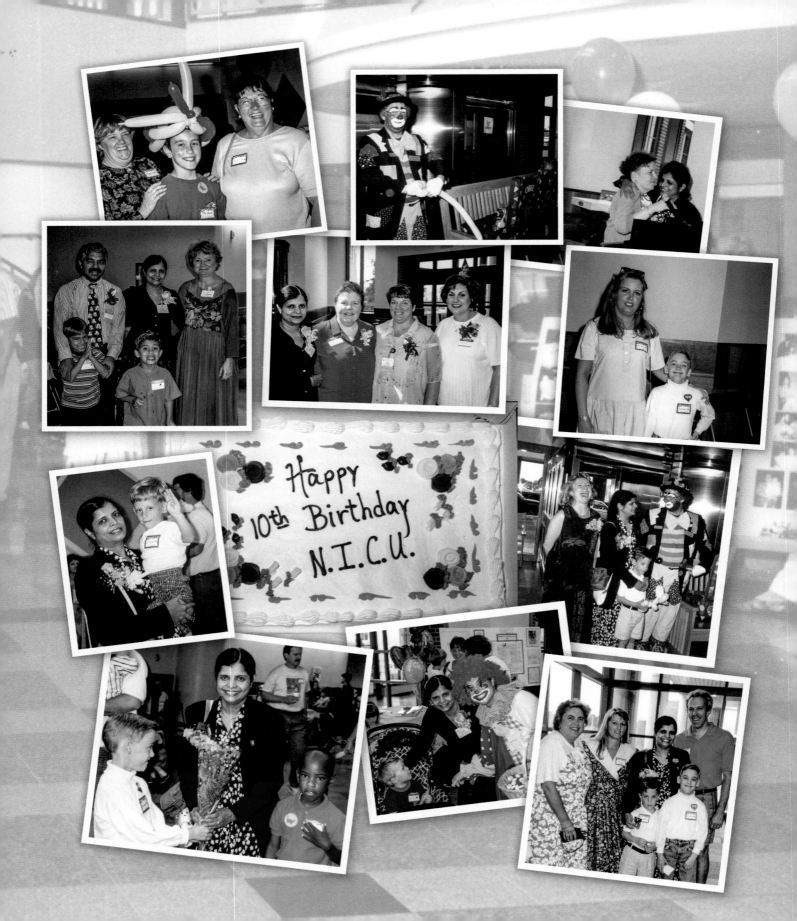

Happy
10th Birthday
N.I.C.U.

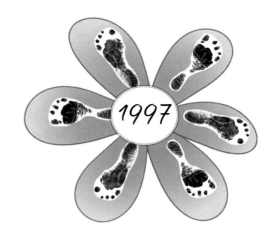

The neonatal unit continued to flourish, and in 1997 the *New Era* ran an article about our little Irish miracle, Jacqueline, born on St. Patrick's Day at twenty-five-weeks gestation—delivered by cesarean section due to maternal preeclampsia. Who knew that this tiny baby would not only graduate with academic honors but also would be a wonderful musician and actually play the bass at Carnegie Hall?

LANCASTER, PA, NEW ERA   MONDAY, MARCH 17, 1997

Girl born 3 months early celebrates her 1st birthday

by Andrea S. Brown
New Era Staff

Her last name is Hynes, but her ancestors were called O'Hynes. So maybe it's the luck of the Irish. For whatever brought Jacqueline Anne Hynes safely to this St. Patrick's Day - her first birthday - her parents are grateful.

A year ago, they weren't sure they'd have a first birthday to celebrate.

Jacqueline was born to Amy and James Hynes of 1432 Glen Moore Circle three months early. She weighed just 1 pound, 10 ounces and was 14 inches long. "It was very scary," says Mrs. Hynes, 27.

Jacqueline arrived by C-section, scheduled after Mrs. Hynes had spent 10 days in the hospital suffering from eclampsia, an attack of convulsions during pregnancy. Her blood pressure was so high that it was damaging her liver and kidneys, and her baby began losing weight.

That's when the doctors decided they must deliver her, even though Mrs. Hynes was 15 weeks shy of her due date.

Jacqueline, the couple's first child, spent the next 81 days in the hospital and came home weighing 4 pounds, 3 ounces. Until three weeks ago, she had to wear a monitor constantly to make sure she kept breathing.

Once a month, she spends a day at Lancaster General Hospital getting intravenous drug treatment to prevent respiratory viruses. And she gets developmental support at the Schreiber Pediatric Rehab.

But Jacqueline is getting stronger every day. She now weighs almost 17 pounds. She's tall and blonde like her dad and very active, crawling all over the house and chattering happily. On Sunday, her parents took her to Philadelphia to witness her first St. Patrick's Day.

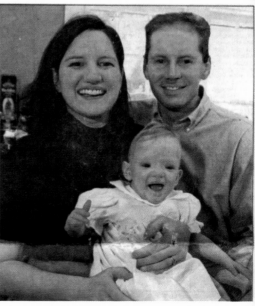

Jacqueline Hynes, born three months premature, celebrates her first birthday today with parents Amy and James at their Manheim Township home.

In December, 1997, the *Sunday News* ran an article highlighting the rapid advances in neonatal medical technology and featuring several of our micro preemies.

"Little feet, big feat" read the caption! Little Jonathan born at twenty-three weeks, and Quinn and Dylan Laughlin born at twenty-five weeks after a long maternal hospitalization earlier that year were included (both stories are featured in this book). Jonathan, one of the youngest babies to survive at LGH at that time, was a cute little eight-year-old; Dylan was portrayed as the social butterfly at nine months of age, whereas Quinn was quieter and laid back. They both remained on home monitors for several months, and in fact one of them stopped breathing and was resuscitated by Mom. This was indeed Mom's feat. All three (Jonathan, Quinn, and Dylan) are thriving today.

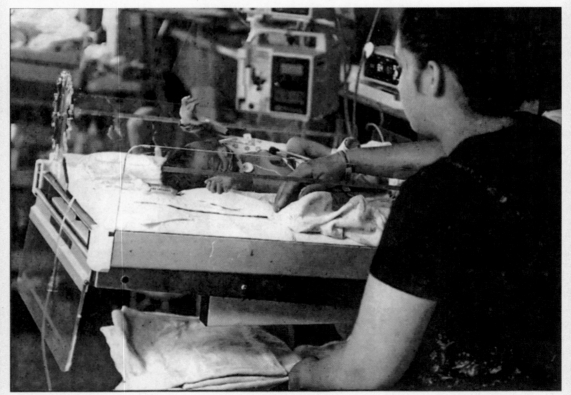

Born too soon, they fight for life

Sunday News Photos/Jack Leonard

A mother keeps vigil all day beside the bed of a baby on the critical side of the unit.

Smallest of Miracles

In the neonatal unit at LGH, babies born before their time fight for life, guarded by doctors and nurses, who get involved.

By Elizabeth Cummings
Sunday News Staff Writer

Dr. Manjeet Kaur's office is down the hall, away from the big machines she uses to treat her tiny patients. Above the books on her shelves are the children, hundreds of pictures in a haphazard montage on the walls.

More goofy-grinned babies than you could count. School pictures of sweater-clad youngsters. A boy about to deliver a karate punch. Another hanging upside-down from a swing set.

The photos are a reminder of what her work is worth. Forty years ago, many of them would have died.

The fast-moving science of neonatology is touching on some of the most complex issues of our time. Abortion. Parents' rights and responsibilities. Teen pregnancy. Euthanasia. Money.

Lancaster General's neonatal intensive care unit or NICU is an example of what modern medicine can do. It is also an example of what it cannot. In the midst of all the high-tech wonders, each child's life depends on the ability of a peanut-sized heart to keep beating.

All the babies the NICU cares for are not premature -some are sick, injured or born with genetic problems. But most were born too small or born too soon.

Many of the reasons why are still unknown, although doctors believe that improving prenatal care will help.

In Lancaster County, the only NICU is in Lancaster General. Each year, between 450 and 500 babies spend some of their earliest moments here on LGH's sixth floor.

On a day early last summer, seven nurses arrive to find a unit even busier than they left it the day before. "Crazy night," says one nurse to another, indicating the two warming beds nearest the door: twin girls, born in the early hours of the morning. The twins are stable—but, in the blunt words of NICU chief Dr. Kaur, very sick. Born unexpectedly at 28 weeks to a patient who had undergone infertility treatments, they are as yet unnamed. The nurses call them "A" and "B," and have already filled pages of notes about them—their "meds" or medications, blood gases, blood pressure, heart rate.

Twin B has not been doing as well as Twin A. In the first 12 hours of her life, she has had blood drawn eight times.

It is only the beginning for both of them. them. And for their parents.

Statistically speaking, they have an 80-90percent chance at surviving. If they do survive, it will be through long, difficult months, full of ups and downs.

Their lungs, deprived prematurely of the life-giving liquid of the uterus, are struggling to breathe. They don't know how to suck yet, so they cannot eat. Their bowels and kidneys are immature.

The new father looks on, his hands dug deeply in his pockets. The nurses begin to explain these patches to help the baby breathe, this tiny circlet around the toe for a blood-pressure reading. Tubes going into the umbilical stump carry nutrition in—and blood out. He nods, wordless. A few hours later his wife arrives, seated in a wheelchair.

...

Dr. Kaur said that during the hard times she draws strength from her faith in God and the people she works with.

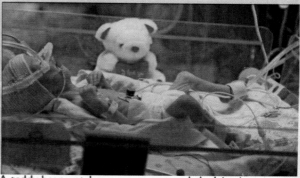

A teddy bear watches over premature baby lying in a nest of blankets, surrounded by tubes and wires at Lancaster General Hospital

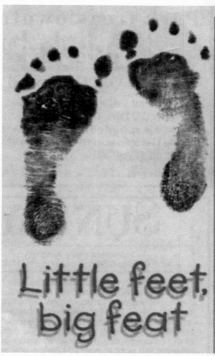

Little feet, big feat

The feet in this logo are the footprints, actual size, of one the newborn twin girls featured in the story.

Some doctors and nurses avoid getting emotionally involved with their patients. Not the ones in the NICU.

"You can only do neonatology well if you feel that bond," she says. "I get pretty emotionally involved with those families, the babies who have been here a longer time. Sometimes it's heart-rending."

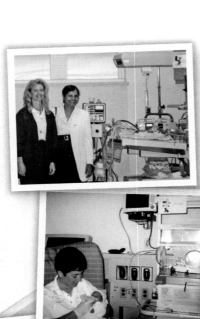
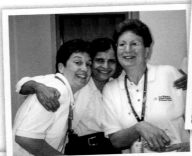
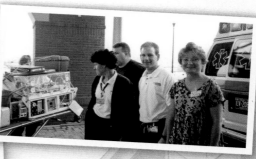
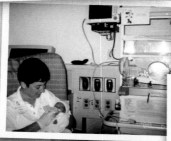
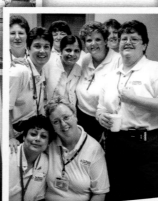
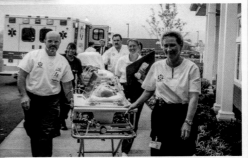
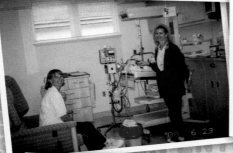
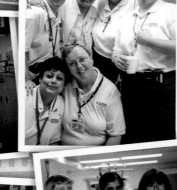
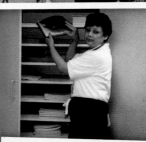
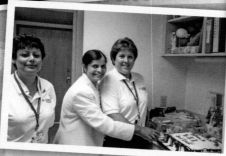
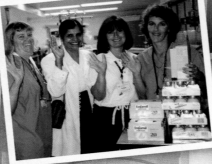
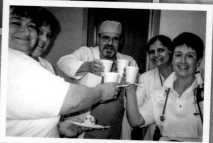
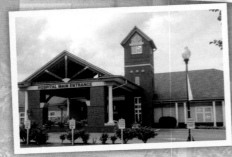

Moving Day

6/28/2000

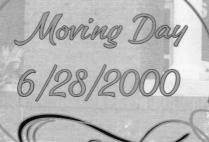
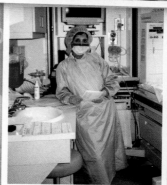

Another decade had gone by. It was the year 2000, the end of the second millennium. There were worldwide celebrations welcoming the twenty-first century and the beginning of the Third Millennium.

Our NICU also celebrated a special milestone at the start of this new century. On June 28, in the year 2000, we moved to a brand-new facility—The Women and Babies Hospital (WBH)—the first 'baby-friendly' designated hospital in Pennsylvania, and one that would not have a hospital-like atmosphere.

The design of the new Neonatal Intensive Care facility was very different and special, with state-of-the-art technology, multiple pods, and isolation, procedure, and overnight rooms for families. This new design provided more privacy to families and quieter housing for our little campers in contrast with the large, open rooms of our prior NICU.

The planning had been a very exciting process, and every detail was addressed. We were thrilled to be

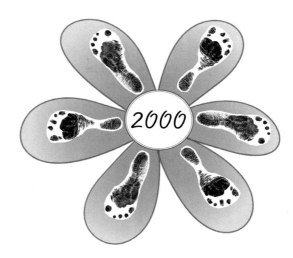

moving into this lovely new facility, yet anxious, since each sick baby needed to be transported safely into the new accommodations.

And, of course, we had cake and a small celebration amidst the chaos of house-moving. The photos on the opposite page give a glimpse into that move in the new millennium on June 28, 2000.

> " … in the year 2000, we moved to a brand-new facility—The Women and Babies Hospital—the first 'baby-friendly' designated hospital in Pennsylvania.

One of the first NICU deliveries at WBH was a meconium-stained infant. I attended that birth with Dr. Diamantoni, who, in 1984, was ironically one of the first residents, often covering the NICU. (He subsequently started his own practice and heads a large, elite family practice group in Lancaster today.)

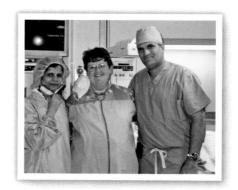

NICU Celebrations 2003—2008

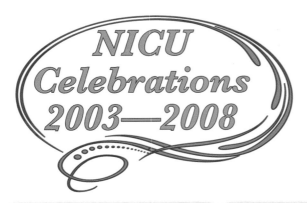

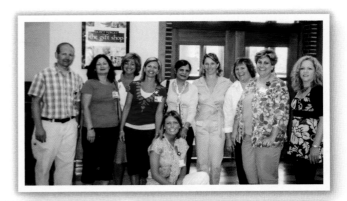

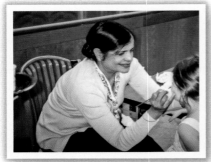

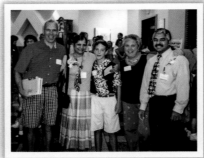

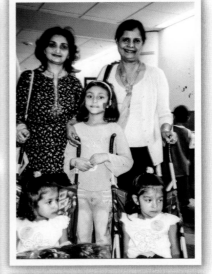

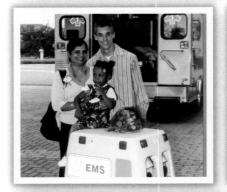

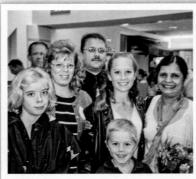

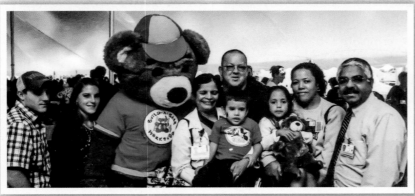

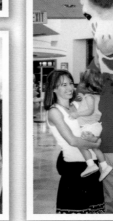

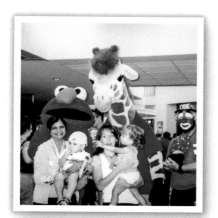 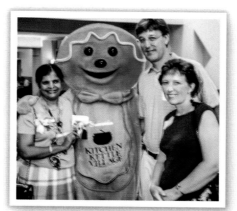 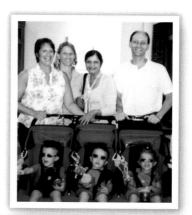

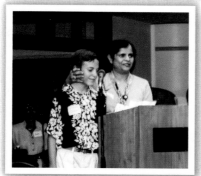 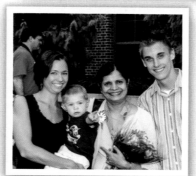 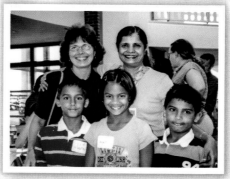

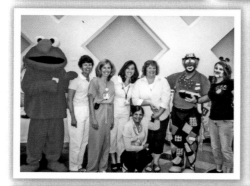 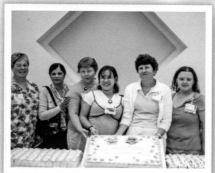 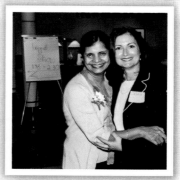

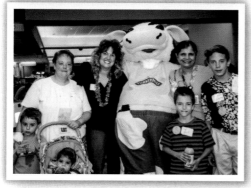 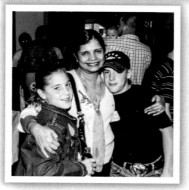 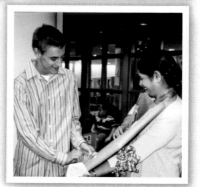

A Celebration of Life

The spinning wheel of time whirls and creates,
A tapestry of luminous beauty allure.
With multifarious colors and hues fabricates,
A marvel of nature, a phenomenon so pure.
Amidst this lustrous bliss prevail,
Chaotic moments , a stormy gale!
Precious instants of hope, yet gruesome despair,
The bells of time ring through to a morrow … …
With celestial intervention, a sublime prayer.
A glistening art, a dream , a connection
On the palette of life … a glorious celebration!
—Manjeet Kaur

A Celebration of Life

Many more little cherubs; many more sagas; many more roller-coaster rides in the NICU arena.

I often tell parents that these babies who had such a tough start must have a special role in life. Though fraught with challenges and some long tough nights, this still has to be one of the best jobs in the world. Photos of my NICU babies and Grads remain some of my most prized possessions—each picture a story, a phenomenon, a celebration of life! What a reward to see tiny infants grow into wonderful human beings. The NICU Grads whose stories are featured in this book have bloomed to become talented individuals: musicians, banjo and bass players; sports men and women—playing lacrosse, basketball, and soccer, one- to two-pound babies now with black belts in karate; photographers and carpenters; high academic achievers—college graduates with majors in biology, economics, languages, and linguistics; drama and theater artists—each one marching to his or her own drummer, each one bound to a unique destiny.

Our NICU expanded with the capability to care for the smallest and sickest of newborn babies. However, for surgery and invasive cardiology we still sent babies to Hershey or to the Children's Hospital of Philadelphia. In 2002 we were joined by a group of experienced and very competent neonatologists who have continued to practice evidence-based medicine and provide loving support to the NICU babies.

~

The stream of time continued to flow; tranquil waters occasionally interrupted by torrential rivulets and rushes. Little boats landed ashore and flourished; some tiny ones did not make it there.

~

The population in Lancaster County had grown, and the number of deliveries at WBH had increased from around 2,600 per annum in our earlier years to over 4,000 per annum. Our NICU expanded to twenty-nine beds so that we could handle more sick babies, and we were now caring for over 350 babies per year in the NICU. Additionally, two of the area hospitals had cut on their obstetric program. Women and Babies Hospital was running full capacity and needed expansion, including the addition of parent sleeping rooms in the NICU.

It was during the construction of these parent rooms that I was stopped by a handsome young man, part of the construction team, who said, "My mom told me to look you up as you took care of me in the NICU in 1988." As he told me his name, I gave him a big hug and said, "Of course I remember you, your mother gives me an update off and on." I could just see young Ross's face light up with a big smile. It was ironical that a graduate of the same NICU would help construct rooms for the comfort of future babies and their families. The very walls of the NICU are a testimonial to our NICU Grads, since one of them was part of the construction team.

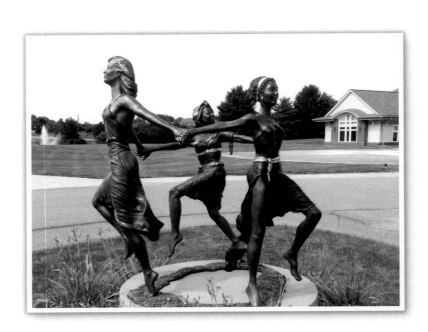

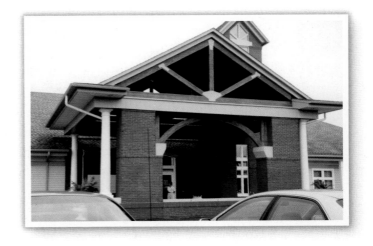

"The very walls of the NICU are a testimonial to our NICU Grads, since one of them was part of the construction team.

Rebirth

Carpenter has special bond to Women & Babies expansion

By CINDY STAUFFER
New Era Staff Writer

Something was on the mind of the slender carpenter installing paneling and chair rail at the Lancaster General Women & Babies Hospital, which is in the midst of an $8.5 million expansion.

Ross Patterson kept an eye on the number of babies listed on the board at the hospital's neonatal intensive care unit, or NICU.

He watched the parents come and go from the unit, which cares for the tiniest and frailest of newborns.

He thought about his own parents.

"I would just look at the babies and, think how much they were worrying about them," he said.

Patterson, 21, of Millersville, is a graduate of the NICU himself, having stayed there for three weeks back in 1988, to be treated for some lung problems.

The Benchmark Construction Co. Inc. employee said he was glad to be able to work on the hospital, which recently opened an expanded NICU and triage area, and is getting ready to open a two story addition with rooms for new moms and two new nurseries.

Someone else was glad Patterson was there.

Dr. Manjeet Kaur, the neonatologist who cared for Patterson when he was a baby, bumped into him as he was working on the hospital expansion.

Kaur has been with LGH since it opened its NICU 25 years ago, at its Duke Street hospital. She was tickled to see one of her former babies, now grown up and out in the world.

"This is the best part of our job," Kaur said, "where you see very sick little ones and now they grow this big."

She put her arm around Patterson, who stood a head taller than her, and recalled how she once boosted him up on her shoulders when he was a-toddler.

"Now, actually, he would be the one carrying me on his shoulder," she said, as they both laughed.

Women & Babies opened in 2000 at the Lancaster General campus on Harrisburg Pike, transferring the hospital's maternity and women's services from Duke St to that new hospital. It is expanding just nine years later for a simple reason.

Lancaster General has gone from delivering 2,800 babies a year to 5,200 babies a year in just eight years. As a result, Women's & Babies has been bursting at the seams, needing more room for moms having babies and the babies themselves

The new expansion includes eight isolettes, or

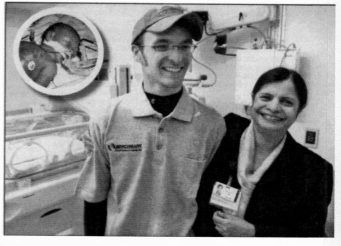

Ross Patterson worked on the Lancaster General Women & Babies Hospital addition. Patterson was cared for in the neonatal intensive care unit at Lancaster General as a baby (inset), by Dr. Martjeet Kaur (right).

specialized incubators, and rooms for them have been added to the NICU, increasing its capacity to 29 babies.

The expansion also added a family waiting area, including a small kitchen, computer area, living room and two overnight rooms. The expanded NICU opened in January.

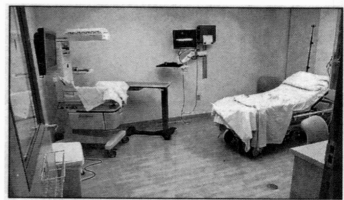

Women will stay in this room in the newly expanded triage unit as they are being assessed for admission at Women & Babies Hospital.

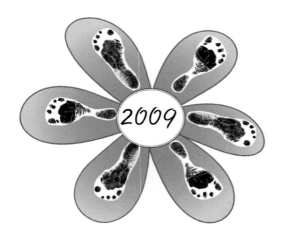

*I*t was now 2009—was it really a quarter century of care in our NICU in Lancaster?

When asked how I would like to celebrate my twenty-five years of service, I immediately answered, "With my NICU Grads from the past twenty-five years, of course!" And, a superb twenty-fifth reunion was held at Women and Babies Hospital.

The celebration of our NICU's silver jubilee was titled "Marking a Miracle" by the *Intelligencer Journal* who reported that over 350 people turned out to attend the milestone celebration at Women and Babies Hospital. Jacqueline, our twenty-five week miracle, and Rebecca were featured on the front page.

Twenty-five years was indeed a landmark! But this was more than a celebration of twenty-five years of service. We had invited babies, some as young as just a few months to others, now grown, and some as old as the NICU itself. Everywhere I looked I saw a miracle! Tiny buds that had now blossomed. It was indeed a celebration of life itself!

We had a wonderful time connecting with our miracles ... both big and small. There was **little Jonathan, born at twenty-three and a half weeks** and now six feet tall; **pretty Jaqueline our musician, born at twenty-five weeks**; and **sweet Rebecca whose Apgar score was 1 at birth**, and whose nursing school graduation I had attended only a couple of days before the reunion. **Katie, Lindsay, and Tiffany, our sick little triplets** now lovely graceful young ladies; **Bud, a handsome young man now,** part of my extended family visiting me off and on especially at Halloween over the years; and **smart young Miles** who had been featured in the newspaper, and who certainly stood two heads taller than me—to name just a few of who that were mentioned in the newspaper article.

And, as well as our NICU Grads there were many other wonderful children at the event. I am sure everyone enjoyed it, but I cannot remember when I had so much fun, running around amidst my blooming garden of flowers. It brings tears to my eyes even today as I recall the melee of lovely children—little angels who were once so sick. What a celebration; a pinnacle of my twenty-five years of service—a labor of love.

These photos are a reminder of that wonderful celebration held at Women and Babies Hospital. What a lovely connection! The news media reporters were in awe of our great turnout. I have never figured out who cherishes these festivities more, our little cherubs while enjoying the pizza and cake or us! I, for one, am certainly in the center of action enjoying every moment of the love of our "little" ones and some "not-so-little" anymore as well as their families.

"Everywhere I looked I saw a miracle!

Marking a 'miracle'

Lancaster General's Neonatal Intensive Care Unit celebrates its 25th anniversary

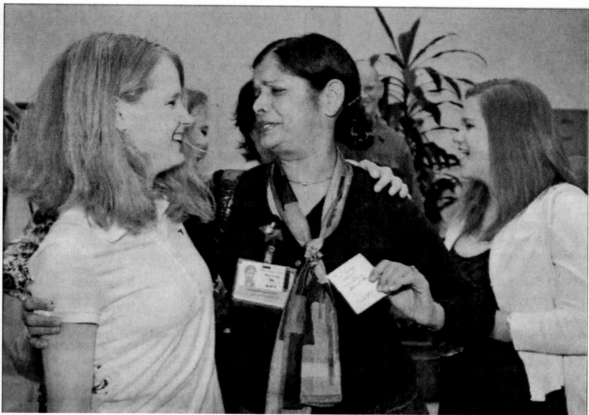

Suzette Wegner / Intelligencer Journal

Dr. Manjeet Kaur, who founded Lancaster General Hospital's Neonatal Intensive Care Unit in 1984, speaks Sunday with 13-year-old Jacqueline Hynes of Lancaster, a NICU graduate, during a 25th anniversary celebration at Women & Babies Hospital. At right is Rebecca Sauder, 20, of Mount Joy, also a NICU graduate and a recent nursing school graduate.

One of Dr. Manjeet Kaur's most prized possessions is a nondescript white binder filled with photos of babies shorter than a ruler and weighing less than 2 pounds.

Kaur, the neonatologist who in 1984 founded Lancaster General Hospital's Neonatal Intensive Care Unit, carried the binder around with her all afternoon Sunday at Women & Babies Hospital, where the NICU is now located, reminiscing about the lives she has encountered in the last quarter century.

Kaur said she believes the thousands of NICU children who have come through LGH are meant to do special things.

"I couldn't have asked for better job if I tried," Kaur said. "This is such a privilege to be a part of these miracles."

More than 35CJ people turned out Sunday to celebrate the 25th anniversary of the creation of the NICU. It's 25 years, Kaur said, that has felt like a lifetime.

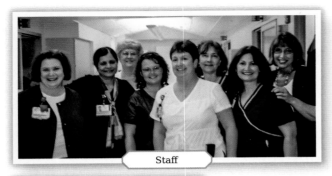
Staff

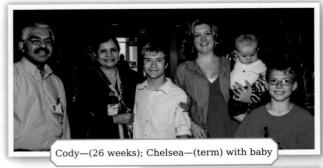
Cody—(26 weeks); Chelsea—(term) with baby

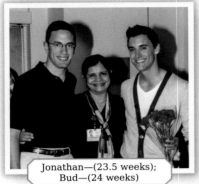
Jonathan—(23.5 weeks);
Bud—(24 weeks)

25
Years

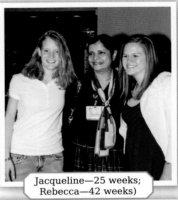
Jacqueline—25 weeks;
Rebecca—42 weeks)

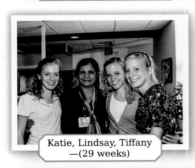
Katie, Lindsay, Tiffany
—(29 weeks)

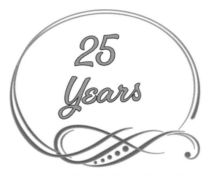
Jacqueline—25 weeks) and family

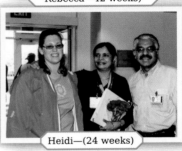
Heidi—(24 weeks)

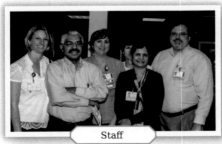
Staff

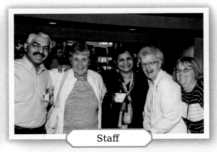
Staff

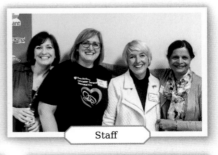
Staff

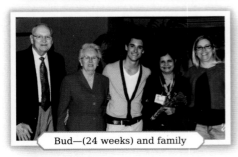
Bud—(24 weeks) and family

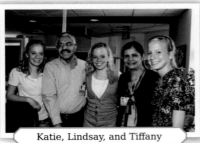
Katie, Lindsay, and Tiffany

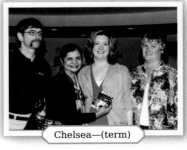
Chelsea—(term)

"Everywhere I looked I saw a miracle!

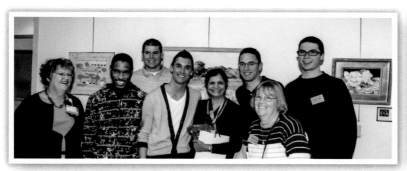

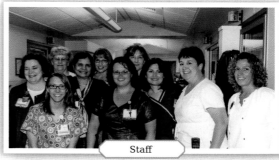

Staff

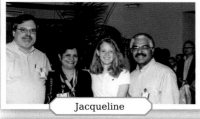

Jacqueline

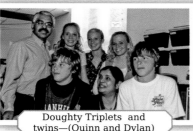

Doughty Triplets and twins—(Quinn and Dylan)

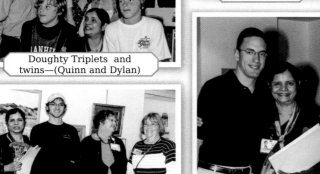

Ross

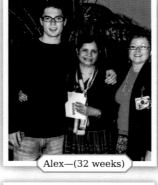

Chelsea

Alex—(32 weeks)

Osmyn—(26 weeks)

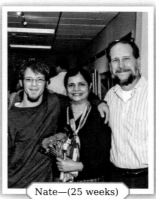

Jonathan —(23.5 weeks)

Nate—(25 weeks)

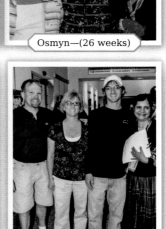

Ross

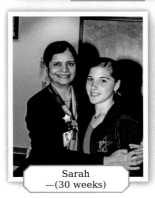

Sarah —(30 weeks)

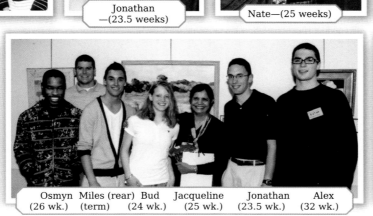

Osmyn (26 wk.) Miles (rear) (term) Bud (24 wk.) Jacqueline (25 wk.) Jonathan (23.5 wk.) Alex (32 wk.)

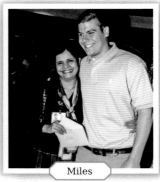

Miles

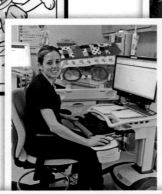

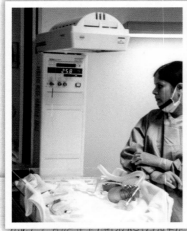

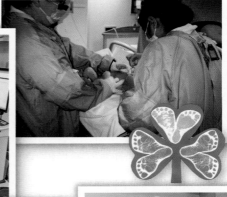

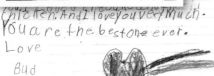

Chicken. And I love you very much.
You are the best one ever.
Love
Bud

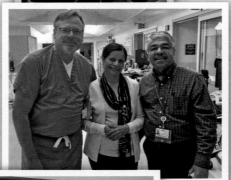

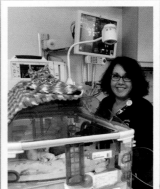

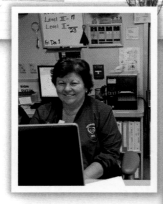

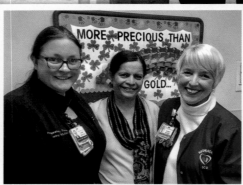

MORE PRECIOUS THAN GOLD...

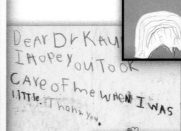

Dear Dr Kau
I Hope you Took
Care of me when I was
little. Thank you.

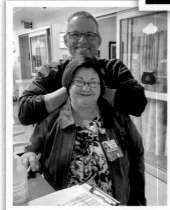

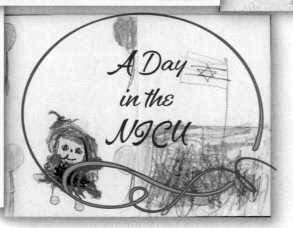

A Day in the NICU

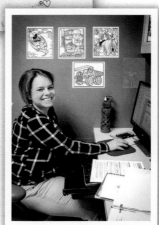

*A*ll neonatologists have their own special stories. These are only a few of my personal experiences and memories and treasured photographs sent to me by families and from my own collection. Nonetheless, each one is special, each dear and unique, each bearing a destiny woven out of that NICU mold, a tapestry interrupted with beeps and wires, the colors enriched with vapors and liquids of varying colors, be they fluids, parenteral nutrition, or transfusions.

The very being of these tiny babies is at the mercy of assisted nutrition and assisted life support, yet amidst this vast ocean of technology, what brings about a meaningful existence are the nurturing arms of the family—both the biological and the NICU ones, love, prayers, and above all, faith, the ultimate healer.

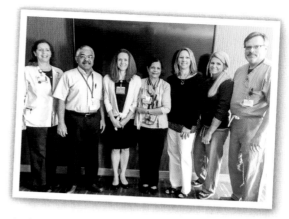

(l-r): Vivian Haughton (Clinical Nurse Specialist), Dr. Anand Mahajan, Dr. Kendra Ardell, Dr. Manjeet Kaur, Julie Leach (CRNP), Heidi Morris (CRNP), Dr. Joel Seacrest

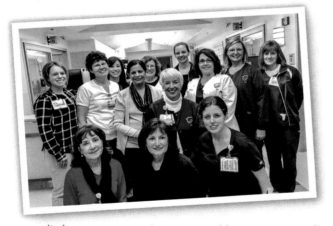

Due to the tremendous growth of the NICU we now have six neonatologists and five neonatal nurse practitioners, two of them trained in Lancaster. We are lucky to have a wonderful and dedicated group of neonatology staff, and our neonatologists now stay in-house at night and are available 24/7.

Front (l-r): Mary Ann Wolpert RN, Debbie Hess RN, Kelly Kubisen RN
Middle: Laura Maurer RN, Kim Stauffer RN, Manjeet Kaur MD,
Margi Bowers Head Nurse, Karen Rausch RN, Judy Minnich RN, Melissa Flora RN
Back: Maria Delgado (Social Services) , Kathleen Warfel RN, Charity Grove RN

"*... yet amidst this vast ocean of technology, what brings about a meaningful existence are the nurturing arms of the family—both the biological and the NICU ones.*

Great Expectations

When I was a little girl
My parents had great expectations
That I'd learn, I'd play, I'd grow
And master this world's grueling show!
When I was a young teen,
My teachers had great expectations
That I'd master my books, equations and glow
And swiftly on the honor roll I would go
When I grew to be a young woman.
A promise in marriage I made
My spouse had great expectations
A wife, a mother would remain
Ever efficient, compassionate and caring
Amidst the chaotic row.
Then as my life grew shorter
I had great expectations
From life and the heavens above
To keep my cup filled to the rim
With love of His children and serve Him
Leave behind a memory, a heritage of love
Did I ever meet those expectations?
Can one ever know, can one ever keep score!
As my life passed through the sieve of time
There was a knock on the door
Lo and behold! Expectations forgotten …
A majestic benediction awaited me,
Celestial blessings galore!

—Manjeet Kaur

*T*his has indeed been a roller-coaster ride for me as well: lows when infants are getting really sick, highs with their achievements both in the NICU and after discharge. The peaks have always been the visits of our Grads and the NICU reunions where we can rejoice with our little ones and their families. The reunions of our NICU Grads that we have every few years always bring much joy to both the families and the staff.

At sixty-five, I thought it was time to stop the twenty-four hour, "in house calls." Teaching has always been my second love. In 2015 I switched my focus to teaching the medical residents at Women and Babies Hospital. Along with teaching them evidence-based medicine, I often punctuate it with anecdotal stories and evidence learned over the years. It is wonderful to be able to share my experiences of Neonatology with future practicing clinicians and continue to connect with my NICU family.

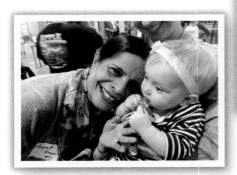

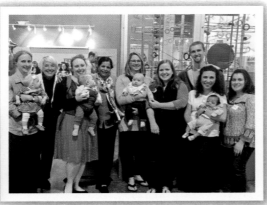

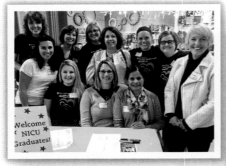

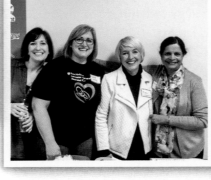

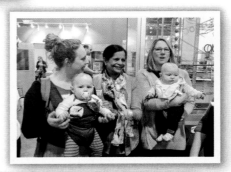

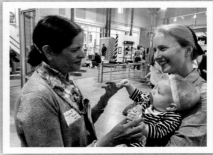

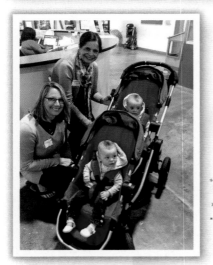

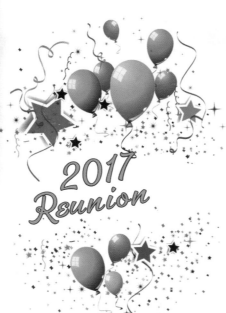

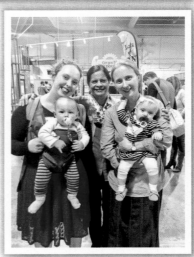

2017
Reunion

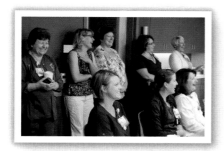

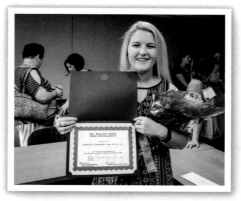

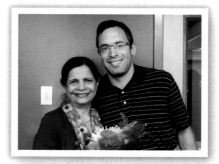

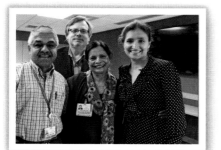

Jessica Carrier RN

First winner of the *Dr. Manjeet Kaur NICU Scholarship* September 2017

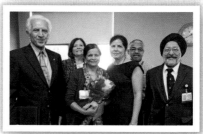

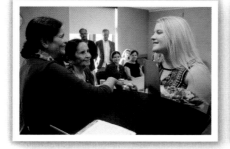

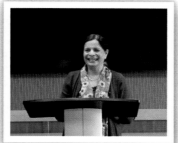

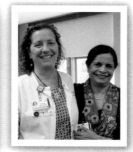

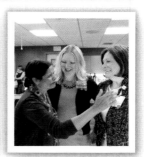

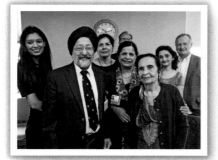

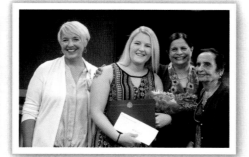

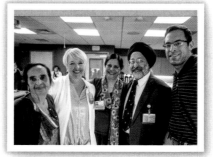

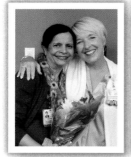

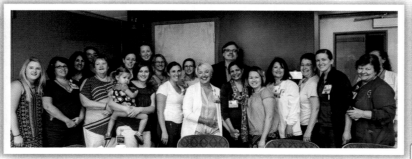

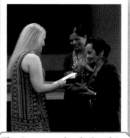

The inaugural scholarship was awarded by Dr. Kaur's mother, Mrs. Parkash Kaur.

Family

"Family," a sweet name of an institution of old,
A lofty pillar, a palatial stronghold.
A dream, a bliss through portals that glow,
Ever loving, ever giving, no matter what's in tow.
Togetherness, a connection, in a challenging vale,
Bringing a sweet conclusion, to a woeful tale.
Rejoicing in exultation with a lyre so bold,
In times of joy as much as the coffers can hold.
A harmony, a melody, a musique, a mission,
For what is an achievement,
Without a family's warm rendition!
—Manjeet Kaur

PART II

Stories of Our NICU Graduates

The following pages describe the experiences of some of the families of our NICU graduates. These stories, told in their own words, are full of hope and optimism for any family that suddenly finds itself with a baby needing intensive care.

Over and over, these narratives describe the fear of the unknown, and how their faith, support, and knowing what to expect were key to helping them to cope with daunting circumstances.

What a celebration of life to see these tiny infants, once so sick and in need of intensive care, now come to bloom as adults leading normal fulfilling lives.

Disclaimer: The stories of our little miracles depict events as their families perceived them, so any medical interpretations in their narratives are parental views only. The medical data provided throughout this book are guidelines only and should not be substituted in any way for recommendations by your physician or medical team.

A Tiny Wonder — Jonathan

*H*ow time flies—was it really twenty-six years ago? Jonathan, when you came with Marisa (your then fiancée) and handed me a folder with photos and a story of your birth sent by your mom, the tall, mature, gentle, and polite young man impressed me once again. It never fails to intrigue me how our NICU Grads seem to be so sweet and polite; maybe they gave their parents too many gray hairs before, and so God now bestows only benedictions on them.

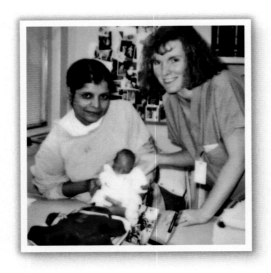

Wonderful Things Come in Little Packages

A tiny package was delivered in the fall,
A sweet, scrawny babe who was loved by all.
It was an instantaneous bonding with a family so slick,
A more caring papa and nicer mama you could not pick.
Our sweet gingerbread boy grew up too soon,
A fine Eagle Scout, tromboning a tune.
This polite young man just recently wed,
A lovely sweet girl to the altar was led.
You'll always remain our luminous little star,
God bless you, Jonathan, as we watch from afar.
—Manjeet Kaur

Jonathan Sherts

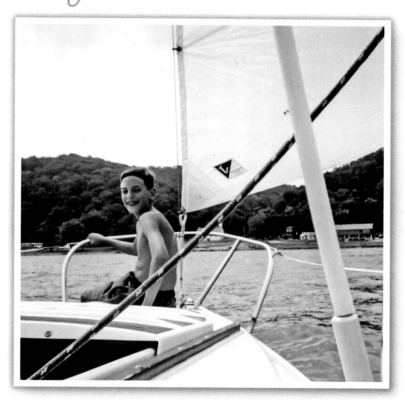

Parents:	Pam and Jeff
Date of birth:	10/12/1989
Birth weight:	1 pound 7 ounces
Medical conditions:	Extreme prematurity, respiratory distress syndrome, anemia, inguinal hernia
Gestational age:	23.5 weeks
Hospitalization dates:	10/12/1989–1/20/1990

"Don't worry, Dr. Kaur, he has strong genes. He will be fine!

I'll never forget your birth at St. Joseph Hospital, now Lancaster Regional. Our NICU team was called in, as a twenty-three-week delivery was imminent and your mom's condition was too unstable to transport her to LGH. We waited and waited, but you, Jonathan, had a mind of your own. Finally, the obstetrician told us that he thought it might be some time yet and that they'd call us back. Of course you wanted to play games even at that early age. No sooner had we gotten back than your mommy's doctors called us, and there you were! We put the needed breathing tubes and IVs in our tiny little one-pound seven-ounce baby.

Whoever would have thought that itsy-bitsy baby would someday be a six-foot-tall handsome young man, and even more surprising, I would be seeing him at twenty-six years of age while writing these memoirs.

We took off to the NICU on the sixth floor at Lancaster General Hospital. We stopped by to talk to your mom, who was on a gurney being transferred to her room, and she said, "Don't worry, Dr. Kaur, he has strong genes. He will be fine!"

So much faith—how could we lose? Following that was a three-month NICU course. I remember a photo of you lying next to a pencil, and one next to a huge gingerbread-man cake that your mother baked for the NICU staff. With her usual sense of humor, she said, "This is you, Dr. Kaur, and that's little Jonathan" (a tiny gingerbread toy next to the huge cake)! We just laughed.

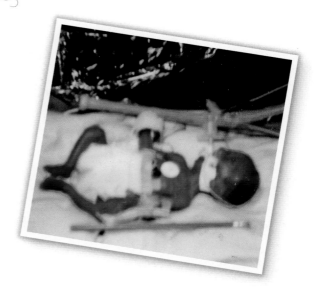

We had to laugh now and then amidst our typical roller-coaster ride of NICU micro-preemies—what some neonatology literature refers to as "fetal infants." Jonathan, you surely had strong genes as your sweet mom said, her prediction reinforced by your dad and a strong faith. You came through all the ups and downs with flying colors and were finally ready to go home after three months.

That didn't cut the cord with the NICU. Your mom and dad kept us posted, and I received cards with your progress reports. I feel I've been a blessed godmother seeing my baby grow. You've been at Christmas parties at my house, and I have a photo of you with your dad at one of them.

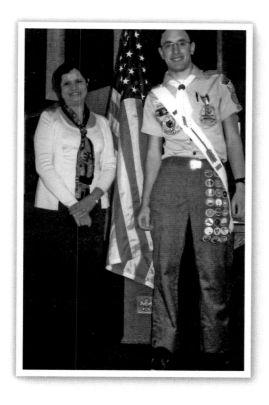

One of my favorite events was your Eagle Scout ceremony at a beautiful church. It was almost as glamorous as a wedding. I remember the quiet, handsome youth with a gorgeous smile who escorted me to my seat and stood by me for photos. I had tears in my eyes watching my "li'l Jonathan" receiving the award at center stage, his scout uniform decorated with medals.

I've heard a lot about your wonderful woodwork, and creations of your carpentry. "This is our twenty-three-weeker," I say, "obviously gifted with the fine motor skills needed for that trade." Seeing you with your pretty, intelligent fiancée was great! More recently I was at your wedding reception. We were seated at the family table, and you wanted to dance with your NICU doctor. You and your sweet wife are so wonderful together. I will always cherish that memory! What a lovely extended NICU family connection. May God always be with you in all your endeavors!

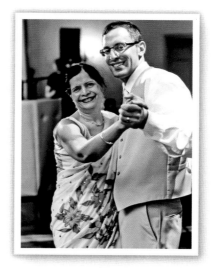

Wedding photo used with kind permission from Brittani Elizabeth Photography, Willow Grove PA.

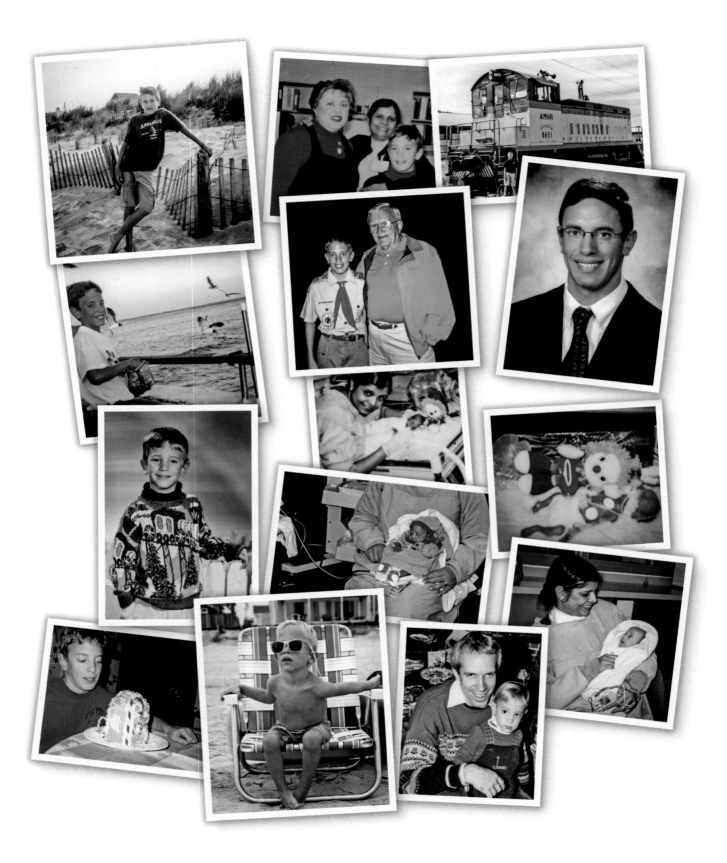

Pam and Jeff's Story

As I begin writing this, I vividly recall that day twenty-four years ago. Jonathan Eugene arrived home from the NICU on Martin Luther King Jr. Day in 1990. It seems Jonathan had a penchant for holidays—his due date was Groundhog Day, February 2, 1990; however, he chose to discover America early, just like Christopher Columbus! October 12, 1989 is Jonathan's actual birthday. But, first things first.

> "He looked at me and declared, much to my dismay, 'There is no way this baby will survive. I can't stop the labor, and the baby is only twenty-three-and-a-half-week-gestation age. There's no hope.'

Upon learning I was pregnant, we were absolutely joyous and immediately shared the exciting news with our five-year-old son Steven. Having miscarried twins three years prior, I remained cautiously optimistic during the pregnancy that all would go well. After the experience of the twins (one miscarried at ten weeks or so, and not knowing I was pregnant with twins, I miscarried the second about eight weeks later), I was apprehensive about carrying any baby to term. Steven had arrived about three hours before his due date, and that pregnancy was a breeze.

While I remained on edge during this pregnancy, all proceeded according to plan until Steven came home from kindergarten with a viral bug during late September. He suffered from the usual high fever and nausea. Naturally, in early October, I too contracted the virus. My fever remained high, and on the family physician's advice I took Tylenol to reduce the fever. I did not know, however, that a high fever could precipitate labor.

As was the Sherts' family tradition, we made plans to go to the Manheim Community Farm Show parade in October. During the parade, Steven wanted to sit on my lap, and I was uncomfortable—something just didn't feel right, but I said nothing and allowed my father to hold Steven. This bit of pain lasted into the next day, so I called the ob-gyn office. They felt that it was just normal contractions, and I agreed, thinking that during this pregnancy I was so attuned to every little nuance. Four days later, the pain remained and seemed to get worse. The Avon lady happened to come by for a visit, took a look at me, and said my color wasn't so good. She asked whether I felt well, and when I explained how I was feeling, she immediately took Steven to a neighbor's home and drove me to the obstetrician's office.

After an exam, it was determined that I was in labor, but it was thought that the labor could be stopped. I was immediately sent—the Avon lady again providing transportation—to what was then St. Joseph Hospital (now Lancaster Regional Hospital).

Upon my arrival, the doctor on duty came into the room to perform an exam. Afterward, he looked at me and declared, much to my dismay, "There is no way this baby will survive. I can't stop the labor, and the baby is only twenty-three-and-a-half-week-gestation age. There's no hope."

Left alone after receiving this news, I began to cry. I called my husband, Jeff, at work and told him to get to the hospital as soon as possible. Then, left with my thoughts in the quietness of the room, I called upon my faith and prayed. I said that if this child would have severe issues, I understood the need to take the baby now. I accepted that, and would be thankful for the healthy child I had, and would accept that we wouldn't have any more children. I couldn't go through this again. If, however, this baby had any chance at all, I needed a sign that all would be well, and upon receiving this sign, I would get this baby all the help I possibly could in order for it to survive.

A few minutes later, an RN came into the room to check on me. She held a stethoscope to my stomach, and to my amazement and hers we heard a really good, strong heartbeat. I asked her to get the doctor immediately. This was my sign—my prayer was being answered! When the doctor arrived, I explained that I didn't care about the cost and didn't want to hear the odds; I just wanted him to deliver my baby and get the team he needed there as soon as possible. I recall telling him, "This baby is going to make it. This baby will survive." He looked at me in dismay, but as we all tease, "Never argue with a woman in labor!"

"This was my sign—my prayer was being answered!

The labor pains intensified somewhat, yet my body didn't want to cooperate. The baby was so small my body didn't realize, I suppose, that it was to push during contractions. Finally, around 10:00 p.m., Baby Boy Sherts was born. He was whisked away from me after one brief glance, and taken by ambulance to Lancaster General Hospital's NICU. I recall Dr. Kaur briefly showing me the baby and wanting to explain his chances for survival. She has never, to this day, been able to share those odds with me. I simply told her, "Take good care of this child. He is going to make it. He comes from good, strong genes, and I have no doubt he'll survive."

With that, the team left, and it wasn't until two days later that I was allowed to see Baby Boy Sherts in the NICU. Nothing quite prepares you for the NICU experience, and perhaps that's just how it's meant to be! How can you describe all the tubes, noises, lights, and activity, plus the gowns, the scrubbing, and all the rest? Yet, when it's your child in the NICU, you're so thankful for all those bells and whistles and the hustle and bustle of the staff. At twenty-three and a half weeks of age, Jonathan's eyes were still fused shut. It was apparent, though, that he heard our voices, as his head turned toward the sound. His color was good for his age. The core team of nurses who cared for him quickly became trusted friends and "surrogate mothers." He was in the best of hands with Vickie, Beth, Susanne, and Sandy. The entire NICU staff, led by Dr. Kaur, was amazing, and instantly put me

"Nothing quite prepares you for the NICU experience,
and perhaps that's just how it's meant to be!

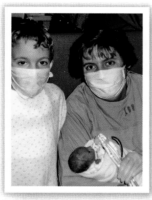

at ease. I knew that my baby was receiving the best care possible. Steven teased that his baby brother looked like E.T. the extraterrestrial.

Jonathan weighed one pound seven ounces at birth. He lost a few ounces, as is normal, so his lowest weight was one pound two ounces. He was twelve inches long. I explain to people that you could hold him in the palm of your hand, and tell them to imagine spreading one pound of meat over twelve inches. That was Jonathan! Keep in mind that this was before the approval of surfactant to help with breathing. Those days I was in labor were a help to Jonathan's little lungs, forcing them to work hard and get strong for what was ahead.

Truly, he was a miracle child. He gradually began to gain weight, and the day he reached two pounds was cause for celebration! Any parent worries when faced with months in the NICU. How could we possibly afford this level of care? I pushed those cares from my mind, just willing Jonathan to gain weight and get better every day. I could worry about all those other things when I knew the outcome of this ordeal. We would take one hurdle at a time.

Life at the Sherts' house was a different story. In the morning I would drop Steven off at kindergarten and go directly to the hospital to spend quality time holding and bathing Jonathan, and talking and reading to him. I had to leave the NICU in time to pick Steven up from school at 11:30. I was home in the afternoon for quality time with him, doing laundry, cleaning, running errands, and returning phone calls, so that when my husband arrived home from work, we could eat dinner and head back into the hospital together to see Jonathan. Wherever possible, I tried to keep some semblance of normalcy in our lives. My parents or Jeff's parents would keep Steven for us, and we were thankful they all lived close by. Life quickly settled into this pattern, and by Christmas, Steven was able to visit and hold his baby brother. I bought a Santa cat costume at a pet store and put it on Jonathan to have our family holiday photo taken so we could send it to family and friends near and far. When I look at that little cat outfit each Christmas and recall Jonathan nearly "drowning" in it (it was way too big for him), we all have a good laugh, and yes, it brings back all the NICU memories!

Of particular help to me at the time were all the people who sent us meals. Almost every evening for months on end, our church, our friends, and our relatives cooked for us. My advice to parents going through this experience is, when people offer to help, take them up on their offer—you need the sustenance to keep up the busy schedule. I truly appreciated having one less thing to think about each day. Now, I jump at the chance to take a meal to a family in their hour of need.

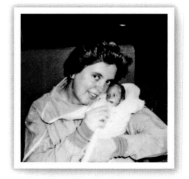

"After this experience, you never again take a day of your child's life for granted.

It's all about the "paying it forward" movement! My husband and I were blessed to have community organizations, churches, friends, and family help us with the cost of Jonathan's hospitalization. People would just randomly appear at our door or send us checks, and I truly thank each of them for their kindness and generosity. I knew the cost of this ordeal was weighing heavily on Jeff's mind, as he was then the sole wage earner. I found I didn't have time to spend worrying about something I had no control over. I knew we'd somehow pay for this special baby, and I wouldn't put a price tag on him or his care. The hospital was very kind and worked out payment plans for us. Finally, by age five, Jonathan was paid in full! NICU parents take note: Of all the things to worry about, let payment be the least of your concerns. I understand it's a worry, but in time, it works out.

Between the great care in the NICU and our daily visits, Jonathan continued to thrive. Only one day did I really question the covenant that God and I had worked out: Jonathan was just not having a good day—his stats were off, his color was awful, and the NICU called us at home, very concerned for him. Dr. Kaur gave him a blood transfusion (one of thirteen transfusions Jonathan received), and lo and behold, Jonathan took a turn for the better.

Our fond memories of the NICU experience include the staff, whose communication was excellent; they were always able and willing to answer our questions, explain a procedure, or just ease our concerns. LGH was a state-of-the-art facility, a first-rate care center, and it remains so today, at its newer location, for premature babies or those who need extra care

at a critical time in their lives. The parents we met and formed friendships with are also memories that I cherish. We were supportive of each other during this experience, celebrating the highs together and comforting one another in the times of greatest stress. After this experience, you never again take a day of your child's life, or life in general, for granted.

I treasure the first time I held Jonathan—tubes, bells, whistles, and all. In fact, looking at photos now, you can hardly see the baby, but oh, how good it felt to hold him! The joy of talking to him and seeing him check me out in response was the highlight of my day. I remember to this day the first time he smiled at me. I grinned right back! When Jonathan moved across the hall to the "bigger baby NICU," I knew we were out of the woods! That was a scary moment. I depended on the doctors and nurses who were so attuned to Jonathan's needs to know what was best for him. Soon there would be no one but my husband and me to care for him. Were we up to the challenge? Would we know what to do when alarms went off? Though Jeff never mentioned his concern over baby Jonathan coming home, I knew he was worried about it, and here is proof. We, along with my parents and Jeff's parents, were required to take a CPR class for infants. Jeff was so intent on doing the procedure properly, he didn't realize that he'd bitten the inside of his lip, and next thing we knew, blood appeared on the infant mannequin! The class was over immediately as the instructor had to clean up the mannequin. Too funny! Fortunately, we never had to administer CPR to Jonathan at home. We did, however, have to rewire our home. We live in a home that's about a hundred years old. While the electric was updated, it wasn't adequate to all of Jonathan's machines, and Jonathan

> "The parents we met and formed friendships with are also memories that I cherish.

could not come home until it was totally rewired, which was completed just in time for Jonathan's arrival. Whew!

When Jonathan was released from the hospital, his nurses were approved to come and provide respite care so I could get out and run errands without having to take him along and expose him to germs and cold air, etc. Unknown to us, Steven came home from school with chickenpox. Of course we didn't know it until the marks began to show all over his body. Nurse Vickie had never had chickenpox, and being exposed to the virus prior to our knowing Steven had it, she came down with the illness herself. Every baby in the NICU and the nursery had to be inoculated to protect them from chickenpox. The medicine not only had to be flown in from the Centers for Disease Control and Prevention in the Carolinas, but also it had to be done twice, because Nurse Vickie contracted chickenpox yet again. There are some things you just can't control, and this was one of them.

I recall Jonathan made an ambulance trip to CHOP (Children's Hospital of Philadelphia) for a hernia operation. You'd have thought they had a celebrity on their hands at CHOP. Night and day, a steady stream of doctors, residents, interns, and nurses came through the room to look at this "Miracle Baby from Lancaster." To see the amazement on their faces (they treat children and babies from all over the world and see it all) when they heard this baby was simply at CHOP for a hernia operation was priceless. We knew Jonathan's care in Lancaster was the finest, but now this world-renowned hospital reinforced our opinion. I share this so that parents will know the quality of the Lancaster NICU. Be grateful for the terrific care you receive in Lancaster, and know that nowhere else is the care better. We truly believe we were blessed with the best, and that accounted for much of Jonathan's success.

At age twenty-four, Jonathan has reached many goals in his life. He became an Eagle Scout, the highest honor a Boy Scout can achieve. He was named Student of the Quarter in middle school. In fact, his teachers from elementary school through high school always said they wished they could have a classroom full of Jonathans. He strived to please, loved to learn, and listened well. He played trombone in the high-school marching and concert bands. He has traveled to Europe and hiked Yellowstone National Park and Philmont Scout Reservation.

Jonathan is a graduate of Thaddeus Stevens College of Technology, and he now works at Keystone Wood Specialties (behind Brubaker Kitchens) in Lancaster. He is a member of the Lancaster Church of the Brethren, and is married to his wife, Marisa. He enjoys reading, model railroading, hiking, yard work, traveling, and designing and crafting fine furniture. Jonathan has such patience, is a happy adult, and has a fine sense of humor. To know him is to love him!

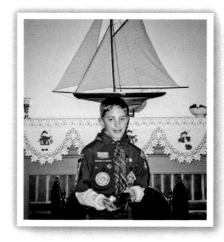

> " My advice to parents going through this experience is, when people offer to help, take them up on their offer.

Twenty-four years after our NICU experience, many of the memories have dimmed and we tend to take things for granted; however, we still correspond with most of Jonathan's core nurse team and Dr. Kaur. It's amazing that when we're out in the community, staff who worked at LGH and St. Joseph Hospital at the time Jonathan was born will see us, recognize us, and comment that they remember the night of his birth. They recall the miracle of seeing one of the youngest babies to survive at twenty-three and a half weeks grow and gain strength in the four months he spent in the NICU. We are truly blessed to have such a wonderful son. *I think NICU babies are some of the nicest, most calm, and caring individuals I've been fortunate enough to meet. Know that your NICU child has a definite purpose in this world!*

Parents going through this stressful time need to know that they will be forever changed and better for having gone through the NICU experience. It's truly a miracle to witness life outside the womb, and is an event you'll never forget. Our children and we are blessed that modern technology and medical advances have enabled our children and us to experience this wonderful event called life. Cherish it!

Jonathan's Story

I don't remember much about my birth other than the stories I've heard and pictures I've seen. I'm very lucky to not have had many issues from my prematurity. I've always been slower in math and comprehension, but had the help I needed to succeed in school. I remember taking speech class in elementary school. I graduated from Thaddeus Stevens College of Technology with Certification in Cabinetry and Woodworking, and am now employed by Keystone Wood Specialties in Lancaster.

I've been very fortunate to take part in the NICU reunions; I like to see all the other children, teenagers, and adults who were in the same situation in the NICU now doing so well. Two articles were written about me in the Lancaster newspapers; they still hang on our refrigerator today. The NICU reunions allow me to see others that went through similar situations and have an extended system of support.

Dr. Kaur and the other neonatologists and nurses who took care of me during my four-month stay have become a second family. Dr. Kaur was there to see me presented with my Eagle Scout award. She and I bonded and we have formed a very special relationship from day one of my life, but I don't think of myself as any more important than the rest of the babies in the NICU. They all deserve the utmost attention and the best care, and they receive it there.

On my most recent visit to the NICU area of Women and Babies Hospital, Dr. Kaur was kind enough to show my then girlfriend (now wife), Marisa, and me a NICU baby who weighed about the same as I did at my smallest. It was hard to imagine now that I was that tiny at one point, especially considering I'm now six feet tall! Dr. Kaur told me that after my birth, she laid a pencil beside me and it was almost as long as I was!

"I've been very fortunate to take part in the NICU reunions; I like to see all the other children, teenagers, and adults who were in the same situation in the NICU now doing so well.

I have nothing but respect and admiration for the doctors and nurses who work day and night caring for these precious babies. I've always been amazed at all the technology they use and the schooling they complete to be able to do so. I'm proud to be a NICU alum and to be able to share my story with others so they know they're not alone and that there will always be support and love, long after your days in the NICU are behind you. While I'm not yet a parent, I want to encourage all NICU parents to not give up hope and to be patient while going through this stressful time. I also want them to understand that their baby is in the most special hands while being cared for by the NICU staff. These men and women are truly tops in their field, and Lancaster is so lucky to have this dedicated group caring for such precious lives!

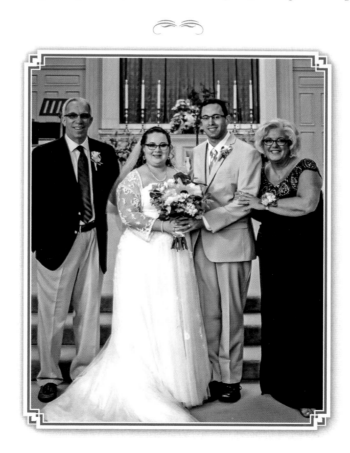

Surviving the Odds with Silver Wings — Heidi

*J*ody—it's been quite a journey! What a heartwarming and heartrending story! It must be tough to talk about a loss of a twin in the same breath as the celebration of a birth. You mourn the loss, yet stories like yours may help bring solace and strength to families in similar situations. You've traveled a rough road, but you've done a fabulous job!

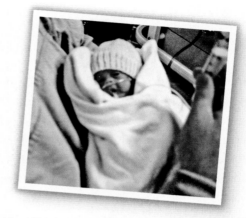

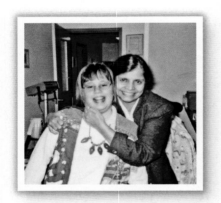

Thanks for the progress reports and the framed photos of Heidi, which I keep in a special place in my home, a place for my NICU Grads. Heidi—every Christmas for years I have looked forward to you and your mother stopping by to visit. The cards with updated photos, and the holiday ornaments, continue to be among my most treasured possessions. In fact every year when we put up our family Christmas tree I hang Heidi's "doctor ornaments," nostalgic celebratory reminders. Those visits and cards mean the world to us who work with the sick little ones in the NICU. Continue the great work! God bless you both.

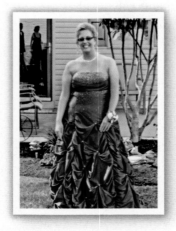

Heidi of the Alps

Oh dear sweet one with silver wings,
Your melodious voice in the meadow rings.
As you climb mountains and traverse steep slopes,
May you achieve your goals and your special hopes.
Like Heidi of the Alps may you happiness bring
To those all around you, like a breath of spring.
—Manjeet Kaur

Heidi Gerhart

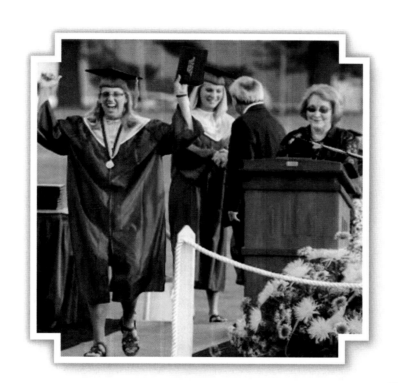

Parents:	Jody and Scott
Date of birth:	1/9/1993
Birth weight:	1 pound 15 ounces
Medical conditions:	Extreme prematurity, respiratory distress syndrome, intraventricular hemorrhage, apnea
Gestational age:	24 weeks
Hospitalization dates:	1/9/1993–3/28/1993

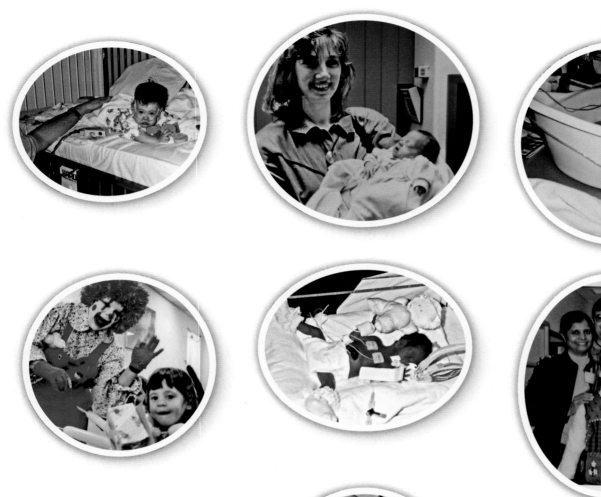
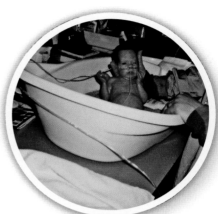
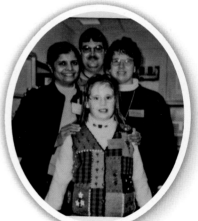
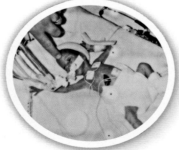
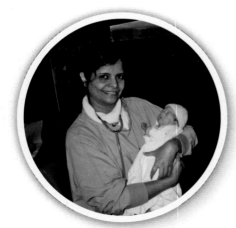
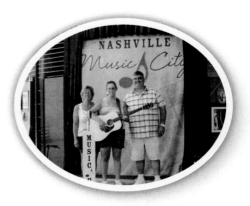

Jody and Scott's Story

In October 1992, when I was three months pregnant, I had spotting and was sent for an ultrasound at Lancaster General Hospital. I was thrilled to find out I was expecting twins. The spotting stopped after two days' rest, and I went on with everyday activities. Everything appeared normal with my pregnancy, and I felt the babies moving. Then, on Friday, January 8, 1993, the spotting started again and I was admitted to Lancaster General. I received injections that made my body shake all over. That was scary, but I'd have welcomed a lot more injections if they'd stopped me going into labor.

On Saturday, January 9, we had visitors, and everyone went home except my husband, Scott, who could stay with me the whole time. A nurse came in to check me late that night, and then came Steve and Julie, NICU nurses, with cribs. Steve spoke very calmly to Scott and me about how things were going to go really quickly. I thought, *How am I going to deliver these babies? I didn't have birthing classes.* Then a doctor came in and said, "OR, stat." They rolled me down the hall quickly as I held Scott's hand, crying out, "I don't want to lose my babies; I don't want to lose my babies."

As they pushed me into the operating room, Dr. Kaur asked Scott questions and wrote the information right on her scrub. I was put under anesthesia and Scott got to sit above my head as they removed the babies. He later said it was really quiet as he handed the babies to Dr. Kaur (Baby A, born at 11:23 p.m., one pound fifteen ounces) and Dr. Mahajan (Baby B, born at 11:24 p.m., one pound four ounces), born at twenty-four weeks. Shortly after, Dr. Mahajan told Scott, "Baby B is not breathing. What would you want me to do?"

"Give her every chance you can," Scott said. "I'm not just going to let her die."

As Dr. Mahajan went back in, Scott asked the surgeon, "Why did he ask me that?"

The surgeon replied, "Some people don't want their babies worked on when they're born very early."

We named them when I was in recovery: Baby A, Heidi Sue, and Baby B, Heather Ann. Scott kept going between the NICU and the recovery room. Before they took me back to my room, they pushed me into the NICU to see our babies. We hadn't been back in the room long when Dr. Mahajan talked to Scott in the hall and said it wasn't looking good for

> " 'Give her every chance you can,' Scott said.
> I'm not just going to let her die.'

81

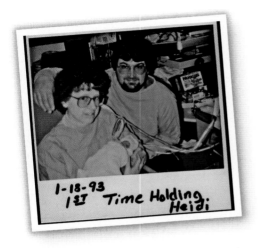

1-18-93
1ˢᵗ Time Holding Heidi.

> "It was nine days before I could briefly hold her; it was another twelve before Scott could hold her.

Heather. We just cried. Scott just lay on the cot and thought, *With all this technology why can't they save these little girls?*

Then they came with a wheelchair and said, "We must get you down to the NICU. Heather isn't gonna make it."

Heather lived just six hours. It was heartbreaking to hold my dead baby. Then, to see Heidi lying there—all wired up and fighting for her life—and not be able to hold her was very hard on us. I'm thankful it was worked out with our insurance to cover me to stay in the hospital for one week.

The day I had to leave the hospital without a baby and leave Heidi behind, knowing she was still very sick, was emotionally draining for both of us. Every morning when he got up, Scott would call the NICU to speak with Steve, Julie, or Susan for an update on Heidi. It was nine days before I could briefly hold her; it was another twelve before Scott could hold her. A lot of stimulation wasn't good for Heidi. She received several blood transfusions and we found our own donors. The NICU was like family to us, always there to support us all along Heidi's seventy-eight-day hospital stay, which was a roller-coaster ride for us.

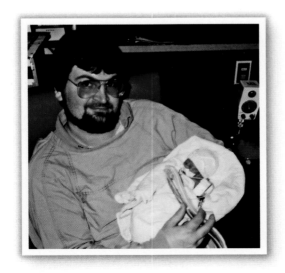

> "The day I had to leave the hospital without a baby and leave Heidi behind was emotionally draining for both of us.

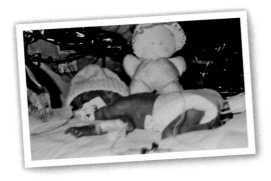

" We were keen to bring Heidi home, but we were scared because we knew we had to be nurses and parents.

We asked a lot of questions about Heidi's outcome: Would she be severely disabled? Could she lead a normal, independent life? No doctor gave us straight answers because they didn't want to give us false information. We understood that. Heidi did have grade 3 and grade 4 hemorrhages (very mild cerebral palsy); we were very fortunate that she didn't develop a severe disability. While we visited with Heidi we tried to get as involved in her care as possible: changing diapers, doing feedings, and checking her temperature. We tried to absorb as much medical information as we could.

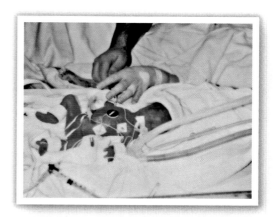

Valentine's Day was a big day—Heidi could breathe on her own. Yay—no more ventilators! Scott and I could hold her more. During the night, after we'd left, they took her off the ventilator, then took a picture of her, and one of the nurses made a heart-shaped frame and put the picture in it for us.

Monday, February 15: Heidi was moved into an incubator. She weighed two pounds five point six ounces.

Tuesday, February 16: The Heparin IV came out; no more IVs.

Thursday, March 4: Heidi got her first bottle; previously she was fed by IV and tube.

Saturday, March 13: A blizzard made it difficult to get there, but we managed.

Tuesday, March 16: Heidi graduated to a crib. Yay! Big-girl bed; weight four pounds seven ounces.

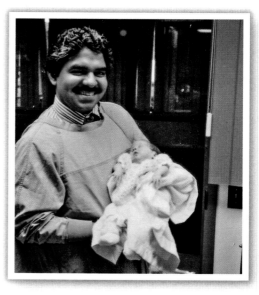

Tuesday, March 23: Mom and Dad had to get training on monitors, oxygen, and CPR.

Wednesday, March 24: Four pounds fourteen ounces; one of the evening nurses bought Heidi her first wagon and took her for a ride—boy, that was fun!

Thursday, March 25: A heartrending day for all. Heidi was to come home, but at 7:00 a.m. she stopped breathing, and they had to bag her. Her blood count was low; she had to get some more blood.

Sunday, March 28: The BIG DAY finally came. Heidi got to come home. It was emotional for us to say goodbye to the nurses and doctors who took wonderful care of Heidi for seventy-eight days. At five pounds one ounce, she came home on an apnea monitor, a pulse oximeter, and oxygen.

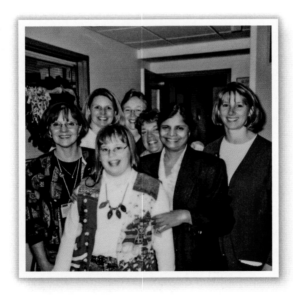

We were keen to bring Heidi home, but we were scared because we knew we had to be nurses and parents. I slept on the bedroom floor next to Heidi's crib for at least a week because I was afraid I wouldn't hear her monitor alarms. Visiting nurses came a few times a week. The only place we took Heidi was to doctors' appointments because we were told her immune system would be low and she could pick up germs really quickly. We had a sign on the door saying, HEIDI CAN'T HAVE YOU VISIT IF YOU ARE SICK.

We were told that preemies could easily pick up RSV (respiratory syncytial virus). Wouldn't you know that Heidi, at just over a year old, had to be hospitalized for a few days when she got RSV. Every time she got sick, it usually ended up in her chest and affected her breathing. Heidi had increased muscle tone from her low birth weight, so a therapist started coming to the house. After an office visit, Heidi's child neurologist said she wasn't making enough progress and had to go to Schreiber Pediatric Rehab Center in Lancaster. I had to drive from Ephrata to Lancaster twice or thrice a week, but it was well worth it. Heidi received occupational, physical, and speech therapy.

Also, they tried to correct her walk so she'd walk toe-heel and walk a little on her left toes. A doctor sent us to Hershey Medical and had Heidi wear a Dafo (dynamic ankle foot orthosis) on her left foot. That was a challenge—we had to buy two pairs of different-sized shoes, one pair to fit her right foot correctly and the other a size larger to get the Dafo in place. That went on for some time but it didn't correct the problem, so I told the doctor I wanted a second opinion. He sent us to DuPont, where another doctor said we could try it without the Dafo for a few weeks and see if it was better. Sure enough, it was, so Heidi has gone without it since early childhood. She went to Schreiber's from infancy until about fourth grade.

Monday, November 1: Roseville Pediatrics said no more apnea monitor. Scott and I were happy, but scared. I didn't sleep well for over a week, worried about not having the monitor.

December 1993: Heidi could sit by herself.

During Heidi's first winter she got a lot of respiratory infections, so Roseville Pediatrics sent her for a sweat test at Harrisburg to check for cystic fibrosis; another wait-and-see. We were thankful the results were negative.

July 1994: Heidi could pull to stand.

August 1994: Heidi could walk by herself!

Heidi had to wear bifocals to correct the movement of her eyes, which had started to cross. We had several visits with Dr. Klombers, who would check her prescription twice a year to try to keep her eye muscles in line. That worked for a while, but then, in second grade, Heidi had to have strabismus surgery at Lancaster General Health. That really helped, and to this day, at age twenty-one, Heidi's eyes are still aligned, but she must still wear a progressive bifocal.

Heidi was mainstream in school, but the Schreiber's staff told us to focus on her schooling because she was borderline and could slip through the cracks. We stayed on top of it to make sure that didn't happen. Heidi did very well in school, but had to work hard to get good grades. In June 2011 she graduated from Ephrata High School with a 3.24 GPA.

Over the years, Heidi twirled baton and marched in parades, took jazz and tap-dancing lessons, got a part-time job at age fifteen bagging groceries, and then worked her way to cashier.

She got her driver's permit at sixteen and then got a driver's license.

It was rough for Scott and me seeing Heidi get into a limo with her prom date, because her sister wasn't there to get in that limo, too.

On Graduation Day, Heidi came home from graduation practice and said, "Mom, the *Ephrata Review* was there taking pictures of seven sets of twins who are graduating in my class tonight. I could have been in that picture, Mom."

It broke my heart to hear that. I'm thankful that a lot of family and friends came to support Heidi and us that night. To this day it's still hard when Scott and I see twins out and about.

After graduation Heidi got a full-time job, with good benefits, as a waitress and hostess, and she loves it. She also upgraded her car to a good, used 2010 Honda CRV. Heidi is dating and doing wonderfully. She lives a typical normal life.

I remember all the hours spent in the NICU, and how encouraging Dr. Kaur was on Heidi's prognosis. If Heidi had a setback, Dr. Kaur would give a hug and always explain everything in a way that we could understand.

Scott remembers the night Heidi was born: Dr. Kaur came out to him, calmly asked him specific questions, and wrote the information on her gown. To this day, if I get talking about that night, I'm still amazed at how calmly Dr. Kaur handled what I thought was a very stressful situation, and kept me informed about what was happening.

Heidi recalls that, as she started to learn to talk and we would visit the NICU, Dr. Kaur wanted Heidi to say her name. The doctor would say, "Dr. Kaur—like you ride in a car." She always said, "Heidi Gerhart, look how you have grown!" I'll never forget the warm welcome she always gave us, and how she remembered Heidi!

A Small Bud Unfurled—Bud

What can I say about you, Bud? You seem to be part of my extended family. From seeing a tiny twenty-four-week-gestation infant whose eyes were fused at birth, to a respectful, well-mannered, intelligent young gentleman, I've watched your special journey over the past two decades with pride and joy.

I remember you soon after your birth, though I wasn't present at the time. A tiny, scrawny, but adorable peanut (we had only one or two that size in those years), with a lovely family, whose cute little sisters came by often. Little did I know that I would so closely see this family grow up. Your problems were the usual ones: issues with pulmonary immaturity requiring ventilator support, gut immaturity requiring parenteral nutrition, apnea, and jaundice, to name a few.

Your mom met with me from time to time and we formed a very special bond. After your discharge she kept in touch via photos and phone calls. As you grew older you came to NICU reunions and for NICU visits. Mom brought you to my house every Halloween, which was such a treat for both of us. My boys knew we had to wait for Bud at Halloween. I had a photo of you that your mom gave me on the mantel at home. At

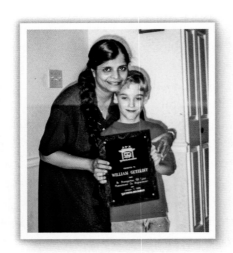

A Bud Unfurled

One summer, not so long ago,
A tiny babe was born,
Bringing his parents a special glow
As his two cute sisters looked on.
When I set my eyes on tiny Bud,
Little did I know
Amidst the paths of tubes, oh Lord,
How dear this sprite would grow.
Not ready yet to see the light,
His eyes were tightly fused.
The little tiger fought a valiant fight,
Leaving both doctors and nurses bemused.
Today we are proud of our karate kid,
And marathon runner, too.
Polite and sweet at every bid,
Cheers to our "NICU Bud!" Keep it up, young man, oh, do!
—Manjeet Kaur

William (Bud) Getzloff

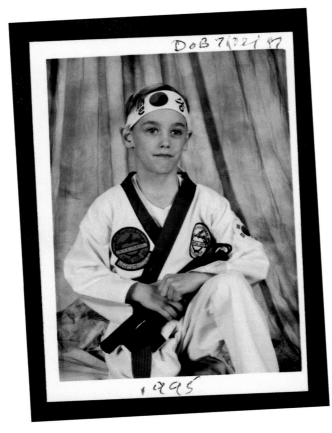

DoB 7/22/87

1995

Parents:	Rita and Tim
Date of birth:	7/22/1987
Birth weight:	1 pound 9 ounces
Medical conditions:	Extreme prematurity, respiratory distress, apnea/jaundice
Gestational age:	24 weeks
Hospitalization dates:	7/22/1987–10/16/1987

NICU puts the accent on care

By Lisa Christopher
Sunday News Staff Writer

When Rita Getzloff gave birth to a baby three months prematurely in July 1987, she didn't know whether it was a boy or a girl. All she knew was the baby was in distress.

"The way we found out the baby was a boy was the doctor came over to us and said 'I'm sorry. He didn't make it.' "

The baby, Getzloff said had no heartbeat. The medical staff tried cardiopulmonary resuscitation but to no avail. For some reason, though, when they pulled an air tube out of the baby's throat his heart started beating on its own.

"He was alive and they told us to just take things one day at a time. That's what we did," Getzloff said.

Today. William Leonard, "Bud" to his friends, who weighed 1 pound, 9 ounces at birth is a first-grader at Sacred Heart Parish School where his favorite topics are recess and lunch he said. This year, he's going to be a green Power Ranger for Halloween.

Bud is just one of the miraculous stories that has come out of the Lancaster General Hospital Neonatal Intensive Care Unit. This year, the unit celebrates its 10th anniversary.

'The staff here is an extended family to us " Getzloff said. "We spent three months with the people here. They gave us more than just medical help. They gave us moral support."

"They keep in touch. It's amazing how they remember me,' said Dr. Manjeet Kaur, chief of neonatology since the department's inception.

Kaur's office walls are lined with bright smiling little faces of the babies she's nurtured at the unit.

There's Adam. Jonathan. Bobby. Jake, Ethan. Amber and dozens more.

"Amber had eight chest tubes in her at one point. Here she is at discharge," Kaur said pointing to one of the photos. We never thought we'd see that day. We thought she'd die."

Kaur is one of three doctors assigned to the unit. But when it opened, Kaur was the only doctor. At the time, she was the mother of a 1-year-old and a 7-year-old and assigned to 24- hour-a-day, on-call duty.

At that time, the unit accepted children 32 weeks and older. Nowadays the unit can handle babies as small as 23 weeks into development. The survival rate of the unit is 55 to 60 percent. The unit can handle 18 babies at one time. Most babies spend about three months in the unit.

"Statistically, we do have losses, but it is always hard to take," Kaur said. "When I get depressed, I come into my office and see all these pictures of these faces of the babies who were once so sick and now are thriving."

Before the LGH unit opened premature babies or infants in need of specialized care ere sent to Hershey Medical Center. Having a neonatal unit in the county saves precious time in the first moments of life and enables immediate medical assistance for a baby in distress.

After 10 years on the unit, Kaur has one wish for its future.

"I would like to see us be able to do pediatric surgery here so babies won't have to be transferred to Hershey or Children's Hospital in Philadelphia," Kaur said.

Kaur said parents and medical staff bond to one another during the baby's stay in the hospital.

"You get attached to the kids here because you are together a very long time through the bard times," Kaur said.

"I think being a mother has made me a better doctor," Kaur said. 'I feel for the parents. I sit and cry with them sometimes, and while I can't get too emotional, I think the parents are comforted by the fact that their doctor feels what they are going through.

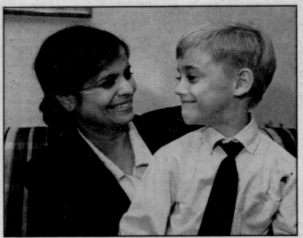

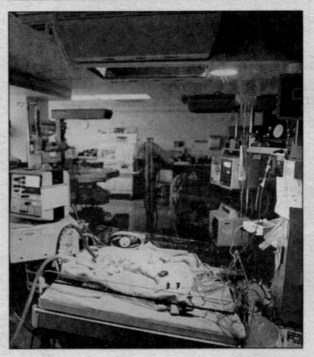

Sunday News Photos/Jeff Ruppenthal

Dr. Manjeet Kaur (top photo) talks with former patient Bud Getzloff. Cody Scheid, above, the son of Keri and David Scheid, Holtwood, is a current patient. He was born 14 weeks premature.

one point, my son—now a pediatrician—felt a sibling rivalry and hid that photo frame. It seemed to him I had three sons, not two, and that didn't feel fair. However, I remember him talking to some friends who asked him why he's chosen pediatrics, and he replied, "My mom is so close to her babies and is always talking about them. I just feel that this field of medicine has to be great!" That was a very touching tribute!

I recall, Bud, when your mom asked me to attend your karate test for a black belt. As I couldn't attend due to my call schedule, you came to my house and broke a wooden block with those special maneuvers. A new role for our fragile twenty-four-weeker who'd been so sick. I still have that wood block, with the inscription **BROKEN BY BUD** written on it. Your mom had a poem embroidered and framed in honor of the NICU and you presented it to me, which remains a cherished memory.

On one occasion, you and your mom actually traveled to Ellicott City, Maryland, where we were having a Lancaster General administrative retreat, as ambassadors of the NICU. You came in carrying a bouquet of flowers and said, "My mom always told me to greet a lady with flowers." What a pleasure it was to introduce you to our administrators. You can't imagine the joy those little acts have given me, your physician and friend.

After your high-school graduation, you came to my house, as I was unable to make it to the ceremony. Your mom emphasized, "Before Bud went out with his girlfriend, he had to come see you and your family." What a compliment!

And, now you are a marathon runner and have a full-time job. As I write this, I feel a sense of pride in these memories, as with God's grace we have such a wonderful young man, far from that one-pound nine-ounce micro-preemie. That's the beauty of my job as a neonatologist: to see a little bud, despite his premature entrance into the world, flower into such a gracious young man. Your mom has always been supportive of the NICU, and has been a special friend participating in NICU celebrations. God bless you, Bud. You and your family have brought me much joy!

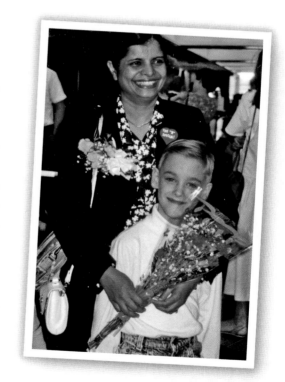

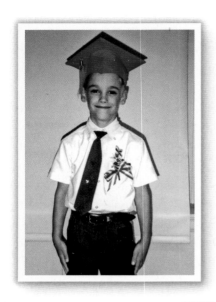

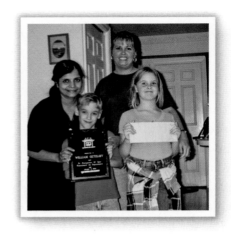

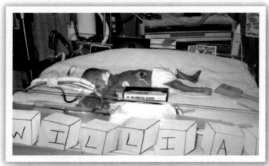

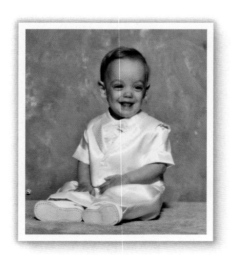

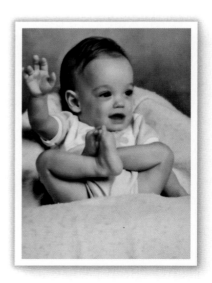

Rita and Tim's Story

*B*ecause part of the placenta was not attached to the wall of my uterus, the placenta was born first and then Bud was pulled out. We're thankful that Bud had suffered no medical conditions due to his early birth. "Shock" would be the best word to describe our emotions around the time of delivery. We were frightened because we didn't know what was going to happen. I remember the doctor trying to explain, but he was talking way over my head. Not being medically trained, I had no idea what he was saying most of the time. Only after a while did I start to understand some of the terminology and the numbers.

The nurses—the guardian angels of the NICU— definitely helped us the most. I don't know what I would have done without Vicki, Steve, and the others. It was so painful to see my son cry when the IV was replaced or they had to prick him to test his blood gases. Seeing the pain on his face but not hearing a sound from him, due to the respirator, broke my heart.

When Bud was born, the NICU team was right there in the delivery room. They started to work on him immediately. A few minutes later the ob-gyn doctor came over and told us that Bud hadn't made it. Right after that, the NICU team ran back to the unit with him. They took my husband, Tim, and me

> " We were frightened because we didn't know what was going to happen.

back to the delivery room. Tim left soon after that to go see why they'd run if Bud hadn't survived. A short while later, Vicki, the head NICU nurse, told me that when Bud was born he had no heartbeat and wasn't breathing. They put a breathing tube down his throat and did CPR, but his heart wasn't beating. That was when the doctor came and told us he hadn't make it, but when they pulled out the breathing tube, Bud's heart started beating, and that was when they ran back to the NICU.

Vicki asked me if I wanted to see him, and I told her, "I don't know—I don't know what a baby that premature looks like." She assured me he looked like a very small baby. When I first saw him I was overwhelmed with emotion—happy that I had a son, and afraid that I might not have him long.

Bud has two older sisters, Reagan, who was eight when he was born, and Amanda, who was fourteen months. We created a schedule: I would take Amanda

> " When I first saw him I was overwhelmed with emotion—happy that I had a son, and afraid that I might not have him long.

> "Having a baby in the NICU is like being on a roller coaster: you have good days and bad.

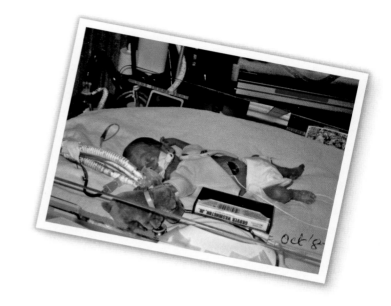

to the babysitter and then go into the hospital to see Bud before going to work. Tim would get Reagan ready for school, take her there, and then go in to see Bud. We would both go in over lunch. I would pick the girls up, go home, do homework, have dinner, and get them ready for bed. Tim would go see Bud after work and then come home, so I could go in to kiss him goodnight. We would take the girls in whenever we could. Sometimes it got a little overwhelming for Reagan so she would read books into a recorder and ask if we could play them for Bud.

The first time I got to see Bud's whole face without that clip holding the respirator tube down his throat is my most precious memory of the NICU. I walked into the NICU, and Bud's nurse told me he had pulled his respirator tube out again, for the third time. I was so excited that I couldn't remember my home phone number to call Tim so that he could see his son's beautiful face.

Having a baby in the NICU is like being on a roller coaster: you have good days and bad. The hardest thing for me was having Bud's heart rate drop when I held him. It seems every time someone touched him it caused pain, so he associated touch with pain. I was afraid I was going to kill Bud, so I didn't want to hold him. The nurses assured me that wouldn't happen, and they were correct.

Our faith played a vital role. I prayed for Bud all the time, but I did find it hard to hear his name at church, when they were praying for the sick.

He won a black belt in karate. In high school Bud played basketball and football, and ran track. He now runs marathons, reads constantly, and is a big sports fan. Bud works for Praxair, the same company where his grandfather and I worked. Bud wants to follow in his granddad's footsteps.

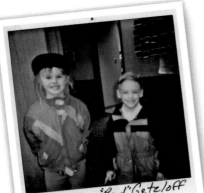

Amanda & "Bud" Getzloff
5½ yrs   4 yrs
"Hello" from William Getzloff

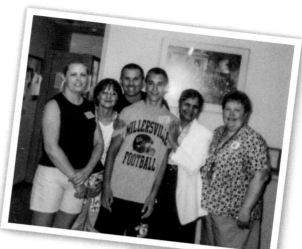

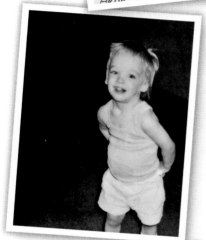

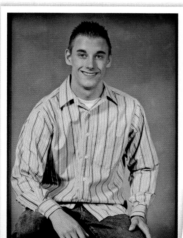

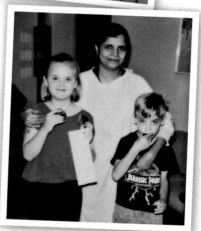

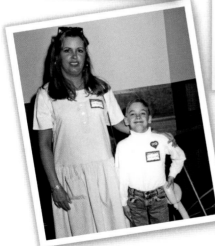

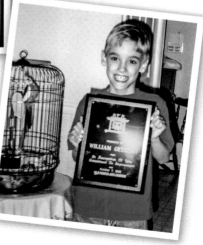

A Precious Musician Is Born—Jacqueline

Jacqueline, my musician, we have another strong bond right there, as music is very dear to me as well. The memory of seeing you at our twenty-fifth-year reunion is very vivid, and of course you were a fabulous star in the paper the next day. Seeing photos of you over the years and at reunions has made me feel a wonderful inclusion in your life's journey. Music is truly food for the soul; your connection through music started early, and has culminated in your playing at Carnegie Hall. Such a marvelous achievement!

Both your academic and musical accolades make us feel proud of our "twenty-five-weeker," now such a beautiful young woman. May God bless you with a wonderful career and a wonderful life!

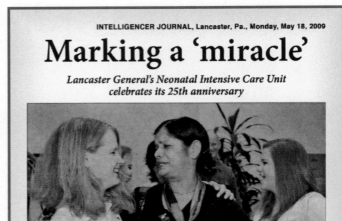

INTELLIGENCER JOURNAL, Lancaster, Pa., Monday, May 18, 2009

Marking a 'miracle'

Lancaster General's Neonatal Intensive Care Unit celebrates its 25th anniversary

Suzette Wagner / Intelligencer Journal

Dr. Manjeet Kaur, who founded Lancaster General Hospital's Neonatal Intensive Care Unit in 1984, speaks Sunday with 13-year-old Jacqueline Hynes of Lancaster, a NICU graduate, during a 25th anniversary celebration at Women & Babies Hospital. At right is Rebecca Sauder, 20, of Mount Joy, also a NICU graduate and a recent nursing school graduate.

On Music

Music brings sunshine, music brings spring,
Music brings tears and a thousand wings.
Music is love, little Jacqueline, love is music,
Music is healing, healing creates music.
Music connects, music rejoices, music numbs, music beams,
Music, like a brook, brings a bubbling meaning to life's stream
Music is life. Life is music!
May your music bring happiness and solace
To those in need, to those in pain!
—Manjeet Kaur

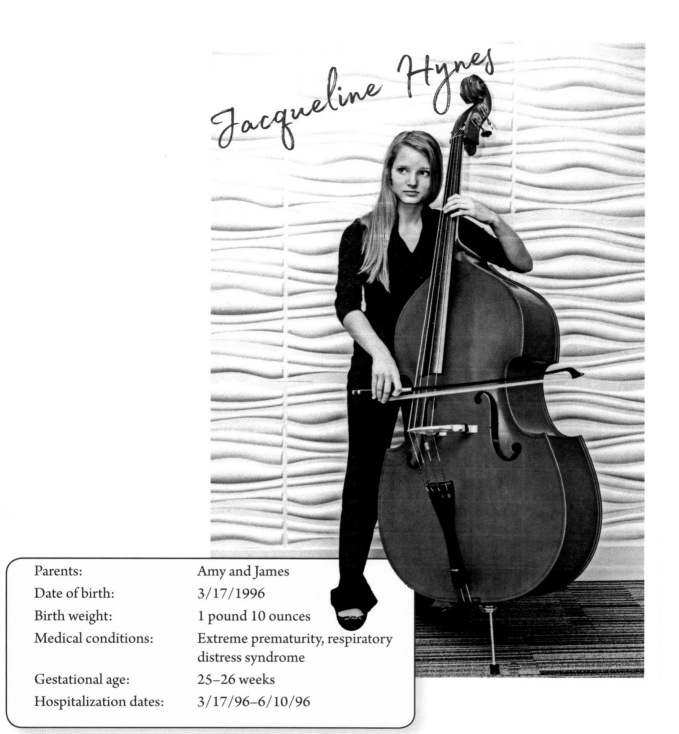

Jacqueline Hynes

Parents:	Amy and James
Date of birth:	3/17/1996
Birth weight:	1 pound 10 ounces
Medical conditions:	Extreme prematurity, respiratory distress syndrome
Gestational age:	25–26 weeks
Hospitalization dates:	3/17/96–6/10/96

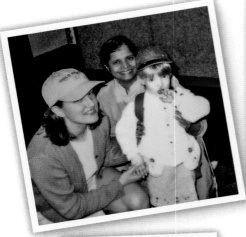
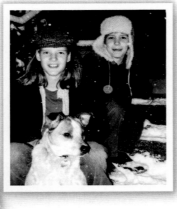
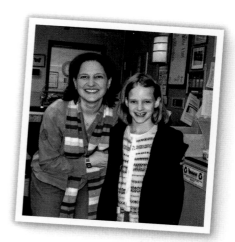
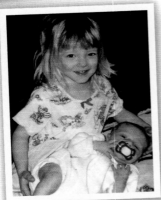
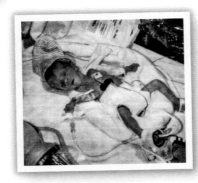
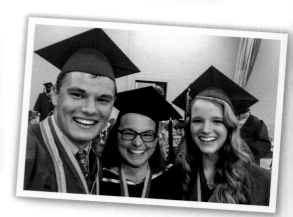
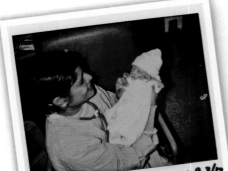
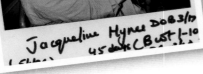

Jacqueline Hynes DOB 3/17
45 days (Best 1-10

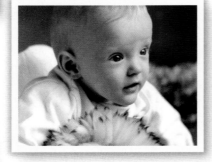
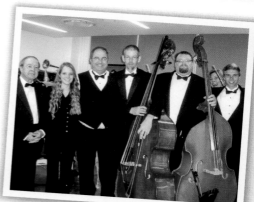
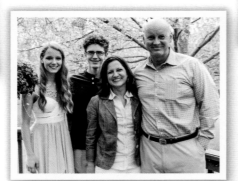

Amy and James' Story

We were very blessed that Jacqueline was born without ailments or in need of surgeries. She had an almost-textbook course in that when she was at a certain week of gestation we were dealing with the standard activities a normal micro-preemie would go through at that point. There were nights when her status wasn't the best, but nothing that she didn't respond to in the grand scope.

To this day Jacqueline has a slight heart murmur and is lacking a little flexibility in stretching. These are things she would never even think of as making her unable to partake in any activity. She has run track, played soccer, and loves rock climbing, all due to the great care she received and the continued physicians' care and follow-through.

Due to toxemia/eclampsia that came out of left field, our hospital visit at twenty-four weeks was not the hospital trip we expected to be taking. We were at Lancaster General Hospital with Dr. Martini, a man of grace and compassion. We had a few days of trying to keep Amy's toxemia and extremely high blood pressure under control, and we even went home for a twenty-four-hour period with Amy under medication, thinking that bed rest would relieve her symptoms. This did not have the desired result, and we were back in the hospital, knowing that we needed to use steroids in anticipation of delivery. The doctor set up a visit for James to go to the NICU to meet

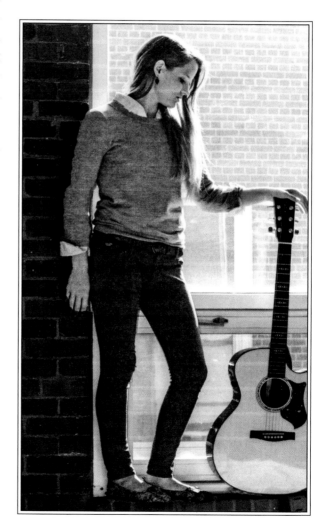

some wonderful RNs—BJ, Sandy, Julie, and Mary Kay—who showed him what we might be expecting and then, with the reality of Jacqueline actually being there, came to our room to speak to me.

I was terrified, and felt like a visitor from another planet: alone, but not alone; scared, but strong; guilty, but realistic. I can still feel all of these emotions today, the guilt probably most, because I second-guessed everything. The "what-ifs" were jarring and very real, but were quickly dispelled by the support system that surrounded me in the hospital. We knew that we needed to focus on the delivery and stay calm and supportive of each other. I think "focus" is the word that best describes our emotions. We stayed focused on all that we took in and all that was going to happen, and we asked many questions that helped us make sure we were part of the plan.

> "I was terrified, and felt like a visitor from another planet: alone, but not alone; scared, but strong; guilty, but realistic. I can still feel all of these emotions today, the guilt probably most, because I second-guessed everything.

On the night of Saturday, March 16, it was decided that we could no longer wait, as Jacqueline was showing signs of distress and was ready to fight. She was delivered via C-section on St. Patrick's Day, and surprised everyone by being tinier than expected. The world of the NICU was there, waiting for Jacqueline with the compassion of a million hearts.

From the moment she was laid in their hands, they never let go. She had a fighting chance with them, with steroids that toughened her lungs, and surfactant, which had just begun to be used in the NICUs throughout the country. We were ready!

What helped us most in the NICU was embracing the community of nurses and doctors, learning all that we could, and staying focused on the current and not our fear of the what-ifs. This was 1996, before the Internet, blogs, texts, and Facebook, so we had the benefit of not having an information overload and listened only to the knowledgeable doctors in front of us.

James and I were blessed to live very close to the hospital, but we weren't prepared to walk out and go home and try to figure out how we were to feel and how others might react. There's no answer; those feelings just need to happen and we needed to deal with them in order to stay focused. Emptiness needs to be filled with hope, so we just decided to make the NICU our home and join the family. Focus and hope. All other emotions take a backseat; letting in only those that are a positive force in your life is the best remedy. There was no social media to help us communicate with family and friends. We see friends who've had a preemie in this age of social media, and

"The world of the NICU was there, waiting for Jacqueline with the compassion of a million hearts.

the support systems are absolutely amazing! Social media seems to have taken over the "journaling" that was part of our daily support, and to this day, we continue it once a year for Jacqueline. We started it the day she was born, and we looked forward to jotting down our thoughts and emotions each day and then closing it to the world. Our journal was a place to get it all out and then stay focused on Jacqueline.

Oh my! The unknown can be so fearful, and there were so many things going on that it was hard to understand exactly what "NICU" really meant. First it was an acronym, and then it was a place, and then it was home. But the fear of getting there was real. We didn't want to accept a lot of the things that were going on, but that was the reality. All that I thought would be happening in my pregnancy was to happen in the hands of the NICU instead of my own body. That's a big step, accepting that the love in the NICU is real, though they don't even know you yet. I remember James going with Jacqueline the moment the NICU team took her from the delivery room, and how lovingly he brought me her first photo. I knew that our love was going to get us through.

I have so many precious memories of the NICU: the rocking-chair conversations, the personal friendships we developed, the time the staff took to communicate and teach us, and their compassion and commitment. If I had to choose a moment though, it would be Dr. Kaur and her complete faith that Jacqueline just needed to grow and that she was ours. These seem to be simple things, but the doctor's support each day was the cord that held it all together for us. Her staff extended this to even the littlest things,

like hiding the wires as best as they could under the blankets when family came, and getting as excited for us as we were when tubes were gradually removed one at a time as Jacqueline improved! Those were always big days!

The day one of Jacqueline's eyes first opened a few weeks after she was born and the day we were able to hold her for the first time were amazing. My father-in-law came from England to visit soon after Jacqueline came home. Until then the only way we

"Our journal was a place to get it all out and then stay focused on Jacqueline.

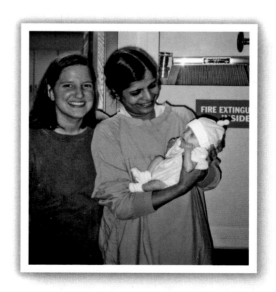

"NICU—First it was an acronym, and then it was a place, and then it was home.

could communicate with him was by phone, which was difficult at the time. When he arrived, we took him to visit the NICU so he could meet all of the great people whom James had told him about during their conversations. It was truly a perfect moment to see Jacqueline's grandfather hold his granddaughter, and see him stand next to the NICU staff.

As Jacqueline grew and improved, it became so hard to leave each day. We felt that we could take better care of her if only we could take her home. This was unrealistic, of course, but milestones were happening, and at those times we were still in the NICU, the moment to go home so close—but not yet. The waiting was the most difficult thing to endure. It was hard to find a happy balance between the feeling that we were there enough and the worry that we weren't.

Our faith was a great help to us. Decisions needed to be made, and the reality was that every day brought something new, so we needed to embrace both our own spiritual beliefs and our belief in those around us. Our faith was also evident daily in our love for each other, and as we looked down at Jacqueline on her warmer bed, we knew that our faith would keep us strong enough to be her strength.

Each moment when she would wrap her fingers around ours, even with all that she was going through, our faith grew more powerful.

Leaving the NICU was a hard step because it was all we knew, and we couldn't help thinking, *How will we survive without a nurse or doctor with us?* Then "living" happens. Jacqueline just grew, and her strength is amazing. How did we go from a one-pound ten-ounce preemie to an eighteen-year-old? Each step, each day, each year has been filled with her milestones, just like any child's. Even after her early delivery, we were blessed to be able to give Jacqueline what she most wanted when she was three—a brother—and they have an exceptional bond! Jacqueline is a very special daughter, granddaughter, niece, cousin, and friend; she is surrounded by love and support.

"This was 1996, before the Internet, blogs, texts, and Facebook, so we had the benefit of not having an information overload and listened only to the knowledgeable doctors in front of us.

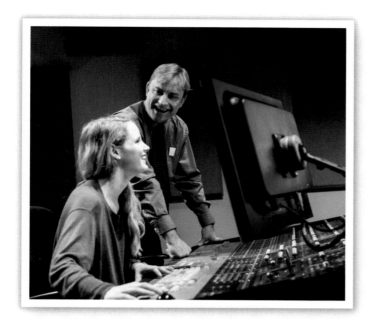

Jacqueline was accepted into Millersville University for Music Technology/Performance and also plays double bass in the Hershey Symphony, which played in Carnegie Hall in April 2014. She began to play stringed instruments in first grade and never looked back—all that music therapy she received from the S. June Smith Center was undoubtedly an early inspiration. She plays violin, double bass, guitar, and piano; was part of the National Honor Society; and graduated from high school with academic honors. Jacqueline also offers her time to Music for Everyone, a nonprofit organization that helps keep music in the schools. She walks each year for March of Dimes, (an organization that works towards preventing birth defects, premature birth, and infant mortality), and has twice been their local ambassador. Where would we all be without their commitment to healthy babies in this preemie world?

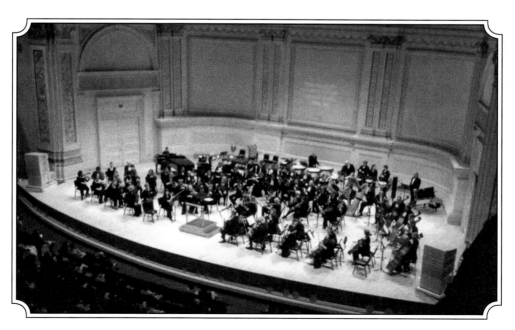

A Scrawny Little Braveheart — Nate

Nathan, I remember you in the NICU at LGH. We had just started keeping little ones your size instead of transferring them to Hershey, as another neonatologist had recently joined me. Because of your family history, I made a folder on Aarskog syndrome, which would be unnecessary in today's world of "Internet everything." It was great to take care of a little one with such a wonderful and supportive family. You certainly had a strong personality even back then. It's been fun seeing you periodically over the years. We are proud of the sensitive and caring young man that you have become, always ready to help people in need, just like your family.

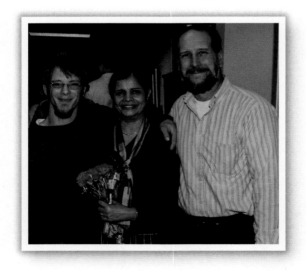

A Little Rock Climber

A winsome tyke was born in June,
Destined to have everyone dance to his tune.
This sick little cutie, who was to know,
Would one day go rock climbing, camera in tow?
Nathan, you were a determined braveheart, we knew,
A valiant fighter when anything went askew.
Now a young man of great repute,
We from the NICU are happy to salute.
Keep that compassion going strong
For those in need when things go wrong!
—Manjeet Kaur

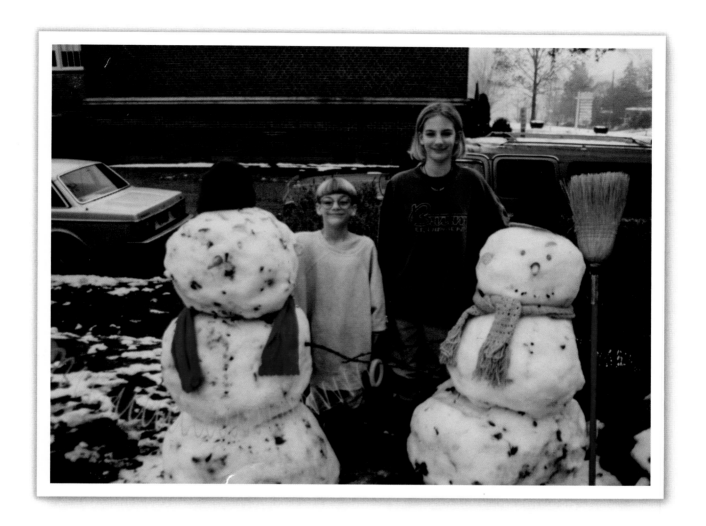

Parents:	Susan and David
Date of birth:	6/18/1987
Birth weight:	1 pound 10¾ ounces
Medical conditions:	Extreme prematurity, respiratory distress syndrome, pneumothorax anemia, inguinal hernia, cranio synostosis
Gestational age:	25–26 weeks
Hospitalization dates:	6/18/1987–9/14/1987

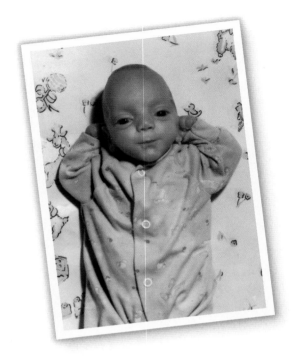
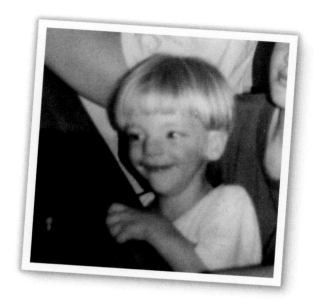
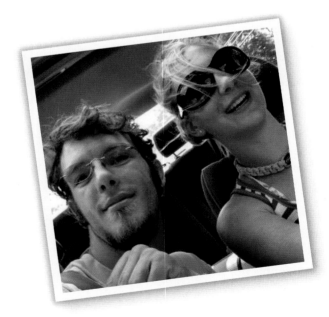
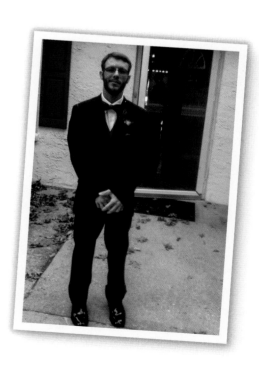

Susan and David's Story

Nathan had respiratory immaturity. His alveoli weren't completely developed, so he needed a tube and a vent. He also had arrested eye vascularization, an underdeveloped intestinal tract, and was severely underweight. He suffered three pneumothorax episodes (those scars still look pretty to me, though Nate gets asked about them when he has his shirt off), and he needed many blood transfusions.

Later, after his discharge from the NICU, Nate had surgery for craniosynostosis done at the Children's Hospital of Philadelphia. The doctor said the NICU staff should be praised, for their work saved Nate hours on the operating table. He still weighed less than ten pounds at one year of age. When he saw a nurse coming with an IV needle, it took three nurses and myself to hold him down so another nurse could get the line in, after which he was like a lamb. They couldn't believe he fought so hard before the needle was in and didn't try to rip out the needle afterward. We said, "He's a NICU baby. He knows if he yanks it, you'll just put another one right in."

Irregular vascularization in his left eye caused Nathan vision problems, but we didn't realize it until he was older and began to take piano lessons. We noticed he'd lose tracking from one line of the score to the next. It turned out he had nearly no depth perception, and the muscles of his left eye made it difficult for him to track. Nathan played baseball, ran the steps, did gymnastics and balance beam, and drove go-carts, so who knew? Eye surgery helped him.

Nate also has a learning disability. We don't know whether it's hereditary, or because he was a preemie, or it's just him. Nate has 20/20 vision, and sees whole letters, but his brain perceives only bits and pieces of the lines. As a young child, he also found it extremely difficult to sequence. I thought he would never conquer shoelaces, and it took him till he was five to swim hand over hand, which was long compared to Meggie, who was swimming at just past two years old. Meghan was very quick to learn to read, and Nate seemed a little slow, but I just thought, *Eh, he's a boy.*

I kept seeing red flags, though, and had Nate tested before he was six. I had been homeschooling and doing some specialty teaching with him. We used cutting-edge computer programs and good curricula, along with a specialist in reading and disabilities. When he reached the end of fifth grade we were told, "Nathan has an extremely high IQ, and the vocabulary and comprehension of an eleventh grader, but you should try to teach him to write his signature so that he won't have to make his mark on documents as an adult."

We found a wonderful woman who was an educational therapist and consultant to work with Nate. She was a bit unorthodox at times; making tailored instruction for Nathan is an understatement. He went to conventional school for the eighth through twelfth grades, graduated from Lampeter-Strasburg, the Career Technology Center, and went to college for a year.

"I remember being in continual prayer for help. … 'You've gotten us through an hour; please help us make the next one.'

With his ear physiology, Nate was for all intents and purposes deaf, but we didn't know. He had acquired language, and made appropriate sounds when he pointed at pictures of animals. When his condition was discovered at DuPont, the doctors were amazed that Nate was speaking at all. It was a marvel to them that he had acquired any speech, and they couldn't believe he was talking above his age level (David says the children learned to talk in self-defense because I'm a talker). After the first set of ear tubes was put in, Nathan and I sat looking at a book. I pointed to a bird and said, "What sound does the bird make?" He replied, "Tweet-tweet, chirp-chirp, and, Mommy, I hear one now!" It was the first time. He had never before heard any of the birds in our backyard. We never knew, because he had compensated so well for his deafness.

Aarskog-Scott syndrome is present in our family, carried by females but more severely affecting the males, manifesting in a pleasant personality, ears smaller and a bit lower set, a pointier chin, a slightly higher incidence of cleft palate, looser joints, and comparatively longer torso for leg length. Dr. Scott, a geneticist at A.I. DuPont, asked permission to see Nathan periodically until he was eighteen. In that process, it was Dr. Scott who, quite accidentally, found Nate's deafness. He crumpled up some papers he wanted to throw in the trash, and saw no response

from Nathan. He thought that was odd, because paper crumpling has such a high-pitched sound that even children with partial deafness show some kind of response. We pursued with tests and found that Nate couldn't hear well.

Nate also needed surgical repair of a double inguinal hernia, which was later redone to reduce scar tissue so his testicles could descend properly. In addition, he needed skin grafts, and later, several reconstructions over his left hip and the underlying muscles—Nate was in an accident at age three when a chunk of the muscle on his left hip was cut off. It's miraculous that he retained the ability to walk. It really doesn't impede him. Before the ambulance arrived, Nate kept telling us he wanted a doctor, and in the ambulance, he held out his arm for the IV. The EMT started wrapping a lot of gauze around his arm and the board. We told him, "Don't bother. Nate was a NICU kid and won't rip it out." He didn't believe us, and applied at least a two-inch-thick layer of gauze. In the ER, a phlebotomist in a white coat came in. Nate held out his arm and said, "Here, take the blood," then looked at me and said, "Mom, he's not a doctor; he's just someone from the lab. Get a doctor to come fix me." He was very glad to see Dr. Arthur. To this day, Nate isn't keen on stepping into a hospital, even to visit someone who's a patient.

Susan's NICU Story

I was across the street in PT with our daughter, Meghan (Meggie), who was about twenty months old, when Nathan decided to be born. I don't remember how I got across the street, but I think David came and got us. I remember they wouldn't let him in with Meghan. He had to leave to take her home. That was the hardest separation from him I've ever endured. We didn't have anyone to leave Meggie with, so David left her with a neighbor, a good Christian woman whom we could trust. She took Meghan without question. Poor David! He was such a brick. I didn't know until later how much he suffered over the baby and me.

Initially, I thought this was just a complication, and I'd go home, maybe restricted to bed rest. I was thinking my mom, who was in Florida visiting my aunt, would need to come to Lancaster to take care of Meggie, and wondered how soon she could get here. When the doctor started talking about therapeutic abortion, I knew things were serious. I was furious—they knew how adamantly opposed I was to any kind of abortion. I told them to just do the best they could for the baby and me. All I wanted was for them to give us the best chance.

I was told I was so early that if I went into labor they couldn't stop it. They would try to give me steroids to mature the baby's lungs, but it probably wouldn't have time to work. The doctor started antibiotics immediately, as he suspected hemolytic strep infection. Thank God, he didn't wait for the culture.

I remember being in continual prayer for help. Looking at the clock, I would say, "Okay, God, you gave this baby one more hour inside, one more hour for that steroid to work. You've gotten us through an hour; please help us make the next one." It was all so overwhelming that I couldn't think of more than an hour at a time. I remember thinking of 2 Samuel 12:22–23, about David and Bathsheba's first child. David sought the Lord for the life of the child in fasting, sackcloth, and ashes at the altar. When the child died, his advisors feared to tell him, but David perceived what had happened, and said, "While the child was alive, I fasted and wept: for I said, Who can tell whether God will be gracious to me, that the child may live. But now he is dead, wherefore should I fast? Can I bring him back again? I shall go to him, but he shall not return to me."

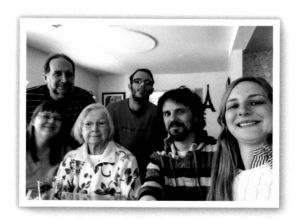

I knew that, impossible as it seemed, God loved this baby more than we ever could, and that if He took the child, it was to spare it from something worse, and that one day we would see the child again in Heaven. King David was sure; he was inspired by God when he wrote that scripture, and it was a great comfort in our time of uncertainty.

When I went into labor, I remember having a feeling that God had forsaken me. Wow, was I wrong! Having Nathan so early by C-section saved his brain. He was later diagnosed with craniosynostosis (no fontanels, just solid skull). The neurosurgeon said that if Nathan had been born full-term, his brain

> "I knew that, impossible as it seemed, God loved this baby more than we ever could, and that if He took the child, it was to spare it from something worse.

would have been crushed inside his skull and he'd have been a living vegetable. His early arrival allowed for a surgery to put in fontanels, giving his brain room to grow. How gracious God is!

Labor was excruciating, though I don't remember the pain. I recall praying for God to help me; I didn't want to scream anything except for God. Later I asked my husband what I was yelling, and whether I was nasty to anyone. He said I just screamed for God, though I answered the nurses a bit curtly, which, he said, was understandable.

I remember telling the obstetrician the baby's head was down, the bottom was up, and it was in the right position, so why was he not doing the C-section? He said he needed a sonogram to be sure. The sonogram confirmed what I knew, so finally to the OR and the sweet smell of the anesthetic. Roused in recovery to put fingerprints on documents, I was told I had a son. I kept thinking, *Impossible, impossible—my thumb print was larger than his footprint.* David was there when I finally woke up with no anesthesia fog. I didn't know how much time had passed, and I asked to see the baby. The nurse said I couldn't till I could get in a wheelchair by myself. I told her to get one and I'd get in it. Oh, the look on David's face as I struggled and he could not help me. I got in, and then to the world of the NICU!

So tiny, so perfect. I remember when Meghan would be playing inside me at this gestation and I wished I could see what she was doing. Now, here was my window. How thankful to God we were that

he was still alive and in a place where they were going to fight to save him, our tiny Nathan, gift of God. He was one pound ten and three-quarters ounces, and twelve and one-eighth inches long, the smallest to survive at LGH at that time.

While I was at the hospital, my mother flew from Florida, and my sister brought her down from Allentown. They actually saw Nathan before I did. The doctors didn't expect Nathan to live the night, so they let them scrub and go in to see him. Scrubbing became routine to see Nathan, and to this day, Meggie remembers having to scrub "forever" to go in and see her brother.

Many people began praying for Nathan's life. Hundreds and hundreds of people, some we knew and most we didn't: our church, my brothers and sisters, my mom's family, my husband's family and their churches, and friends of theirs and their churches. Churches all over the East Coast were praying for that baby, for his life, and later that he might have his sight and not be tied to an oxygen tank all his life. God answered those prayers! Nathan just has the scars from three pneumothoraces, no oxygen tank, and he has 20/20 vision with glasses.

We certainly took my mom for granted. She had been a pediatric nurse for over fifteen years and had retired not long previously, but she was just my mom. I had a background in biology and chemistry, so a NICU nurse who'd just graduated in May gave me her textbook to read. It took me about three days cover to cover. My mom was just a rock. I'd come home and talk blood gases, "sats" (oxygen saturation levels), lab results, settings—and she understood it all. She took care of Meggie, and when I just had to see the baby at 2:00 a.m., she'd say, "Make sure you have a cup of tea and are awake to drive before you go. Don't worry about Meghan or David for tomorrow morning." Mom's walk with the Lord is extraordinary. She was a Barnabas to us.

I know it was very hard on my mom and my sister, because with their medical knowledge, they knew how serious Nathan's condition was, but they never said so until years later. At that time they just were there, listened, and asked what his status was each day. We know it was hard on the rest of the family too, but at the time we were so involved with Nathan and Meghan that I'm not sure we fully realized what it was like for all of them. Maybe it was easier for those who didn't have much medical knowledge.

> "David and I sat and held each other and started to cry and pray. In moments, Dr. Jirka came out and said, 'Don't worry, it's only normal serious,' and then disappeared back into the NICU.

Recollections of the NICU

Nurses Marion, Inez, Judy, Steve, et al.—I remember thinking I wasn't a prejudiced woman, but I thought, *Oh no, a male nurse is taking care of our baby!* Steve is an excellent nurse. I told him a long time afterward what I had thought and he laughed. We had a little stuffed bear with Nathan, and it was named Steve. Nathan still has Stevie bear.

Marion was the best at getting blood. For several years afterward, when Nathan needed bloodwork we would call and ask Marion to come to the lab and do the draw. She said it wasn't nice because every time Nathan saw her he thought he was going to get stuck, but one time someone else did it, and then Nate was glad to have Nurse Marion come.

When Nathan was a few days old, a woman from the insurance company came and asked Dr. Jirka, right in front of me, how long he expected the baby to live and how long the company would have to pay on this claim. I can still see the red creeping up the doctor's neck to his face. He told her that she had no compassion, no sensitivity, and how dare she in front of a parent, and did she think he was God that he would know? I don't remember what else, but he let her have it good! I knew then he would fight for my baby.

"The hardest thing ever was to walk out of LGH after my C-section and not take Nathan home. I felt as if I couldn't bear it.

In one of our first visits, I was still in the wheelchair. We'd come down to see Nathan, and we weren't allowed in. They quickly closed all the blinds. David and I sat and held each other and started to cry and pray. In moments, Dr. Jirka came out and said, "Don't worry, it's only normal serious," and then disappeared back into the NICU. How thoughtful, though we weren't quite sure what he meant.

My fingertip filled his entire hand.

"Two steps forward and one step back, standard recovery with some plateaus in there." If we had a nickel for every time we heard that, we might have been able to pay our bill without a payment plan. Yet how true it was. Often we'd look at Nathan's chart and see a digression. We were told, "It's just a step back—don't be discouraged. The two steps forward are coming." We were glad to know the pattern.

A rep from the insurance company came each week to see if it was justified for Nathan to continue in the NICU. Once, one came and wanted to physically examine Nathan. She was a big woman with an authority complex. The nurses actually formed a line and locked arms at the elbow, blocking the door to the scrub room, and told her that she'd have to go through them to get in to even see Nathan. That was the end of that! How wonderful to see the nurses protect Nathan as one of their own.

I remember the first time I held Nate. When he stretched, his head was at my elbow and his feet barely went to my wrist, and I know he was more than two weeks old, I think almost three.

For Nate's first haircut, for an IV, they taped the hair on a little 3 × 5 card and wrote on it: NATHAN'S FIRST HAIRCUT. It was funny, because Meghan hadn't had a haircut yet. We tease her that Nathan had one first.

We made a Walkman tape for Nate. We read books that we'd read to him before he was born, and Meggie and I sang songs, and we all talked on the tape. Meggie's favorite was "Jesus Loves Me." She sang it to the baby every morning when she got up and talked to him. They would play the tape when they had to do something nasty, or Nate's sats were low, and he would settle or else his sats would go up. I remember a NICU mate's family was fond of sports. At their house they had a game of some sort on all the time. Their tape for their baby was all sports games, with yelling and cheering and announcers—he would hear that and calm down and his sats would go up.

In a science magazine of mine sometime previously, I had read about surfactant and its use with preemies to help ease their breathing. I asked Dr. Kaur why little Nate wasn't given this when he was working so hard to breathe. She was surprised that I knew of it, said it was experimental and in trials in only a few hospitals, and that she couldn't get it no matter how she wanted to. I went home and cried. Surfactant is in common use now.

I recall seeing one of the beds empty, and there'd been no discharge. I remember how personally the staff took it. I felt agony for the parents, and hoped I'd never see Nate's bed empty until he was moved to the other side of the NICU.

Nathan hated to be intubated. He would get his hands up and rip out the tube. Then he'd alarm because he went without oxygen or breathing. They finally put the tiniest little cotton bracelets on him, with little tethers safety-pinned to the bed to keep his hands just out of reach of the tube. He used to get so mad he'd arch his back and toss his head until he'd dislodged it (and set the alarms off again). That should have been a clue he was going to be stubborn—our family says that bit of mule in him helped him to survive.

The dolphin sound, as I called it, occurred when the intubation tube was getting small and Nate's vocal cords partially touched. It sounded like "Flipper." It crushed my heart when Nate would cry and there'd be no sound. It still brings tears to my eyes to think of it.

The worst time was when Nate had a brain bleed, and we had to wait to find whether there was probable damage. Nate was always okay. It was a huge help that Dr. Kaur was so much a doctor, and yet so much another mom as well.

The nurses rocked Nathan near the end of his stay. When he came home, he wanted a new mom to rock him every twelve hours. Some people say he's still spoiled. We blame the nurses for that good head start. The nurses didn't let Nathan lie on his side of preference, but rotated him and made him lie on the other side. This saved him hours of time on the operating table later on, because his head was symmetrical from their diligence.

> "You think you go to have a baby, and a couple of days later you go home together … not three months later.

I got shingles, and they had to scrub down the NICU and give the babies gamma globulin. I was mad that someone who knew we had a NICU baby would even think of having me in their home when they had chickenpox. I felt awful about the extra work for the staff, and that I couldn't go in for so long.

The hardest thing ever was to walk out of LGH after my C-section and not take Nathan home. I felt as if I couldn't bear it. You think you go to have a baby, and a couple of days later you go home together … not three months later.

When we got to bring Nate home, I was afraid he was too small for the car seat. When we got home, Meghan had a "nest" waiting for him. She took blankets from all the beds and the cedar chest and made a circle on the living room floor with them, and lots of soft blankets for padding in the middle. It was to be his safe place. Meghan did that for years, after each of his many surgeries.

Not long after Nate was home he had an infection despite our quarantine. He couldn't keep anything in at either end, and still weighed less than five pounds. Dr. Tifft, our pediatrician, said he'd give Nate until 6:00 a.m. or he'd need to go to the hospital. I called my mom to pray. At the time, she had a Sunday-school class of ladies in their eighties and nineties, and Mom said she'd call and ask them to pray too. Those ladies did pray, and by 6:00 a.m. Nathan did not have to go to the hospital.

At various times, Nathan had IVs stuck all over his arms, legs, and head. They left little white dots, which were almost invisible then. After I got him home and he got some sun, the scars became really apparent. At first I thought he had some sort of rash. That very day I read an article by a preemie mom talking about how precious all those IV scars were. It saved me a trip to the doctor. Nate's scars can still be seen, especially when he's tanned. Just recently someone accused him of having been on drugs. Nate laughed and told them they were from IVs and started showing off his scars. He likes to amaze people with his survival story.

Preemie clothing was nonexistent back then. I found a few extra-small newborn pieces, but actually used Cabbage Patch Doll clothing till Nate could wear newborn clothes. Diapers were too big; outside of the hospital, no preemie size was available. We folded a cloth diaper in quarters and then folded it as a regular diaper until he grew into the "T" diapers.

We will always be thankful for the extraordinary care of the NICU staff for their personal care not only of Nathan but also us. We trust that though the unit changed physically, and so has the staff, the caring remains. We can't say how much it meant to us that the staff trusted us to read the notes and Nate's chart (not to "flip out" or take things the wrong way), though we knew that wasn't strict protocol. For us, the more knowledge we had, the more we felt connected, calm, and prepared to handle whatever came.

Nate was always small for his age, and didn't even get onto the height/weight chart till he was twelve, and then just barely on the edge of the chart. When he was three, he was the size of a one-year-old, but he had all the sass of toddlers his age and then some. We had to be very careful how we spoke to him in public, because people thought we were being unreasonable if we scolded such a tiny child.

❧

David's Remembrances

The doctors tried to keep the baby in the womb as long as possible. After labor started, Susan wanted what gave the baby the best chance to survive, and it was decided to do a semi-emergency C-section.

I was unable to go in for the C-section because I hadn't taken a class for it (that wasn't on the radar for this pregnancy). I had to watch from the outside as the doctor performed the procedure, during which some blood spurted into the obstetrician's eye. You could see he was worried—AIDS was a serious concern then, with guidelines just being established for the protection of healthcare workers. I later tried to reassure him that there was no need to worry because we were and always had been totally monogamous. I watched as Nathan was rushed to the NICU. At this point I was torn between being in the NICU with the baby and with Susan in the recovery room. It didn't hit me right away that I actually had a son!

Eventually I wound up shuttling back and forth to get and give reports and call our parents. Susan wanted so much to see the baby, but was told she'd first have to get into the wheelchair on her own. I winced as she got into that chair, but I knew there was no stopping her from seeing our baby and finding out all that was going on. It was always amazing how her voice, touch, or singing would calm and settle Nate. Meanwhile the physical therapists were keeping an eye on Meghan across the street. I was over there at least once before taking her home when their office was about to close. We had recently moved to Lampeter and only knew a few people. I asked a neighbor if she knew of anyone who could watch Meg. She recommended a stay-at-home mother who lived down the road. When I explained the situation, she graciously took Meg for the evening, noting that they would pray for Susan and the baby. She also watched Meg till Susan's mother arrived the next day. They remain good friends and neighbors to this day. Susan's sister, Joy, even gave blood (this is a woman who passes out at the sight of a drop of blood, so they draped her arm with a sheet so she couldn't see anything). Thanks to her and many other family, friends, and coworkers who donated, Nathan's needs were covered.

When the opportunity arose, I talked with Dr. Jirka. He wouldn't give me the odds of Nathan making it, but he did say that if we went twenty-four hours there would be a good chance for survival.

We were thrust into an entirely new world of wires, tubes, and all kinds of alarms going off. We learned quickly, and the staff was always willing to explain. We also had a visit from Becky, a friend and a parent who had had a child in the NICU. She told us what we might expect and made herself available for support. A few years later Susan did the same for other parents of NICU babies.

Dr. Kaur, Dr. Jirka, and all the nurses were fantastic! Nathan was born on Thursday, June 18, 1987. When I came in on Sunday the twenty-first, I found a card made by the nurses, with a photo of Nate and Father's Day wishes. I was so blown away by all that had happened in the past few days that I hadn't even realized it was Father's Day.

We had total access. We could visit or call twenty-four hours a day. There were many middle-of-the-night trips to LGH, when getting to the hospital took just twelve minutes, and if we drove at the right speed we could make all the lights down Duke Street and out King Street to get home. We were so grateful that the NICU team was there and Nate didn't need to be transported to another hospital.

> "For several years, I worked with social services at the hospital, counseling other NICU parents and grandparents. It wasn't till I got involved in counseling that I realized what a double whammy it is for grandparents. They not only feel helpless about the NICU grand-baby but also feel unable to help their adult children.

After Nathan stabilized we would take Meg in to visit. First came the scrub, all the while telling Meg that if she put her thumb and fingers in her mouth she'd have to come back out. Her visits were usually on the very short side.

At that time, we had been getting our socks from Frank "The Sock Man" at Root's Country Market for years. When he found out we had a preemie, he special-ordered preemie socks for Nathan. Our personal relationship with God, and our prayers and those of others, was our biggest support. We knew that it was not our will but God's will, and we knew that God had given Nathan to us to love and care for. At work I kept updated pictures of Nathan posted by my workbench, and wrote information updates—weight, etc.—on a dry-marker board. Many coworkers would ask how he was doing, especially those who had given blood.

With Nathan coming home on a heart monitor, Dr. Tifft urged us to self-impose a quarantine. The doctor said he would keep me from going to work if he could. I recall sitting on the sofa, my elbow on the arm, and rocking Nathan in the palm of my hand. Nate learned that if he made the monitor alarm go off, someone would come running to give him attention. At one point after I'd fed him he spit it back up, so I refused to feed him. He was on nutramigen; it didn't smell good at all, but he would guzzle it down, and it sure didn't smell any better when it came back up. After Nate graduated to solids, there was a time when he couldn't keep much down and began losing weight (he'd come home at only four pounds four ounces). We found that Michael's (Homestyle Breads Bakery) cinnamon-raisin bread was the only thing he would eat and keep down. That kept him out of the hospital.

The scariest time after discharge was when Susan thought something wasn't right when she woke to feed Nathan. She got Meghan's Fisher-Price stethoscope, listened to Nate's chest, and heard him wheezing. She called the doctor and got Nate to the hospital right away. He had RSV and was placed in a tent. Because it was caught early Nate made it through. The doctor said that if we'd waited even another hour, it probably would have been too late.

Nate went on to have other procedures, and when we were at other hospitals you could always tell the NICU children from the others because they didn't pull out their IVs. There was also a battle between the insurance company and the hospital. I think it was two years before things were settled. It wouldn't have mattered if it cost a million dollars; I'd have worked the rest of my life to pay it off.

We got everything settled just a few days before Nathan's second birthday. An administrator from the insurance company called to thank us for all we had done to help resolve the matter so quickly. They said a child is usually six or seven before things are settled.

Nathan is now thirty. He's still no giant in height or weight, maybe five feet six inches and 115 pounds when he's "fat," but that is deceptive. Nate is quite strong. He works part-time at CVS, helps out a friend in construction/ remodeling/ demolition when needed, and freelances in mostly architectural photography, but does other fields as well. He likes to rock-climb, slack-line, hike, and tent. He loves to explore cities, buildings, and places with his camera, especially Chicago, Philadelphia, New York City, and Washington, DC, but finds he likes small towns, villages, and nature as well. He's just happy shooting with a camera. He likes to play games on his PlayStation 3 and enjoys current films and old black-and-white movies.

I think I would really like him even if he wasn't ours. He's just a great young man. He has tremendous compassion for those challenged in any way, but he still hates to go into hospitals, even to visit someone, though he does if they need a visit. When he was seventeen he said to Susan, "Mom, I'm finally older than the number of surgeries I've had!"

Meghan has become an EMT with LEMSA and runs BLS and ALS with the medics. At the time of this writing, Meghan is in Paramedic School, hoping to graduate in a few weeks. We think part of the reason why she's so interested in the medical field and helping people is because of all the time she spent in hospitals with Nate, and getting all the update messages from Grammy while waiting for Nate to come home.

I know that God is why Susan and I didn't wind up in the statistical norm and get divorced. Having a preemie increases your chances, but God helped us before we were married, before Meghan or Nathan was born, and graciously continues to do so.

Susan adds, "For several years, I worked with social services at the hospital, counseling other NICU parents and grandparents. It wasn't till I got involved in counseling that I realized what a double whammy it is for grandparents. They not only feel helpless about the NICU grand-baby but also feel unable to help their adult children. Though I no longer officially counsel NICU parents, I've had opportunities to offer support to parents of preemies both in and outside of our own family. David and I are pleased to be able to tell parents of preemies that we had a baby much smaller than yours, and everything turned out well. The doctors can do so much more nowadays."

Our daughter, Meghan, was also a complicated pregnancy, and we had a high risk of losing her. Nowadays, she would be considered a routine pregnancy! God has allowed us to have great doctors and nurses to give us two precious children. They will always have our deepest gratitude and thanks.

⟿

From Nate

I don't think it has really affected me. I've just grown up being me, except I think I wouldn't mind being taller, but I don't think that being short is bad or resulted from being a preemie. None of my uncles or aunts or cousins on my mom's side are very tall, so I think being short comes from them.

I've had the opportunity to talk with people who've had preemies. My cousin had one. Looking at me gave her hope that her baby could make it too, because he was big compared to my size when I was born. Recently, a customer at work was talking about her preemie grandchild. She was worried and upset, and I told her, "Look at me. I was really preemie, and I'm big and strong now." She said her grandbaby weighed only three pounds. I said, "Wow, he's big. I was only one pound and a bit." That really gave her encouragement.

⟿

From Meghan

“ I never really thought much about Nate's being preemie. I remember the nest-making thing, but the rest was just growing up with my brother.

A Little Survivor—Osmyn

How lovely to get a card from "Osmyn J. Oree Photography." I know our little NICU babies are destined to do special things. You have a wonderful family, Osmyn—supportive and dedicated. I recall your grandmother coming to the NICU, too, and to the NICU reunions.

Having had a tough NICU course, you've done an amazing job. You started out weighing only two pounds; you had many of the problems usually associated with lung immaturity, and you required respiratory support and a home monitor. We sent more babies home on monitors back then; we're more selective today, and monitor them a little longer in the hospital. Even evidence-based medicine changes over the years. I have several photos of you growing up, Osmyn. It's always been a pleasure seeing you and your family. Good luck with photography, and God bless!

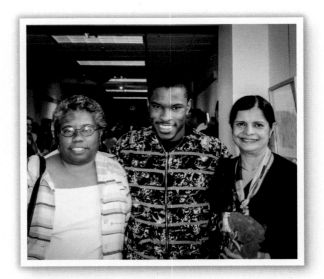

Treasure of Memories

A cute tiny babe was born in the fall,
His swift arrival none could forestall.
Landing in a cradle of tubes, lights, and beeps,
He brought anxiety, prayers, and a love so deep.
Through the eighty-eight days of his NICU abode,
A daily vigil mama and grandma did uphold.
Now a sportsman, a photographer in your glory,
We are proud of your achievements, Osmyn Oree.
As you create lovely memories in your art anew,
May you bring joy and pleasure to all your crew!
—Manjeet Kaur

Osmyn Oree

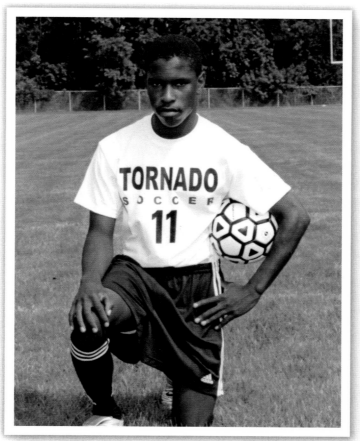

Parents:	Janice and Omarr
Date of birth:	8/19/1988
Birth weight:	2 pounds 5 ounces
Medical conditions:	Lung immaturity, respiratory distress syndrome, apnea
Gestational age:	26 weeks
Hospitalization dates:	8/19/1988–11/14/1988

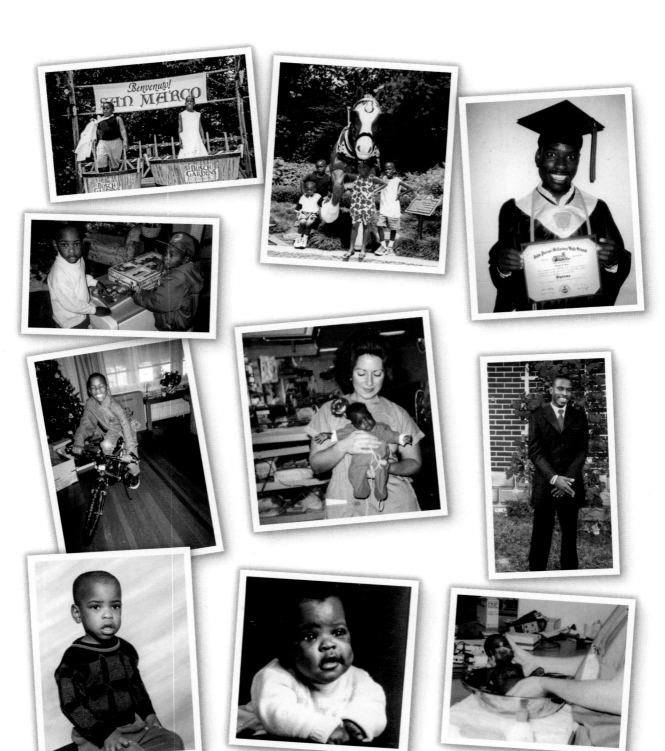

Janice and Omarr's Story

My family thought my contractions were under control. I was alone in the hospital, as it was close to midnight. I'd been there two days. When I realized that I wasn't just using the bathroom but that it was my baby that I was about to drop in the toilet, I was actually pretty calm. What helped the most was my faith in God, my trust in the doctors, and the support of my family.

Osmyn was in the NICU from the beginning. The doctors and nurses were always honest and open about everything that was going on and what to expect. If there were any surprises, they were good ones, because I was always prepared for the worst.

My family is very close and supportive. I had two other sons at the time. My mom and my two sisters helped with getting them to and from school and daycare when needed.

The first time I held Osmyn was my most precious NICU moment—and also my most anxious moment. This was during his second week, when everything was going bad. While I was holding him, I was thinking I was probably going to lose him and this might be the only time I'd get to hold him while he was alive. It was a moment I'll never forget. I didn't cry then, but it brings tears to my eyes when I think about it now and how far Osmyn has come.

The most difficult time was his second week. Every day, when I went to visit, the machine was doing a greater percentage of his breathing for him, until it was at 100 percent. When I saw that, I thought, *What's going to happen when I come in tomorrow?*

When I hear the question "Do you believe in miracles?" my answer is "I live with one." My faith is strong, and my prayers are continuous to this day. My faith and prayers are what got me through that difficult time. I still pray for Osmyn and thank God for him every day.

Osmyn is currently working full time and works as a photographer on a part-time basis. He continues to look for a full-time position as a photographer in a major city or to travel as a photographer.

It's an honor and a privilege that you've selected Osmyn as one of the participants for your book. I must say that we were blessed with three wonderful doctors during Osmyn's stay in the NICU. All of the nurses and staff were just wonderful.

A little background on Osmyn's birth: I was at work on a Wednesday, and I wasn't feeling well, so my boss said, "Go home." I told him I had to finish something, and would then be on my way. I called the doctor, and drove the forty miles to their office where I was examined and sent across the street to the hospital to be put on a monitor, as it appeared I

> "When I hear the question 'Do you believe in miracles?' my answer is 'I live with one.'

was having contractions. Little did I know that I was going to be admitted. At 8:00 p.m. on Friday, as my mother was leaving my room, I heard the doctor tell her that my contractions were under control. Shortly thereafter, I vomited all over myself. I thought, *This isn't good, as it had also happened right before the birth of my other two sons.* I then told the nurse that I had to go to the bathroom and didn't want to use the bedpan. She said I wasn't allowed to get up, and she didn't think that I had to go to the bathroom. She said, "Every time you say that, you're having a contraction."

Her shift ended at 11:00 p.m. and a new nurse arrived. I told her I needed to go to the bathroom and preferred not to use the bedpan. She looked at my chart and said she would get another nurse to help us, as she'd already given me my sleeping pill. The two of them walked me to the bathroom and stood at the door, talking. I stopped them and said, "I think it's the baby."

"No," the nurse said.

"Yes," I said.

She reached up under me as I sat on the toilet and she "caught him." Everything came out—the baby was still in the sac. The nurse ran from the bathroom, and immediately the room filled with doctors and nurses. I wish I could relive that moment, as I remember seeing so many people and the nurse who stayed with me in the bathroom, but I can't recall seeing "my baby." I just remember sitting there and praying till the room cleared. The nurse then cleaned me up again and put me back into bed. A couple of hours later, a doctor came in and told me I had a son, that he was on a ventilator, and his condition was critical.

Osmyn's condition improved over the next week. Week two was a different story. His weight fell from two pounds five ounces to two pounds one ounce. You [Dr. Kaur] told me that the ventilator was doing

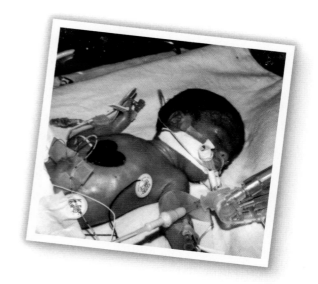

100 percent of his breathing. It was during that week that I first held Osmyn. You told me that his lungs were undeveloped and that he had pneumonia. He was started on treatment for it and began to improve. Of course, he had a few setbacks along the way, but I knew he was in good hands. He was in the hospital for eighty-eight days. I visited every day. My mother, who sang to and visited all of the babies, was there eighty-seven of those days. My husband didn't like all the attention or activity that occurred during the day, so he'd visit late at night, stand at the window, and just look in for a few minutes.

Osmyn went home on medication and with a monitor for nine months. He had no problems at all. After the first year, his development was followed by the S. June Smith Center. At age five, he started to play soccer, which he played through high school. He never seemed to have the stamina of the other players, and he experienced some shortness of breath. The soccer league rules were that starting at age five every child got equal playing time. Osmyn would start the game, and when he'd had enough, he would just walk off the field and sit on my lap. The coach would ask if he was coming back in—I'd shake my head "No."

"We didn't know it then, but we were all special—not better than anyone else, but we were survivors. We made it through a hard time in our lives and we were able to live out our futures.

Osmyn has no physical or developmental problems at all. He was always a good student and is a member of the National Honor Society. In 2006 he graduated from J. P. McCaskey High School with a partial academic scholarship to Lebanon Valley College. He attended Lebanon Valley for only one year, then left to pursue a degree in photography at the Pennsylvania College of Art & Design. He graduated in 2011 with a Bachelor of Fine Arts degree in Photography. His work has been featured at many venues in Lancaster and locations in Philadelphia, Virginia, and Los Angeles.

Osmyn's Story

I don't recall much of anything from my time in the intensive care unit aside from photos that were shown to me when I was older. I remember thinking, *Wow, I can't believe I survived.* I'm still surprised at how healthy I've become, and that I've made it as far as I have in life. One thing that really stuck with me has been what my grandmother told me about her experience. For eighty-seven days she was there by my side, taking care of me like I was her own child. It was incredible to hear for the first time, and it still amazes me that she was so caring.

Now that I've grown up, I've only been to one reunion so far. The experience was a little overwhelming at first. There were tons of other kids who were just like me, maybe even worse, when they were born, and they were all alive and well. I felt like we were all supposed to make it through that tough time in our lives. We didn't know it then, but we were all special—not better than anyone else, but we were survivors. We made it through a hard time in our lives and we were able to live out our futures.

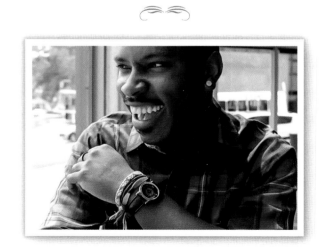

A Special Connection—Cody

*I*t seems to me that a number of the stories I've chosen were transports from St. Joseph Hospital. Born at St. Joseph's, one pound three ounces at twenty-six-weeks gestation, you were certainly a trouper. It was lovely reading the day-to-day account your grandpa left. How good you must feel to know that your grandparents loved you so much. You had your usual problems: very low birth weight, extreme prematurity, respiratory, and feeding issues. You needed prolonged respiratory support and received transfusions, but the one thing you always had besides dedicated NICU staff and the technology of the 1980s was a loving family with very strong faith.

Soon after, you were in a lovely article in the newspaper. Only recently I attended your Eagle Scout ceremony. To see you up on the stage, receiving the award and giving a speech, gave me a sweet sense of achievement. It's been a privilege and a blessing to have remained connected with your family for over two decades!

What a heritage! And I love that your grandfather has written a story! He has put a beautifully written day-to-day and week-to-week account of the NICU experience in lay terms. It will help other families to read about the progress and the milestones of a very low birth-weight infant. Recently I received a note from you from the bank where you work. What a wonderful connection after twenty years, and what a joy to know that today you're an intelligent, healthy, and athletic young man.

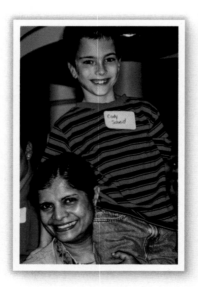

An Ode to a Grandparent—
"That Special Connection"

That special link, that special bond,
A nurturing prayer, a connection so strong.
Warm hugs and kisses, a steadfast hand,
A guiding star in the galaxy's milky wonderland.
Sweet music, that melody beyond the hill,
Seeming afar, yet close to me still.
Morn or noon, eve or night,
To honor and love, and hold on tight.
A caressing look, with its mellow glow,
From the ocean of love, forever shall flow.
From the heavens above, to the meadows below!
—Manjeet Kaur

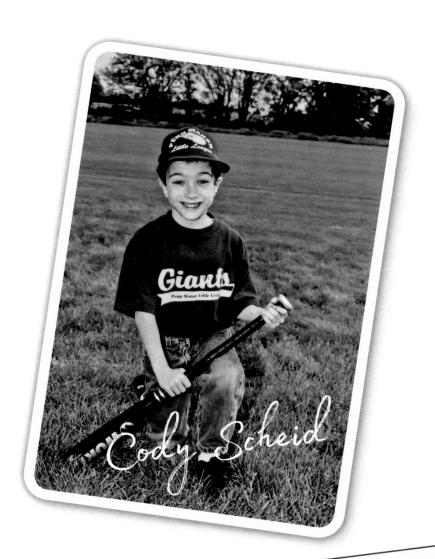

Cody Scheid

Parents:	Keri and David
Date of birth:	9/26/1994
Birth weight:	1 pound 3 ounces
Length:	11½ inches
Medical conditions:	Extreme prematurity, respiratory distress syndrome, anemia
Gestational age:	26 weeks
Hospitalization dates:	9/26/1994–12/22/1994

A child is born

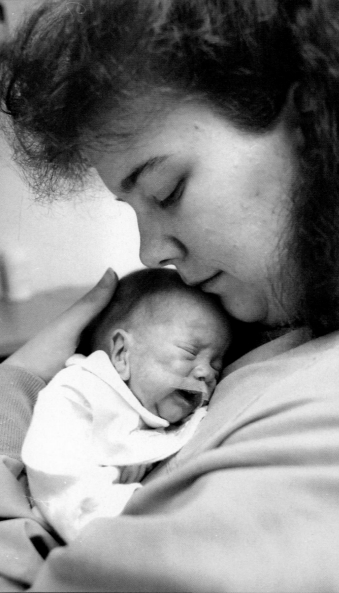

For nearly three months, Keri and Dave Scheid donned hospital gowns and scrubbed their hands before they could even get close to their newborn son.

To hold him, they unraveled the tubes that stretched from his body to beeping and flashing monitors.

To feed him, they held syringes full of formula and breast milk, allowing the solution to drip through a tube in their son's nose.

Cody Scheid didn't come into this world in the best possible way. Twenty-six weeks after he was conceived, he began to threaten his mother's health. Keri was rushed to St. Joseph Hospital for an emergency Ceasarian delivery as her blood pressure skyrocketed.

According to doctors, Keri was allergic to being pregnant. The only cure was to bring Cody out — much earlier than expected.

"The night he was born, it was pretty doubtful, pretty hairy," Dave said.

Cody weighed 1 pound, 3 ounces at birth, and was shorter than a No. 2 pencil.

"I was expecting small, but not anything that tiny," Dave said of his first child.

Cody was then whisked to Lancaster General Hospital's Neonatal Intensive Care Unit.

In the rush, the Scheids didn't even find out the sex of their baby.

"It was two hours before we knew it was a boy," Keri said.

Keri stayed at St. Joseph Hospital to recover from the delivery that brought her baby into the world at the end of September instead of his New Year's Eve due date.

"This little guy was determined not to wait," Keri said.

Impatience has a price. With only six months to grow inside their mothers' wombs, the lungs of premature babies aren't developed, the brains aren't fully formed and the eyes are fused shut. And they can't fight infections.

"It's amazing the ones that are living now," said Judy Ecenrode, one of Cody's three primary-care nurses. "It's really something you never lose that awe of."

Babies with extremely low birth weights, like Cody, have a national survival rate of 50 to 60 percent. At Lancaster General, the rate is 66 percent.

"The main problem that kills them is lung immaturity," said Dr. Manjeet Kaur, chief of neonatology. "They're missing surfactant, which keeps the lung sacs open." A synthetic version of the chemical, which became available three years ago, now helps save the lives of the tiniest babies.

Still, the effort of breathing can be too much.

Until they can breathe on their own, premature babies need a ventilator. Such a unit, an endotrachial tube hooked to a respirator, was part of the tubing network that surrounded Cody after his birth.

As his body is able to handle more functions, the tubes are removed. They are a visible gauge of a baby's progress.

"We tell the parents, one tube at a time," Dr. Kaur said.

The first to go are the umbilical catheters that monitor blood gases and give fluids. Next are the intravenous lines that provide proteins and fats. When babies can digest food, the IV is replaced with a nasal-gastric tube.

"It tickles his nose to put it in," said Keri, who, after spending more than 85 days in the intensive care unit, is adept at feeding her baby through the tube.

Babies younger than 7½ months don't know how to suck or swallow, so they can't use a bottle. They drink about an ounce of 24-calorie milk every three hours, working up to about two ounces of 20-calorie milk every four hours before they can go home.

"I still think we need to grind some cheeseburgers up in his bottle," Dave said.

Before babies can leave the hospital, they must be able to drink the higher-quantity/lower-calorie milk from a bottle at every feeding.

"His whole focus right now is eating. Right now we want him eating and growing," Ecenrode said. "By the time they're ready to go home, they're just like any other baby."

The problems don't end there though.

Dr. Kaur said new obstacles can develop in the first year, from jaundice, to low platelet counts, to apnea (when babies "forget" to breath), to long-term lung problems.

When they take their baby home to Holtwood, the Scheids will also take oxygen and a monitor to measure his heart rate and breathing pattern.

"In a way, we'll have a better time than most first-time parents," said Dave. "We have a monitor."

Like most new parents, the Scheids decorated a room to serve as their baby's nursery. But to prepare for Cody's arrival, they also learned CPR and practiced administering oxygen, just in case the alarm sounds, indicating he has stopped breathing.

When Cody was first born, the Scheids jumped at every noise in the intensive care unit. That fear followed them home as nightmares.

"You have many sleepless nights when all you hear is that alarm," Dave said.

But after so many weeks of buzzing and beeps, the Scheids have become seasoned.

"Parents learn so much what to do here, they don't need us because they've dealt with it for months," Ecenrode said.

It wasn't so easy in the beginning.

"The first week I was a basket case," said Dave, who juggled his time between visiting his wife in one hospital and his baby in another. What made it especially difficult was the physical separation from his newborn son.

"Especially in the first three days of life, we have to be so very cautious," Dr. Kaur said. "They just don't tolerate being moved."

For the Scheids, that meant limited snuggling with their baby. Although many friends and family wanted to visit the newborn, Keri reserved the few opportunities to hold him for herself.

"Right now I'm just a little selfish," Keri said. "I want my holding time."

When machines and nurses and doctors limit contact with their child, families cope by personalizing their baby's area in the hospital. Cody's first presents were a plush football emblazoned with the Pittsburgh Steelers logo from Dave and a tiny Steeler hat knitted by his great-grandmother.

"It's a strange environment and a noisy place," Ecenrode said. "That's why we allow stuffed animals, allow parents to dress them up. It gives them a sense of control."

What also helps the Scheids is giving Cody his weekly bath. The daily contact they have with their son, however brief, helps them to notice subtle changes that could signal larger problems, like a momentary lapse in breathing.

"You got a little gray there, kiddo. You can't be doing that," said Keri, jostling Cody to remind him to take his next breath.

Both she and Dave talk to their son, telling him, over and over like a mantra: "You must breathe, you must eat."

Keri said she stopped worrying that her son wouldn't survive his early entry into the world.

"There was only one bad time for me that I thought he might not make it. It was about the fourth day, and it just hit me," she said. "But I've been fine since then. I never had any doubts."

Ecenrode said Cody's prematurity shouldn't distinguish him from babies delivered on their due date.

"They're a little delayed because they spend so many months just trying to breathe and grow," Ecenrode said. "But a lot of times they catch up and you'd never know they were a premie."

Keri is optimistic about Cody. "He's a feisty little guy," she said. "He had quite a few strikes against him when he was born, but he's licked them all."

He's done so well that he may come home for Christmas, said Dr. Kaur.

It's a Christmas wish the Scheids are counting on.

Their wish was granted. Cody came home from the hospital Thursday evening.

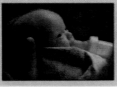

Story by
Daina Savage

Photos by
Dan Marschka

Grandfather's Story

The arrival of Cody Allen Scheid, as told by his grandfather, Donald A. Raugh:

Cody Allen Scheid was brought into this world at 11:01 p.m. on September 26, 1994, at St. Joseph Hospital in Lancaster, Pennsylvania. It was a cool fall evening and, unexpectedly, turned out to be quite an eventful one.

Your mother had quite a time with this pregnancy, Cody. For the first several months, all went well, if you exclude the usual morning sickness. Then some complications set in, which eventually confined your mother to bed for the remainder of the time she was supposed to carry you. Since you weren't due to arrive until December 31, three months of complete bedrest awaited her.

Your dad had his hands full, too. He had to work, try and take care of the house, coach football, and do all kinds of running around, but help was never far away. Grandma and Grandpa Raugh were right around the corner. Your Grandma Raugh was down early every morning, helping take care of your mom. Great-grandmother Bingeman helped out, and so did your paternal grandmother. Your mother's closest friend was always on call and did whatever was necessary—be it sitting with your mom, taking care of the dogs, or anything else. Our whole family was involved. Uncle Steve and soon-to-be Aunt Kristi were there also, doing what they could to help. Grandma Raugh would cook supper for all of us at your parents'

home. This went on for several weeks just before you were born. Then came the evening of September 26.

Monday, September 26, 1994, about 6:00 p.m. – Your dad called to tell us he was taking your mom back into the hospital. She had been complaining of back pain for several days, and he'd just found her in their room having a lot of pain again. They came up to our house and away we went to St. Joe's: your mom and Grandma Raugh in the backseat, me driving Grandma's car, and your dad following in his car. After one brief stop in Willow Street, where your mom got sick, we proceeded to the hospital and straight to the maternity ward on the fifth floor. They were expecting us. The doctor came and examined your mom. He told us she was suffering from a hernia and that they would keep her overnight just to make sure she was okay, and she could go home in the morning. They also did a blood test. The doctor predicted that you were going to be a girl, and told your mom and dad not to buy a lot of blue things (we all know how that turned out).

We went home. Your dad went home, expecting to return in the morning to take your mom home. This was about 8:00 in the evening.

About 9:15 p.m. I answered the telephone to hear your dad telling me we needed to go back to the hospital right away, that you were going to be delivered. It seems your mom had developed something called toxemia and had very high blood pressure, so the doctors had no choice but to bring you into the world, ready or not. We arrived shortly thereafter and you came into our family at 11:01 p.m. We were all surprised by your size, just one pound three ounces and only eleven and a half inches long. The

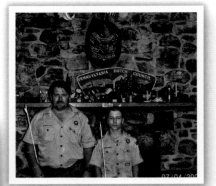

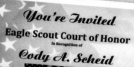

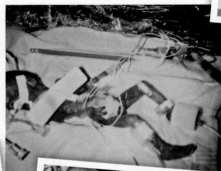

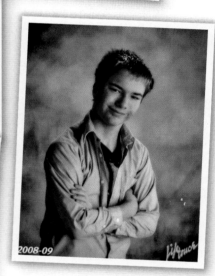

2008-09

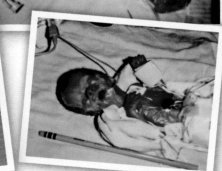

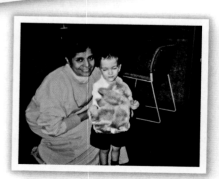

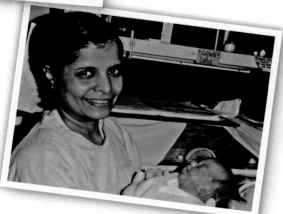

second surprise was finding out that you were in fact a boy, not the girl the doctor had predicted.

I can tell you that you were loved instantly. Our minister, Reverend James Haun, was there with us, and led us in prayer that both you and your mom would be okay and that the Lord would look over both of you and bless you with his care. He must have been listening.

At about 2:00 a.m. on September 27, you were taken in for your mom to see you, and then you were transported to the Lancaster General Hospital Neonatal Intensive Care Unit. We said goodnight to your mom, as she needed to get as much rest as possible, and then Grandma and I went over to Lancaster General to make sure you were okay. Things seemed to be going well.

Tuesday, September 27, 1994 – We've gotten little rest thinking about you and your mother. We got up in the morning and wasted no time in getting back to the hospital to see both of you. We'd stop and see your mom and then head straight off to Lancaster General to look in on you. I have to tell you, Cody, that you are a fighter. You were kicking your mom constantly while you were in the womb, and you've been kicking ever since you were born. Your tiny arms and legs just keep going. You even managed to pee on one of your nurses shortly after you came into this world.

Your progress continues even though you're less than a day old. They have reduced the amount of pure oxygen you're receiving from 100 percent to about 40 percent, which is a really good sign that you're doing well. You have so many tubes and wires on you that we can barely see all of you, but you don't seem to mind; you just keep breathing and kicking away.

Your mom is really tired today, and they have restricted visitors to just your dad and your grandparents. When we visit her we don't stay long, as she needs her rest in order to get strong again. Every time we see her we tell her about you, and she wants to see you very badly. It's hard on her being at St. Joe's with you across town.

Your dad got a good night's sleep tonight for the first time since Sunday. He needed it, as he has been on the go staying with your mother and then running across town to be with you. He doesn't seem to mind, though, as each time he sees one of you he knows all is going well.

Wednesday, September 28, 1994 – Not much change in your condition, which is good. They now have you in about 25 percent oxygen, and that shows real progress on your part. Keep it up, little guy. Your parents have received flowers and cards from friends and coworkers, and that brought a smile to your mom's face. People from all over keep asking about you and how you both are doing. Grandma Raugh even talked to her sister in Ireland today, and they all have you in their prayers.

Your mother was able to get out of bed today, and they told her she could probably go home from the hospital tomorrow, which made her very happy. Her first stop with your dad will be to see you at Lancaster General. She can't wait. We come to see you every day.

Thursday, September 29, 1994 – As expected, your mother was released from the hospital today, and she and your dad made a beeline to see you in the nursery. Your mother became very emotional in the elevator up to your floor with the pending excitement of seeing you. She showed only a mother's love from the time she first laid eyes on you and gently touched your tiny arms and legs.

You're doing quite well today yourself. You're still kicking away, and they took you off the regular respirator tonight at about 7:00 p.m. They might have to put it back on if you get too tired from breathing on your own. At 10:00 p.m. your dad called to tell us that all is well and that you're still off the respirator.

You've had several visitors over the past days. Your paternal grandparents have visited, and Grandma Raugh and I have been in often also. Uncle Steve and Aunt Kristi came to see you, so have our neighbors, Dave and Dawn. Along with several others, they have donated blood for you, as you'll need transfusions often while you're this little.

I don't know how your weight is doing, as I keep forgetting to ask your mom and dad. Your Aunt Sheila and Uncle Jay both called from Ireland today to check on your progress and that of your mother.

Friday, September 30, 1994 – It's unbelievable but you're still off the respirator. I keep telling people that you're a feisty little guy, and you're proving me right day by day. Keep fighting, little guy, we all love you and want to see you grown and home with us. Mom and Dad are spending a great deal of time at your side—as much as they can without wearing your mom out. She still has a way to go to recover fully and can't overdo it yet.

Each day for you is an uphill climb, and each day you seem to make just a little more progress.

Monday, October 3, 1994 – You seem to be progressing pretty well for being less than a week old. Over the weekend your mom and dad told me that your weight is up—now one pound five ounces. They had to put you back on the regular ventilator because the other one was causing you to tire out and you'd set off your alarms.

Your mom and dad visit with you every day, sometimes twice a day. Your mom still has to take it easy, as she hasn't fully recovered from all that's happened in recent weeks. She has really perked up now that she's able to spend time with you.

Grandma Raugh and I were able to get gowns on and say a formal hello to you on Friday night. I can't tell you, little guy, how exciting it was to be able to touch your tiny foot for the first time and tell you we loved you. Grandma Raugh gently rubbed your left foot, but you didn't seem to like that very much, so she switched back to your right one. Grandma and Grandpa Scheid have also put on gowns and have been able to visit with you.

The whole family communicates regularly on your progress. Keep fighting, Cody—you're surely loved, and we want to see you grow and mature as each day passes.

Your Uncle Doug is giving blood for you today, I believe, and your Uncle Steve is going to be tested to see if you can use his blood also.

Thursday, October 6, 1994 – Well, Cody, you're doing great. While your weight dropped a little, as was expected, you've regained it and are back at just a little above your birth weight. Your parents tell us they've started to give you mother's milk, the first time was yesterday. That should help you grow and add weight. We hear you might be featured in the newspaper in the next several weeks. Seems they're doing an article on the neonatal unit at Lancaster General Hospital, and asked your mom's permission to take your picture and put your name in the paper when they do the article. Less than two weeks old and already you're becoming a celebrity. Grandma Raugh takes your mom in to see you almost every afternoon, and your mom and dad visit every evening. Uncle Steve and I made a special trip in to see you last night also. Keep kicking, little guy, we love you.

Monday, October 10, 1994 – You've had quite a weekend. On Friday the nurses allowed your mom to hold you for about one minute while they changed your bedding. Talk about someone being happy—you should have seen your mom after that. The nurses took a picture of her holding you, which I am sure you've seen by now. Grandma Raugh and I went to visit your great-great-aunt and uncle in Bedford over the weekend. We called to see how you were doing, and your mom told us you had gained an ounce on Saturday. When we got home on Sunday she told us you were up another ounce, bringing you back up to your birth weight. If as you read this you get a little confused about your weight, keep in mind that during the first several weeks after you were born, your weight went up and down numerous times. It was nothing we didn't expect, as this is natural with newborns, so you might read that I have your weight up on one day and the next it might be down. Anyhow, as of last evening (Sunday) you were just over one pound three ounces. All is going well, and each day we thank God for your continued progress.

Wednesday, October 12, 1994 – Grandma Raugh and I were in to see you last night. This is the first time since Friday that I've been able to be in there.

" That's exactly what they wanted to see you do—
start gaining weight and keeping it on.

Grandma goes in with your mom every day. The nurses were working with you a lot last night. They must have been having trouble with one of your monitors, for they kept trying different things with the wires attached to you. You held in there like a trouper. Your mom and dad say that they're giving you antibiotics because your white blood-cell count is up. You've also been having some trouble with mucus in your mouth. The nurses don't seem too concerned about it, so we hope everything will continue to go well. One of the nurses told us last night that you're a fighter. Hang in there, little guy, we want you home for Christmas.

Monday, October 17, 1994 – Three weeks old today. We were in to see you last night and you continue to do well. Your white cell count is doing okay also; the antibiotics worked as well. You put on a good bit of weight this week; you weighed in at about one pound seven and a half ounces on Friday. You've lost some of that, though, but this going up and down in weight is to be expected—for a while anyhow.

They've taken you out of the special open bed and put you into a regular incubator. You look more comfortable now, and you're not being disturbed by all the noises around you in the nursery. They also put you on a larger ventilator, which means you don't have to work so hard breathing. Your one nurse is named Judy. She's a really nice person and takes great care of you. She said she worked one whole shift the other night without your monitors setting off an alarm even once. You're really cute when you yawn and stretch. Your little forehead wrinkles as you spread out your arms and legs, and then settle back down into a cozy position. I can't wait until we actually get to hold you for the first time, but that will come. The important thing right

now is for you to grow and get stronger each day. We love you, little guy.

Monday, October 24, 1994 – Another whole week has gone by. You're four weeks old today and still going strong. Mom-Mom (Grandma Raugh) and I (Pop-Pop) were in to see you again last night. Your nurse told us she thought they might remove your ventilator today and see how you do breathing on your own. You're already breathing just room air with no oxygen being given to you, and they expect you'll do well. Speaking of doing well, boy, have you taken to food. Your weight has been at one pound seven ounces for several days and yesterday reached one pound eight ounces. That's exactly what they wanted to see you do—start gaining weight and keeping it on. The extra calories they're giving you are helping along those lines also. You're starting to fill out. Your little arms and legs are getting rounded instead of being so flat. Your hair shows up real well in photos, too, and your little body is growing just a little as each new day passes. Keep up the hard work, little guy. Before you know it, most of the tubes and wires will be gone and you'll be growing a mile a minute. It's hard to believe that four weeks have gone by since you first came into our lives.

Monday, October 31, 1994 – As you can see, I've started to make entries just once a week unless something special happens. Speaking of something special, you turned one month old last Wednesday, October 26. The nurses put a special sign up on your isolette, proclaiming your reaching this milestone. You've been fighting the nurses somewhat with your ventilator. Twice over this past weekend you decided you didn't want it anymore and pulled the tube out yourself. They're trying to decide if you can do without it or if they should put it back in. It does seem to help you to breathe easier, but

"We were both wondering why she wasn't calling for someone to help.

I guess that's how they're taught to do what they do: special training, remaining calm, stabilizing you, and then asking for other assistance to perform checks to determine the cause. We can thank God for people like Judy.

maybe you're getting to the point where you've decided you don't need it. Time will tell. Your weight is doing great: Another two ounces this past week. I keep telling people we'll have to take you off eating cheeseburgers—you're gaining too fast. Ha-ha! I could see a big difference in you when we were in on Saturday. You're rounding out and starting to take on a puffier, baby-like look. Keep going, little one, you're doing great and making us all proud.

Sunday was special too. Although it wasn't a great picture, you were in the *Lancaster Sunday News* this week—one month old and already a star. We've kept several copies of the article for your scrapbook.

Wednesday, November 2, 1994 – What did I say in the paragraph above? Something special happens! Well, Cody, let me tell you that you scared your dad and me out of our wits last night. He and I came in to see you. You seemed to be just waking up. Your dad held you for a few minutes, and then decided to have the nurse put you back in the isolette because of the C-PAP that was attached to you to help you breathe. All went well for the next five minutes or so. All of a sudden your monitors started to go off. First, the one called your SAT started to fall. Nothing unusual in that, except that normally it never goes below seventy to seventy-four. This time it just kept

going down. Seconds later the monitor checking your heart rate also began to drop and kept falling.

Your dad and I could do nothing but watch a calm nurse react to these alarms in a very decided and methodical manner. First this and then that, and finally "bagging" you, which brought everything sort of back to normal. As your dad and I discussed later, we were both wondering why she wasn't calling for someone to help. I guess that's how they're taught to do what they do: special training, remaining calm, stabilizing you, and then asking for other assistance to perform checks to determine the cause. We can thank God for people like Judy.

While she reminded us that it's not unusual for this to happen with premature babies, it was of little comfort to be standing there helpless as it was going on. We don't want to lose you, Cody; you've become very precious to us. We'll have to see if they put you back on the ventilator. You seem to do much better when you're on that, though you don't like it. Just a note: your weight is up to one pound twelve ounces.

Thursday, November 10, 1994 – A banner day in your young life. At weigh-in this morning you topped the two-pound mark for the first time. Quite a milestone, little guy. While you didn't pass it by much (2.02 pounds), you did finally reach it. We're all so

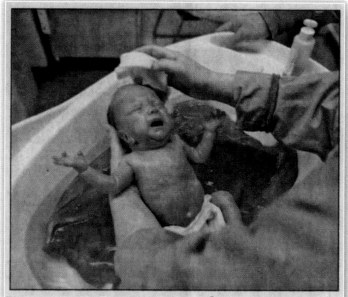

The shock of water on his skin makes Cody wail at bath time. a weekly ritual for his parents.

" One month old and already a star.

proud of how you're progressing. They didn't put you back on the ventilator either. I think maybe, unknown to us, you're setting some of your own goals. You just decided you didn't like that ventilator and wouldn't keep it in. You also had your eyes examined yesterday, and they seem to be in pretty good shape. One eye measured stage one and the other stage two. On a scale of zero to four, the zero is good and a four would mean that you could have problems. The doctors seem to think that the minor thing with your eyes could correct itself over time. At the very worst, it might mean you'll have to wear glasses at an earlier age. Only time will tell, and we'll know by the time you're reading this anyway.

Your mom and dad get to hold you more often and for longer periods. You look really cute in the little outfits they put on you. Your mom called me last Saturday afternoon to come into the hospital and take some more pictures of you. I'm sure you've seen them by now. And yes, I know that boys don't like to be called cute, but there's no doubt about it, at this point in your life you're cute.

Tuesday, November 15, 1994 – Another milestone, Cody. Yesterday the doctors decided to remove

you from the intensive care list and put you on the intermediate care list. While that in itself may not sound like much, it means they feel that you're past the most critical times as far as survival goes, and expect that you'll continue to grow and improve as each day passes. They've taken you off of any kind of breathing assistance also, another sign that you're doing well. Mom-Mom and I were in to see you last night just before your mom and dad came in. You're filling out as you continue to put on weight—up to just under two pounds four ounces now.

Tonight another first, as your mom is going to attempt to give you your first meal from a bottle at your 6:00 p.m. feeding time. Babies as small as you normally have to learn to both breathe and suck at the same time. Sometimes all goes well, and other times it takes a week or two to learn the process.

Wednesday, November 16, 1994 – You weigh in this morning at two pounds five point six ounces. That food they're giving you must be working. Speaking of food, you did try out your first bottle last night at 6:00 p.m. They tell us that a lot of babies your size normally take in about two to four cc of formula the first time they try a bottle. You did a lot better—

you took eleven cc before you started to get tired. Tonight was another important event, maybe not so much fun for you, but your two grandmothers got to hold you for the first time today. Mom-Mom cried when they put you in her arms.

Monday, November 21, 1994 – You're up to two pounds twelve ounces as of this morning. Mom-Mom and I were in to see you again last evening. You're really filling out and each time we see you we are more excited about your progress. At the rate you're going now you will hit the three-pound mark on Thursday, which just happens to be Thanksgiving. Boy, do we have a lot to be thankful for, and you're at the top of the list. The nurse asked us if we wanted to hold you last night, and as much as I would've liked to, your mom and dad don't want us to unless they are there. I guess they think we'll break you or something. Ha-ha! Oh well, I'll wait my turn.

Wednesday, November 30, 1994 – You waited till Saturday to hit three pounds in weight.

Another week has gone by. This morning your weight is just under three pounds five ounces. On Monday evening you had all kinds of visitors: your mom and I came in after work; your cousin Becky brought her grandmother in to see you also; in addition, a very good friend of mine who was in the hospital because of a heart attack came down from the seventh floor with his wife and two sons to see you. That's Al and Debbie and their sons, Eric and Mark. Soon after they left, your great-grandmother Scheid; her daughter, Mim; and Mim's daughter and granddaughter were at the window to see you. You're getting to be quite a popular guy.

Your mom and dad have been getting your room ready for you at home. It's really cute. Last night your dad and I put down the new carpet that Mom-Mom and I bought for your room. You'll have quite a place when you finally come home.

On Monday night another first, at least for me, as I got to hold you for the first time. I can't express how I felt as I held your tiny body in my arms. You're a real fighter, Cody. We all just love it when you're awake and looking all around. We love you, little guy.

Thursday, December 8, 1994 – Today you weighed in at three pounds thirteen point six ounces. They told your mom the other night that you'd probably come home the week of Christmas. What a celebration that will be for all of us! They've removed you from the isolette and have you in an open crib. You continue to do really well and grow a little more each day. I haven't been able to get in to see you until last night, after almost a week and a half. Not that I didn't want to, but I had a cold and didn't want to take any chances of giving it to you. I even wore a mask last night, though I'm pretty well over the cold. We want you home, and as well as you've been doing, you don't need any setbacks. You're going to be quite a Christmas present.

Thursday, December 15, 1994 – You decided on Tuesday that you were ready to hit the four-pound mark for the first time. We thought you'd get there a day or so sooner, but, as with the three-pound level, you made up your mind to gain the weight when you were ready, not when we wanted you to.

“Babies as small as you normally have to learn to both breathe and suck at the same time. Sometimes all goes well, and other times it takes a week or two to learn the process.

" Tonight you get to come home. No Christmas present could ever top this.

Tonight your mom and dad, along with Mom-Mom and me, are going to the hospital to see you. In addition, we're going to take the required infant CPR course so we'll be prepared when you come home, should you have any problems. Today at work, your mother's coworkers are giving her a big baby shower during the lunch hour. While she has some idea that this may be happening, I think Lori made enough changes to the plans this morning that your mom should be surprised. Your room is just about finished and waiting for you to come home.

Thursday, December 22, 1994 – This is a big day. Tonight you come home. No Christmas present could ever top this. You are awaited by parents who love you, by grandparents on both sides of the family who love you, and by aunts and uncles, cousins, and friends who love you and are ready to see you home.

You've fought an uphill battle from day one. I can honestly say, now that you're okay, that to see you on the night you were born I wasn't sure you'd survive, but Cody, you have done it all! You've beaten all the odds, taken all the tubes and needles, and showed us all that you have a willpower and determination as strong as any could be. Tonight marks a very important second step in your young life—that of being nurtured and cared for by the parents who brought you into this world. They're both a little apprehensive about this, but only from the point of wanting to be certain that you get everything you'll need care-wise. They won't sleep tonight, I'm sure, with you being in the next room, but they'll adjust as you continue to grow and prove to them that you'll be okay. Your room is ready; your parents are ready, and you are ready.

God has seen fit to bless you, Cody. On the second day of your life, Mom-Mom and I placed a little ceramic heart inside your isolette. On it are the words "Each day is a gift from God." It certainly is, and if you ever in your life reach a time when you don't believe in miracles given by God, read this story again and look again at the photos of you up till this point. I love you, grandson, and may the good Lord keep you always nestled in His arms.

A Pretty Rag Doll—Brittany

*B*rittany Elise, a strong and lovely name for a beautiful young lady. As I write this, I can envision your devoted mom, dad, and grandparents. I recall meeting your grandparents not long ago outside the hospital; they seemed so delighted to see their grandchild's physician, and they couldn't stop raving about your achievements. Believe me, I feel like a godmother, wishing to do the same.

I've come to trust that our NICU babies have something special in them, an inner beauty, a resilience, a strength, possibly born out of the fortitude and prayers of their families. Your career path certainly is another testament—a valedictorian proceeding on to a great career.

Your NICU course was the usual one for a preterm infant, with immature lungs requiring ventilator support, immature gut for which you needed nutritional support, and apnea and bradycardia, which infants ultimately outgrow.

You can't imagine what immense pleasure it brings us to see our little ones flourish. I certainly cherish those moments of reunions with our NICU Grads. God bless you, my child. I hope you have a wonderful career in linguistics.

This verse is such an appropriate culmination of events:

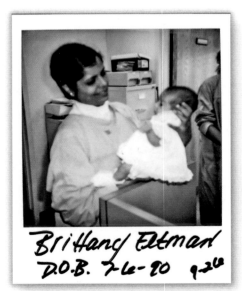

Brittany Eltman
D.O.B. 7-6-20 9-26

The Semantic Brook

Beneath the azure skies, amidst the golden hills,
A bubbling brook merrily flows, unable to hold the water still.
May you, Brittany, excel and shine, in linguistics, as in life,
As joyous as the bubbling brook, melodious as the robin's rhyme.
May you conquer every strife,
Even as a babe, you were a star.
With love and blessings all around, you are destined to go far.
A valedictorian and scholar now, may you achieve every success,
May your strength and compassion
Help the needy ones. God bless!
                                        —Manjeet Kaur

Brittany Eltman

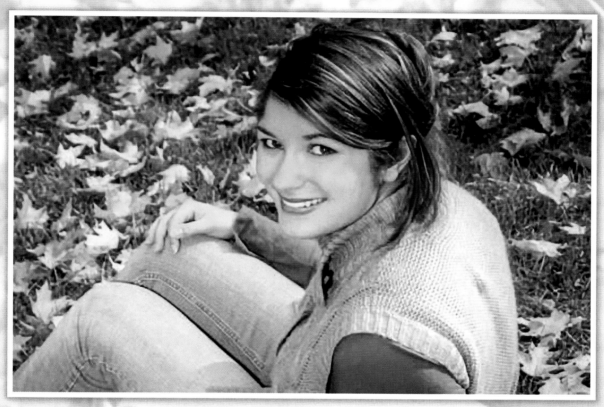

Parents:	Kimberly and Kerry
Date of birth:	7/6/1990
Birth weight:	3 pounds 0 ounces
Medical conditions:	Prematurity, respiratory distress syndrome, patent ductus arteriosus, apnea, bradycardia
Gestational age:	30 weeks
Hospitalization dates:	7/6/1990–8/28/1990

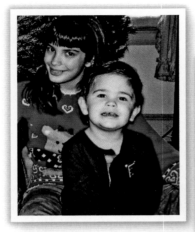
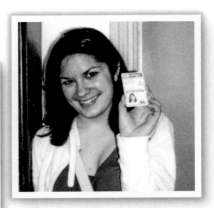
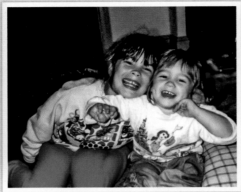
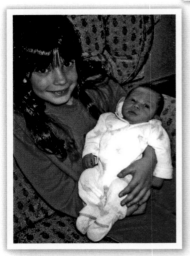
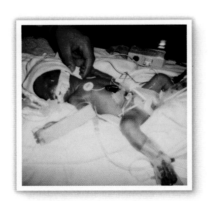
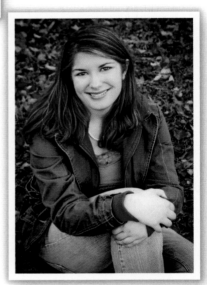
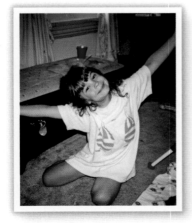
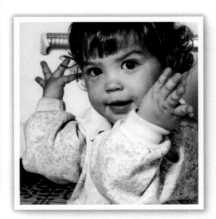
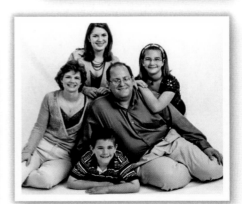

Kimberly and Kerry's Story

When we first brought Brittany home from the hospital, she would stop breathing up to fifteen times a day. She had difficulty remembering to breathe while swallowing, and was experiencing sleep apnea. She was on oxygen and heart/respiration monitors, and was on theophylline to help her breathe and help her underdeveloped lungs, which were stressed from being on prolonged ventilator support. With each day, the episodes of "forgetting" to breathe became less and less frequent. Brittany was off oxygen by six months, and off her heart monitors by twenty months. By the time she was two years old, the only side effect left from her premature birth was childhood asthma, which she outgrew by the time she was twelve.

My husband and I were young, and Brittany was our first child. We had no warning that I was going into preterm labor. I remember feeling miserable, having painful cramps, and telling my sister that if this was anything like labor, I didn't think I could do it. I had no idea that I had been in labor that night and into the next day. I was visiting my parents, and my sister kept noticing me wince every so often and convinced me to go to the family doctor to just get checked out. I knew that something wasn't

right, but figured they would give me a medication and send me home since my due date was two and a half months away. I remember the scared look of the doctor and his nurse's face. He exited the room and I heard him make a phone call, saying, "I have someone thirty-weeks gestation about to give birth in my office—what do I do?" It finally registered they were talking about me.

I went by ambulance to Lancaster General Hospital and remember talking to the crew and nurses, apologizing, thinking this was probably a mistake. I remember pretty emphatically telling the doctor that I was not having this baby now because I wasn't due. I was scared our little one wouldn't make it, being born too early. It was only after he convinced me that the baby was in distress that I agreed to push. My sister called my husband, and he was with me in the delivery room. We were in disbelief and denial at first, and then that quickly turned to fear of the unknown.

When our little girl entered the world, she was a lifeless little gray rag doll. The doctor immediately handed her off to Dr. Kaur and her medical team. I can't explain the surge of emotion, fear, and desperation going through me. The thing that helped the most, which I remember so clearly twenty-three years

"We were both in disbelief and denial at first, and then that quickly turned to fear of the unknown.

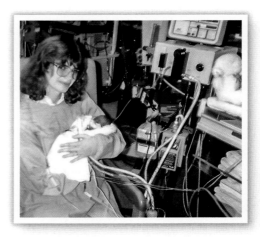

> "When our little girl entered the world, she was a lifeless little gray rag doll.

later, was Dr. Kaur's calm, compassionate, reassuring voice saying, "Mom, you have a beautiful baby girl, and I am going to take very good care of her." I can never explain how much that one sentence meant to me when I felt so helpless. She called my precious baby "beautiful," when the rest of the world may have seen her as gray, lifeless, and black and blue from a rushed birth. Dr. Kaur acknowledged my fear, and was calm and reassuring when I was near hysteria. She spoke those compassionate words, all the while skillfully intubating our tiny daughter, stabilizing her enough to whisk her away to the NICU.

My husband, Kerry, went along with Brittany while the delivery doctor finished up with me and gave me something to calm my nerves, which ended up sedating me for hours. It was frustrating when I came around because I didn't know what was going on, and I was scared. After the first day of being so groggy, I camped out in the NICU. After I was discharged from the hospital, Kerry would drop me off on his way to work around 7:30 a.m., and I'd stay by her side until my parents came to visit and we'd go to the cafeteria for a bite to eat. Then Kerry would arrive around 5:30, and we'd stay till the change of shift at

> "The thing that helped the most was Dr. Kaur's calm, compassionate, reassuring voice saying, 'Mom, you have a beautiful baby girl, and I am going to take very good care of her.' I can never explain how much that one sentence meant to me when I felt so helpless.
>
> She called my precious baby 'beautiful,' when the rest of the world may have seen her as gray, lifeless, and black and blue from a rushed birth.

> "When things went well, we'd pray. When things took a turn for the worse, we'd pray. Our family spent countless hours on our knees when Brittany was born, and she is a beautiful answer to our prayers.

midnight. This became our daily routine. The NICU nurses and doctors allowed me to be with Brittany as much as possible. I saw firsthand the compassionate and skilled way they treated her and the other little ones in their care. They allowed me to take part in her care as well, and this was reassuring and calmed my anxiety.

We were fortunate to have tremendous support from all of our family, immediate and extended. For the months that Brittany was hospitalized, my eldest sister took time off work so she could drive my mother to and from the hospital to visit. My father would stop in on his way home from work. I don't believe my parents missed a day. Kerry's family was incredibly supportive as well. We had no other children to take care of, so I was able to focus all my energies on Brittany. I always felt so sorry for other mothers who felt

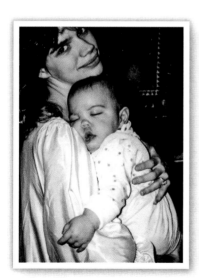

torn between being with their NICU babies and caring for little ones at home.

My most precious memory of our NICU experience came five days after Brittany was born. My sister was just down the hall giving birth to her first child, their son Brandon. I remember my mom coming down the NICU hall, saying, "It's a boy, and he's okay." I was truly happy for my sister, yet it was so hard looking at our little girl struggling to breathe. I walked down the hall to meet my nephew, and it was overwhelming to see his parents hold him when I had yet to hold our little one. We had quickly developed a rapport with all the NICU staff from spending so much time there. I think they knew my heart was hurting, and when I came back from seeing my new nephew, they told me it was time I got to hold Brittany. At first, I refused because I was so worried they were rushing it for my sake; I didn't want to do anything to cause Brittany distress. They assured me she'd remain stable for a little while. The pictures you see of the three of us were from the first time I held our daughter.

Our NICU journey had lots of ups and downs. We were told our daughter might become blind from the amount of oxygen she was receiving, or suffer brain damage or lung scarring. One of the most

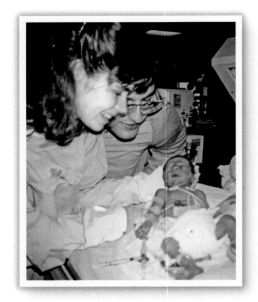

" My most precious memory of our NICU experience came five days after Brittany was born.… I walked down the hall to meet my nephew, and it was overwhelming to see his parents hold him when I had yet to hold our little one.… I think they knew my heart was hurting, and when I came back from seeing my new nephew, they told me it was time I got to hold Brittany.…

The pictures you see of the three of us were from the first time I held our daughter.

difficult days was when they tried to take her off the ventilator. We were so hopeful that this was progress; we knew the longer she was on the ventilator, the harder it would be for her to come off.

I learned a lot about nursing during my time in the NICU, and quickly learned which were "good numbers" and "good signs"—and which weren't. The tubes were taken out and Brittany was under an oxygen hood. It was exciting to see her expressions and not have her face taped so heavily. Most importantly, seeing those tubes removed meant she was getting progressively better, moving toward the day she could come home. This attempt proved to be

too soon, however; she was struggling, and when the decision to put her back on the ventilator was finally made, I lost it. My tears wouldn't stop coming. I think it was a combination of fear, heartache, and exhaustion. One of the nurses asked me to please go home, regroup, and come back the next day.

Without our faith in the Lord, I don't know where we would be. When we felt helpless, we'd pray. When things went well, we'd pray. When things took a turn for the worse, we'd pray. Our family spent countless hours on our knees when Brittany was born, and she is a beautiful answer to our prayers.

While we are indebted to the incredible doctors and staff at LGH NICU, we know who gave them their skills and who is ultimately in control. At one point during our stay, Brittany developed a heart murmur that was going to need surgical repair. She was scheduled to go to Hershey by ambulance the next morning for the operation. We sent out prayer requests to our church and our families' churches, and asked our family and friends to pray. By the next morning the hole in Brittany's heart had healed itself, and there was no need for surgery. Three different doctors came by and listened to be sure. The last one shrugged his shoulders and said, "There's no explanation, but the hole isn't there."

We smiled, thinking, *Yes, there is an explanation—God, who is in control, chose to honor our prayers.* Our daughter's name, Brittany Elise, means "Strong One, Consecrated for God." We didn't know when we chose her name how appropriate it would prove to be. Reading God's word helped as well. Finding scripture that described not only our emotions but also promises from God Himself that He would walk right alongside of us during our journey, often carrying us with His mighty right hand, gave us strength when ours was depleted.

It's good to revisit Brittany's beginnings and remember what we went through. It reminds us to be thankful. Our daughter not only survived, but also she thrived! She had no problem catching up to her peers. When she entered kindergarten, she was already reading at the fifth-grade level. This precocious little girl grew into a beautiful young lady who ended up graduating Valedictorian of her high school. She went on to double major in Biology and Psychology with a minor in English, and received her degree from Messiah College, summa cum laude. She worked for Georgetown University in their Neuroscience department for a year and a half before deciding to go back to graduate school. She had multiple full-ride scholarship opportunities, but chose to go to the University of Pittsburgh for their Applied Linguistics graduate program.

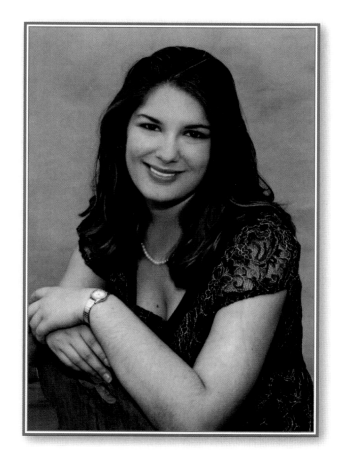

Our First NICU Baby — Lauren

My very first NICU respirator baby, my first "NICU godchild" at Lancaster General, how do I write about you? Our NICU itself was in its neonatal period as I came to Lancaster in May and officially started with the Lord's blessings, with a prayer and ribbon-cutting ceremony by the chaplain in September 1984 on the sixth floor of Lancaster General Hospital. We had a state-of-the-art ventilator and very enthusiastic staff who were recently trained.

I remember speaking to your mom and dad along with Dr. Tifft, who was your pediatrician, about the choice of keeping you here or sending you out to Hershey. The decision was to keep you in Lancaster, and I vividly recall Dr. Tifft saying, "I would trust Dr. Kaur if it was my child." That meant so much to me at the time!

You had a classic textbook course with respiratory distress syndrome, the first days being the critical ones. I must say you were very cooperative. The staff at Lancaster General was excited. This was a brand-new NICU—you were our very first baby in Lancaster to be on a respirator, so you got "Cadillac service" in terms of time commitment. We were constantly at your side, and updated your mommy and daddy frequently as well. Your family was a pleasure to work with. As I close my eyes, I can replay the sequence of events though it was twenty-nine years ago.

I feel as though I have personally seen you grow up. Your parents are great communicators and send me cards and letters from time to time. My favorite photo is one of you, our little Lauren, tying a shoelace as you sit by a dog much larger than you. I have a newspaper clipping of you with an artistic "jute sculpture doll," which you had made that summer. And, of course, I have one from when you graduated from Clemson in May 2007.

What an amazing journey, and what a privilege to have been a part of it. God bless you, my child, now a beautiful young lady!

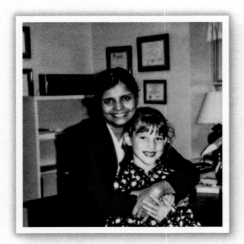

A Pioneer

A cute alluring babe was born in nineteen eighty-four,
Lancaster General had just then opened its NICU door.
This feisty infant scored very well, so goes the local lore.
With loving care and media to boot, she received applause galore.
Now a benevolent mom herself, she rejoices evermore.
Smart and bright with might to cite, and every height to soar
You have our blessings, Lauren, dear, our pioneer of yore!
—Manjeet Kaur

Lauren Sturla Womack

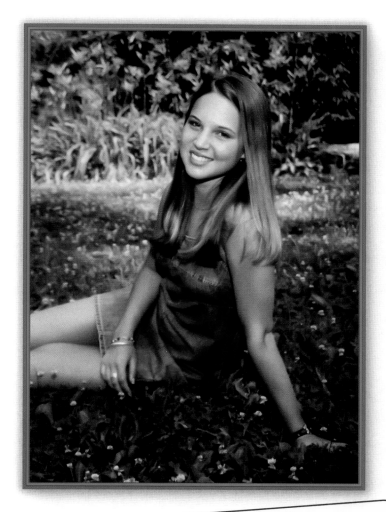

Parents:	Ann and Jeff
Date of birth:	11/12/1984
Birth weight:	4 pounds 6 ounces
Medical conditions:	Prematurity, respiratory distress syndrome
Gestational age:	32 weeks

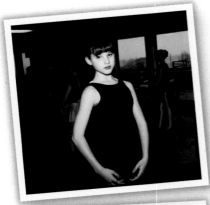
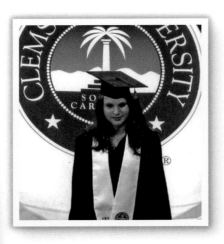
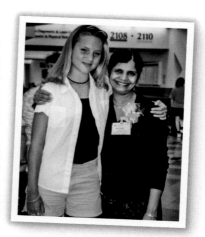
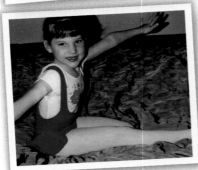
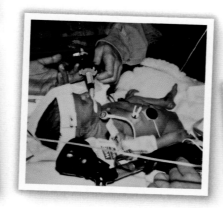
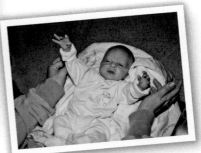
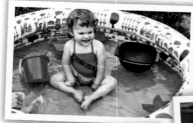
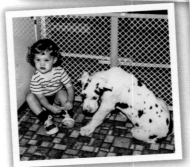
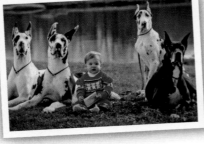
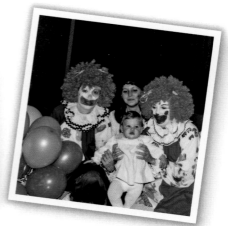

Ann and Jeff's Story

It started on the evening of November 11, 1984, with cramps that got worse as the night went on. By morning I was bleeding, and the doctor's office said, "Get to the hospital as soon as possible." The tests I had done showed that my placenta had torn, and the best chance for my little one was to continue with labor and deliver this baby. My original due date was at the beginning of January 1985. I was taken to the delivery room, and all of the doctors and nurses were very nice, trying to keep me calm. Baby Girl Sturla was born at 5:27 p.m. and, after a quick look from her parents, was whisked off to the NICU with Dr. Kaur. We didn't even have a name for her yet, so for the longest time her records read "Baby Girl Sturla."

> "This was my first child, and not knowing what was happening was very scary.

This was my first child, and not knowing what was happening was very scary. The nursing staff did their best to let us know what was going on. Dr. Kaur made several visits to my room to tell us what they were doing to help Lauren. It was so hard to be in a room and see the mother next to me able to hold and feed her baby and learn how to give baths. Family members would come in to see her baby, and everyone was so happy and excited. My arms felt so empty. I just had to lie in that bed wondering what was happening to my baby and if I'd ever be able to take her home.

> "My arms felt so empty.

I knew that she was in the intensive care unit. Even with the nurses and doctors reporting to me, my anxiety level was high. Lauren was the first baby to be born and stay at Lancaster General NICU, and I was scared. Hospitals aren't my favorite places to begin with, and now my little girl was in the hands of strangers, but as the days went on, I learned to depend on these nurses and came to realize they were taking the best care of her. On top of all that had happened, I had to leave the hospital without our baby. Our families were very supportive, but it was different with the baby staying at the hospital. Family could come and see her through glass, but not hold her. My recovery time was very quick, as I needed to be at the hospital as much as possible to sit with Lauren and hold her hand in the days after I went home.

The NICU was a busy place, with nurses tending to all kinds of medical situations. Never did I feel as if I was in the way or that my baby girl wasn't getting

> " The worst time in the NICU for me was when they had to shave Lauren's head to find a new spot for the IV … seeing an IV coming out of my daughter's head made my head spin and I blacked out.

the medical care she needed. They answered all my questions and explained every procedure they were doing. The names of the nurses I remember who helped were Josephine, Miriam, Nancy, Diane, and Betsy. The worst time in the NICU for me was when they had to shave Lauren's head to find a new spot for the IV. Her tiny feet were so black and blue, and they were having problems finding veins, so seeing an IV coming out of my daughter's head made my head spin and I blacked out. She spent most of her time in an open warmer to keep her body temperature

normal. She had jaundice and respiratory problems. So when the day came to take her home, and we named her Lauren Annabelle, a heart and breathing monitor went with us. She was named Annabelle for my mother, who was also born in November.

We prayed all the time. Lauren was so tiny, dropping to three pounds nine ounces. Her lungs were underdeveloped and needed help. We prayed for her tiny body to get strong. We felt so helpless, we could only wait and pray that the good Lord would make her strong and healthy for us to share our lives together.

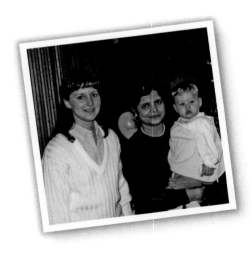

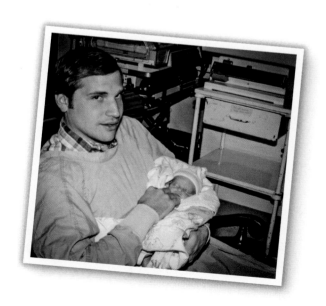

Lauren grew into a very active child and young lady. She loves animals, and grew up with dogs, hamsters, fish, and rabbits.

She was a gifted student, competing in her high-school science fairs. She got along well with her teachers, even baking a cake for her favorite teacher's retirement. Through her junior-high years, she played field hockey, and was a cheerleader and dancer. In high school, Lauren played varsity field hockey. She also played for and helped start the inaugural varsity lacrosse team and was Lacrosse Academic All-American. She was a member of student council and National Honor Society, and was on the homecoming court.

Upon graduating, Lauren went on to earn her bachelor's degree in Graphic Communications at Clemson University. There, she was a member of the club lacrosse team and worked for the student newspaper. She graduated from Clemson with a job at BBDO Atlanta, where she worked for six and a half years.

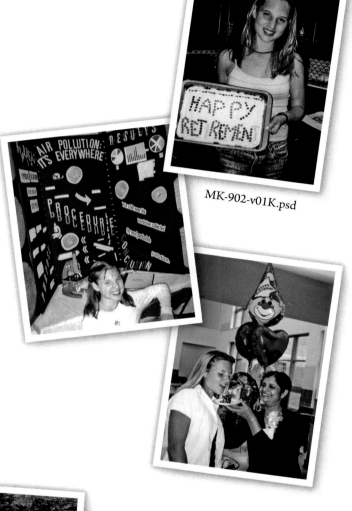

MK-902-v01K.psd

Lauren, now twenty-nine, married Gary in August 2013. Their dog, Rigby, was by their side for the big day. Lauren and Gary (and Rigby) currently live in Chicago, where Lauren works for a branding and design firm. We are so blessed, so very proud of her, and thank the NICU staff for the great care they took of our "Baby Girl Sturla." There can never be enough hugs.

Little Gifts in Doubles
—Quinn and Dylan

What a wonderful testimonial of faith, medical technology, and loving care. As my husband and I were rambling about the walkway a few summers ago, your dad stepped up from a nearby yard and told me how you both had been in the NICU. "Of course," I said, "Quinn and Dylan." I had seen you at reunions before, but now, I thought, *I'll get to see my NICU godchildren grow up in close proximity.*

As we walk during the summers, usually along the same path, I occasionally see both of you playing basketball or practicing lacrosse, a lovely reminder for a neonatologist to see our NICU grads thriving. I feel blessed to have been a part of the lives of such a lovely family.

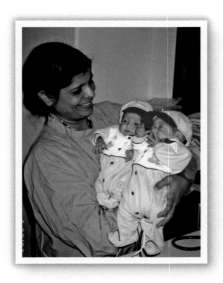

Two Champions

*Lots to achieve, and accolades to claim
Many venues to explore, some elite, some mundane
As you climb mountains and sail oceans galore,
Strive for success and glory furthermore.
There are songs to be sung, Dylan and Quinn, and games to be won.
As your rackets fly 'neath the bountiful sun,
Be kind and caring, rejoice in glee,
In honor of God, your family,
And the loving NICU team that nurtured thee!*
—Manjeet Kaur

Quinn and Dylan Loughlin

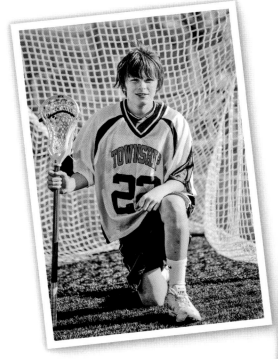

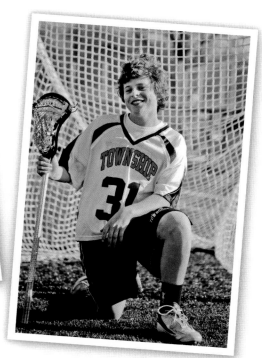

Parents:	Kerry and Ted
Date of birth:	3/3/1997
Birth weight:	1 pound 15 ounces
Medical conditions:	Severe prematurity twins. Respiratory distress syndrome, apnea
Gestational age:	25 weeks
Hospitalization dates:	3/3/1997–5/29/1997

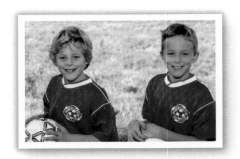
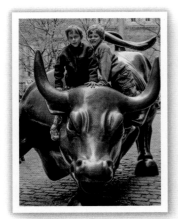
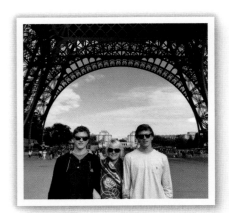
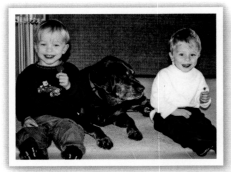
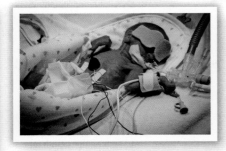
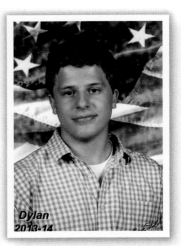

Dylan
2013-14

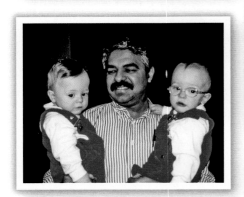
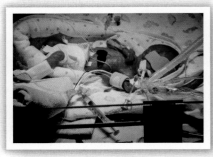
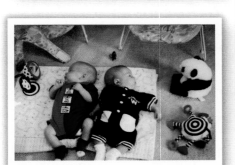
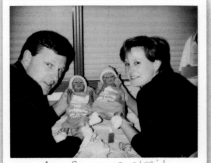

1st family portrait
April 25, 1997

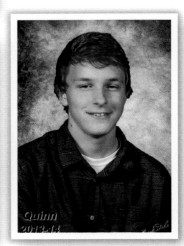

Quinn
2013-14

Kerry and Ted's Story

Sometimes the most amazing moments in life follow the most frightening ones. As Khalil Gibran wrote, "Joy is your sorrow unmasked." I can't think of a better example to illustrate that great wisdom than the day, seventeen years ago, when my husband, Ted, and I brought our twin boys, Quinn and Dylan, home from the hospital for the first time after eighty-seven days in the NICU.

February 7, 1997 – Twenty-weeks pregnant, it started out as a normal day. I readied for work and stood before the bedroom mirror admiring my new maternity outfit—it had only been a week that I moved from stretch pants to full-fledged maternity wear—when suddenly I felt intense pressure and then a rush of amniotic fluid—and then I saw the blood!

Ted drove me to Lancaster General Hospital like a cop in hot pursuit, flashing high beams, blowing the horn, passing cars. A wheelchair met us at the ER, and I was whisked up to the sixth floor where nurses and doctors were waiting. An ultrasound revealed that one of the amniotic sacs had ruptured and lost all traces of its life-sustaining fluid. The image of a child suffocating in a clear plastic bag kept flashing in my mind's eye. With blood and fluid still draining, and contractions coming two to four minutes apart, the doctors prepared us for the worst: our twin boys would most likely deliver today and would not survive.

As magnesium sulfate poured through my veins, I drank pitcher after pitcher of water in hopes of bringing fluid back to Quinn, "Baby A." Ted and I prayed and fought hard to never lose hope, despite the odds.

We made it through the first day … then the second. After three days, my contractions began to subside, and by day ten of full bed rest, much to the doctors' amazement, they stopped. And then the best news of all from the radiologist: The amniotic fluid had begun to replenish itself in the ruptured sac. She allowed us to watch the ultrasound and we saw the "Mighty Quinn" drink from the small pocket of fluid that miraculously formed around his face.

For the next couple of weeks, we happily crossed off the calendar days. Every day a great day, every day a day closer to their actual due date of June 15—more time for their premature lungs and other organs

> "If we could make it to twenty-eight weeks, the survival rate was much better.

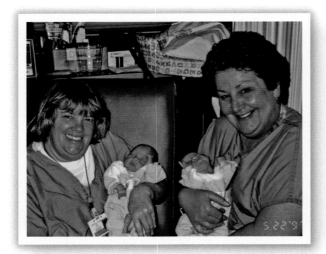

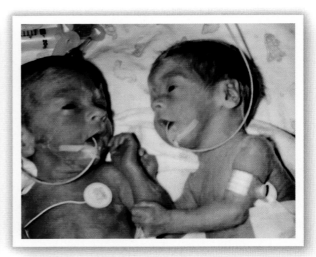

to develop—every day increasing their chances of survival. Twenty-eight weeks became the goal. If we could make it to twenty-eight weeks, the survival rate was much better.

Then, on March 1, two days shy of the twenty-five-week gestational period, progress stopped. That morning I was given the green light to get out of bed for the first time in weeks, and that night my contractions began again. Two days later, on March 3, Quinn was delivered, and the doctor quickly placed a tiny breathing tube down his throat and whisked him off to the NICU. Fifty-eight minutes later they took

Dylan from me by C-section. He too went on a ventilator and straight to the NICU.

Born at twenty-five weeks, each baby weighed only one pound fifteen ounces, and measured just thirteen inches. At twenty-five weeks, their survivability rate was only 40 percent, and even if they did survive, the likelihood of lifelong disabilities was great.

When they wheeled me into the NICU and I saw the boys for the first time, I couldn't believe my eyes. Our babies looked like tiny, shriveled-up old men covered with body fuzz. It made me wonder if old souls are reborn. With no fat on their bodies, they needed to be warmed under Saran Wrap in special

Each evening before we went home, Ted and I prayed aloud to them:

"Lord, look down from heaven above
And touch these special boys with love.
Protect and guide these little ones
Till each and every day is done.
Remind us often that it's true,
Their little lives are gifts from You,
Miracles You've sent our way.
Lord, bless Quinn and Dylan today."

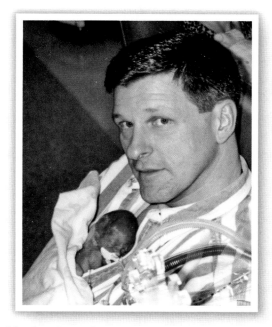

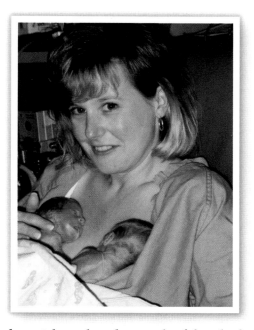

heated beds. Their skin was translucent; you could see all their veins and organs, and so tiny were their hands, so thin their arms, they could fit through Ted's wedding ring.

Our worst fears were somewhat assuaged by the confidence, expertise, and palpable love of the NICU doctors and nurses. Almost immediately, the nurses insisted on our participation in our boys' care, from changing their teeny diapers, to feeding them—albeit through a feeding tube at first—to rubbing the special ointment on their delicate skin. We decorated their NICU nurseries: the nurses drew colorful pictures announcing their milestone dates and weights, and we adorned their cribs with stuffed animals and taped special angel cards to each of their beds. They encouraged us to talk to Quinn and Dylan, read to them, play classical music for them, and be there with them as much as possible. I didn't have other children to care for at home, and was able to quit my job and become a full-time "stay-at-the-NICU" mom. I was grateful for those eighty-seven on-the-job-training days where I learned from the best of the best. One of our greatest moments was the night Ted and I simultaneously rocked Quinn and Dylan, providing "Kangaroo Care," all of us together for the first time. That night we felt like a real family, and Ted and I almost felt like real parents.

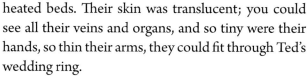

"Their skin was translucent; you could see all their veins and organs, and so tiny were their hands, so thin their arms, they could fit through Ted's wedding ring.

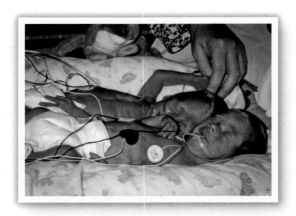

The nurses and doctors became our immediate family, and like family, they shared in our sorrow. One such day was when Quinn needed another blood transfusion and the blood bank dropped our last donated vial, and, again, our worst day in the NICU, when Dylan stopped breathing thrice and we waited while they tested him for cerebral hemorrhage and brain damage. And, like family, they shared in our joys when Quinn and Dylan reached the "big" two-pound mark after having dropped to just over a pound.

Another milestone to celebrate was when Quinn, who'd been struggling for every breath, came off all oxygen and breathing apparatus shortly after the nurses boldly decided to reunite him with Dylan in his warming bed.

In addition to the doctors and nurses, we were blessed to be taken care of by many others in the NICU: the social worker who maintained daily contact with our insurance company and who arranged for Early Intervention support when we took the boys home; the secretaries who patiently and pleasantly answered every one of our daily a.m. calls and the multitude of other "just checking-in" calls; and the speech therapist who so wittily helped us teach the boys how to "suck" so they could take a bottle and eventually nurse. They too became like family members.

May 29, 1997 — Graduation Day. Joy! After eighty-seven days, our sorrow abated; we finally took our twin baby boys home!

Today, almost seventeen years later, Quinn and Dylan are healthy, smart, ambitious, and above all, extremely kind and compassionate young men.

"May 29, 1997—Graduation Day. Joy! After eighty-seven days, our sorrow abated; we finally took our twin baby boys home!

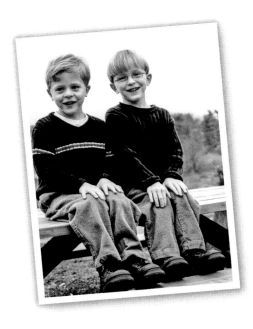

"Looking back at the old photos and stories my parents would tell, I knew I might not have lived, small and sick as I was in the NICU. It was through the care of the doctors and nurses that my twin brother and I lived, and I'm eternally grateful. Dr. Kaur and Dr. Mahajan were the doctors who attended us, and my parents tell me they were excellent doctors and excellent people who were always there for us and cared for us the entire eighty-seven days we were in the NICU. Since then I've been involved in many activities, such as lacrosse and soccer, but my favorite by far is skiing with my friends on the weekends."

—Dylan Loughlin, age sixteen, junior at Manheim Township High School

"My first couple of months I was very sick. The odds were stacked against me, but with the help of Dr. Kaur, Dr. Mahajan, and their amazing nurses, I persevered and lived. I was in the NICU for eighty-seven days and couldn't have survived were it not for Dr. Kaur and Lancaster General Hospital. People said that if I survived I'd have health problems and be unable to function normally in everyday life, but that isn't the case. I survived and I have prospered. I've played many sports, including football, soccer, baseball, lacrosse, swimming, and basketball. My favorite hobby is skateboarding."

—Quinn Loughlin, age sixteen, junior at Manheim Township High School

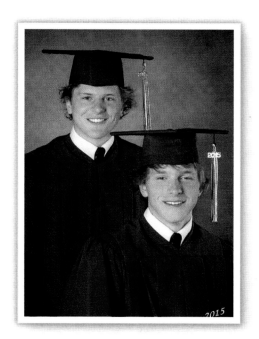

Tiny Pumpkins — Mason and Caden

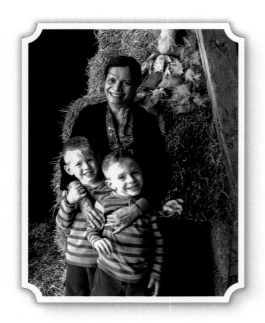

*I*t was a lovely October morning. I had taken my five-year-old grandson and eighteen-month-old granddaughter to pick pumpkins at the Oregon Dairy. A lovely young lady greeted us and said, "Remember these kids from the NICU? Look at them now!"

I turned and saw two adorable children running in and out of the special Halloween corn straw maze. Mom later told me they were doing well in preschool and doing well physically too—running, and riding bikes and scooters. What a joy and a blessing!

Those connections are so precious, the real rewards of being in this special field of medicine we call Neonatology.

Caden was diagnosed with a grade III intraventricular hemorrhage, and the outcome was "guarded," with possibility of difficulties. In my three decades in neonatology, I've always tried to give families the facts as they are, but the feats of the amazing newborns have so often pleasantly astounded me.

Two Little Pumpkins

It was a cool October day on the Oregon Dairy street,
As I reunited with little munchkins, what a feat!
Two sweet cherubs running in and out of a Halloween maze,
A most wonderful sight amidst the late fall haze.
Babes at discharge with a "guarded" fate declared
Dad's wedding band fit an arm of the duo who shared
An adorable vision, a sweet bliss!
Run with that music, sweet Mason and Caden, no goals you should miss.
May you achieve your dreams, may you continue in grace
As you find your potential at your own special pace.
God bless!
—Manjeet Kaur

Mason and Caden Beisker

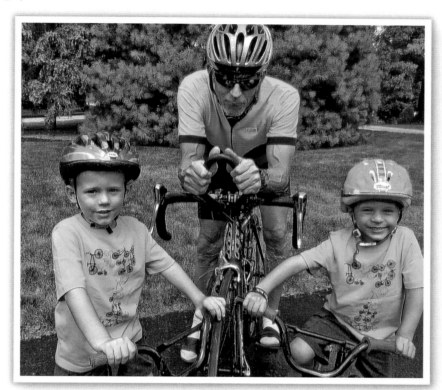

Parents:	Laurie and Nick
Date of birth:	12/27/2010
Birth weight–Mason:	1 pound 12 ounces
Birth weight– Caden:	1 pound 14 ounces
Medical conditions:	Extreme prematurity, respiratory distress syndrome, intraventricular hemorrhage, patent ductus arteriosus
Gestational age:	27 weeks
Hospitalization dates:	12/27/10–3/26/11

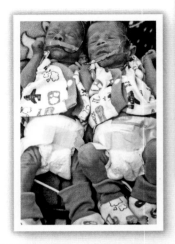

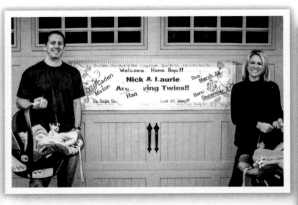

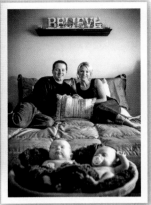

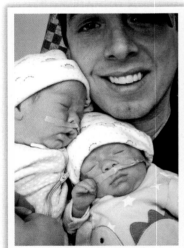

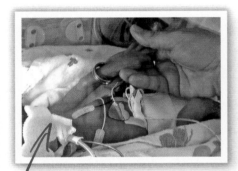

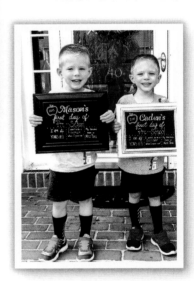

See Dad's wedding band on the baby's arm in these two photos.

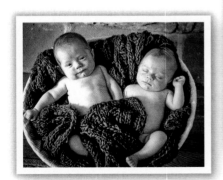

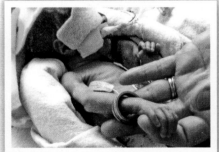

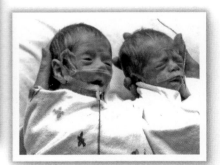

"I recall thinking, *What if they die before I ever get the chance to meet them?*

Laurie and Nick's Story

I remember lying in the recovery room feeling alone. As soon as my twin boys were delivered, a team of doctors immediately took them away. The fear was so paralyzing I couldn't even cry. All our family and friends were there. When they greeted me with big smiles and hugs, it was confusing—I didn't know if I was supposed to be happy. I just remember feeling helpless. The boys were born at 8:32 and 8:35 the night of the twenty-seventh, but I didn't get to see or touch them until the next day because they were so unstable. I recall thinking, *What if they die before I ever get the chance to meet them?*

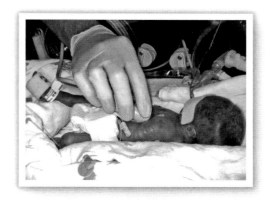

"The fear was so paralyzing I couldn't even cry.

"I mourned not being able to take them home. I never went back to my house after the twins were born. It was too emotional for me to go back without them.

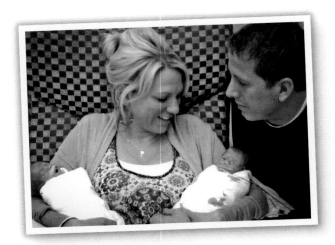

I actually went into preterm labor at twenty-two weeks, so I'd been on bed rest at Women and Babies for weeks before the twins were born. During that time I'd taken a tour of the NICU and spoke with other families that had children there. That brought me some comfort, knowing that my babies would be well taken care of. At the same time, I mourned not being able to take them home. I never went back to my house after the twins were born. It was too emotional for me to go back without them. Instead, I moved in with my parents, who lived closer to the hospital. My husband went back to work, maintained the house, and traveled every day to Lancaster to spend time with the twins.

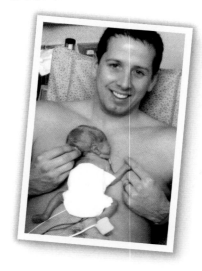

Almost one month after they were born, Mason got his PIC (peripheral intravenous catheter) line removed. Without the IV in him we were able to reach close enough that we could take our first family photo! It was also the first time we could put the boys side by side and reunite them for the first time since the womb. A lot of tears were shed. We just kept saying, "We've waited so long for you, and now you're here!" That moment gave us so much hope for the future!

"We were on our knees, crying out to our Heavenly Father, asking for a miracle.

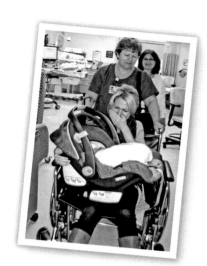

Soon after the twins were born, Caden was found to have a PDA (an open valve in his heart) as well as a level 3 IVH (intraventricular hemorrhage), or bleeding in the brain. This led to many sleepless nights for us as we prepared for the worst. We were on our knees, crying out to our Heavenly Father, asking for a miracle. We had a strong faith prior to this journey, but it was amplified once our babies' lives were being threatened. We found so much comfort and even acceptance in the fact that we couldn't carry this burden alone and that we didn't have to.

"For I can do all things through Christ, who gives me strength" (Philippians 4:13).

Caden and Mason are now in preschool. They'll be five in December, which blows my mind. They have a little sister now, and they love to play with her. They love to ride their bikes, scooter, and anything else that has wheels. If they're outside, they're happy. Life is good … no, life is great!

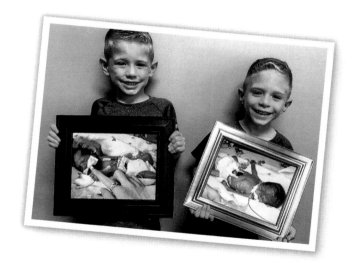

"Life is good … no, life is great!

An Alluring Duo—Ryan and Andrew

*I*n December 1986, our NICU had been open for two years, and Dr. Jirka had recently joined me as a partner when Andrew and Ryan were born. This was the time we started keeping such little ones in Lancaster, as we were now two neonatologists. Born at twenty-eight weeks, both boys were initially on respirators. Even after so many years, I can visualize both Susan and Mark on one particular afternoon when Andrew was really sick. Andrew, you had been on a lot of oxygen and on high ventilator support for a long time. Those were the days before we had surfactant available, a solution given directly via an endotracheal tube into the trachea to help the lungs mature.

Though we had a dedicated staff and the most recent equipment, we had to rely on the technology of the mid-1980s. Pulse oximeters had not yet become available, so invasive monitoring with central lines was required.

At that point, Ryan, you had been extubated (spontaneous respiration established), but Andrew's lungs were still fragile. I've never forgotten those large, beautiful beseeching eyes, so innocent and accepting, having not known any other mode of breathing. As I spoke to your mom and dad regarding your prognosis and the possible long-term need for respiratory support, those beautiful, haunting eyes stayed with me.

Maybe it's that artsy philosopher in me, but those kinds of moments are more memorable and bring me more strength than the tough lessons of that roller coaster.

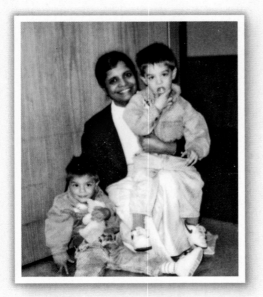

To Ryan and Andrew

Two sweet little babes with minds of their own
Through turbulent times you marched bravely on
Benevolent and kind, ready to greet,
Overcoming struggles with vitality, a laudable feat.
Proud we are of your accomplishments astute.
Writing and poetry, melodious medleys to boot.
Good luck, Ryan and Andrew, our artistic team,
Be fastidious in your goals; may you fulfill your dreams.
God Bless.
—Manjeet Kaur

Ryan and Andrew Huntley

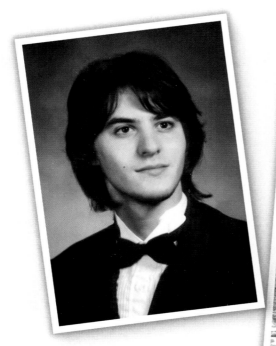
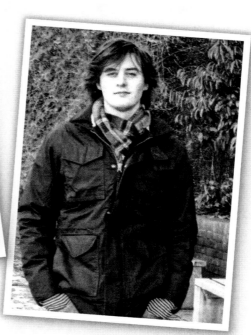

Parents:	Susan and Mark
Date of birth:	12/13/1986
Birth weight– Ryan:	2 pounds 12 ounces
Birth weight–Andrew:	2 pounds 10 ounces
Medical conditions:	Prematurity, respiratory distress syndrome, bronchopulmonary dysplasia (Andrew) requiring tracheotomy
Gestational age:	28 weeks
Hospitalization dates:	12/13/1986–4/23/1987

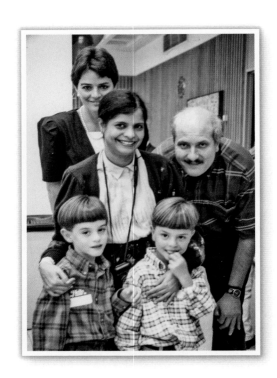

That Dreamy Lure

Those mesmerizing eyes linger
With a special glow.
A gentle dew,
As innocent as a doe.
A special prayer,
Beseeching, communicating.
Reaching out
As though reiterating,
I am strong! I am trying!
I can do it! Truly I can!
Those lovely eyes, … that dreamy lure!
—Manjeet Kaur

Remember, Andrew, even as a baby you were strong, and now that you and Ryan are both such handsome young men, the world is an open arena for your many talents.

A lovely memory! What a blessing!

A Tribute to Lauren*

A pretty maiden, a blithe lass,
A strong little scout came to pass.
Her lively steps, her voice so sweet,
Resounds evermore, clear and upbeat.
As I'd make my daily calls and say,
"Is your mom home?"
Without being told, you'd chime that day,
"Mom! It's Dr. Kaur,"
Lovely cherub, though afar.
Your dear sweet memory lingers on
As Andrew and Ryan the torch carry on.
—Manjeet Kaur

* Lauren was Andrew and Ryan's seven-year-old sister, whose life was
cut short in an accident while selling Girl Scout cookies.

Susan and Mark's Story

It was stressful, with so many ups and downs, especially with Andrew. I knew the boys were early. I told Mark on the way to the hospital to be prepared for two scary-looking babies. I tried to prepare him so he wouldn't be shocked when he first saw them. I guess I didn't dwell on the fact that they might not live.

The NICU staff was the best. Without all of your support, honesty, kindness, and love, getting through the hospitalizations would have been much more frightening. We appreciated the teaching and guidance. You were also so kind to our daughter, Lauren, every time we came to the hospital. My nursing background helped alleviate my anxiety about our babies being transferred to the NICU, but just having the boys there meant they were seriously ill.

Lauren came every day to the NICU and was a trouper, spending hours there because that was where I wanted to be. She was such a good girl. Writing this and looking at photos is difficult. Lauren, who was only seven years old, was killed after both boys had come home. Andrew was still trached then.

He and Ryan went through so much to survive, and then suddenly their big sister was gone. It's neither right, nor fair. She meant so much to them. We're extremely proud of our boys. Andrew had mild learning difficulties due to his prematurity, but he worked hard to be successful and has remained positive. My most precious memory of the NICU is of Lauren reading to him. He's often said that Lauren is always with him. Both Andrew and Ryan are very sensitive and kind.

My most difficult time in the NICU was when I watched one tiny baby girl die. It's very sad seeing other families suffer. Mark's father was an Episcopal priest, and gave us the strength and wisdom to carry on when we got down. I am a very positive person, and remained hopeful that the boys would be survivors and succeed in life. When they finally came

> " I told Mark to be prepared for two scary-looking babies. … I guess I didn't dwell on the fact that they might not live.

home, I told myself I would do whatever was necessary to make sure they remained healthy and had every opportunity to join in activities and cultural events. I often cooked three meals a night to make sure the boys ate what they liked. Andrew wasn't crazy about meat, but he loved pasta and other things. No problem—I just cooked what they wanted. We took them to every kid's activity we could find. When they were little, they took music lessons and swim lessons, and played baseball, soccer, and basketball. When

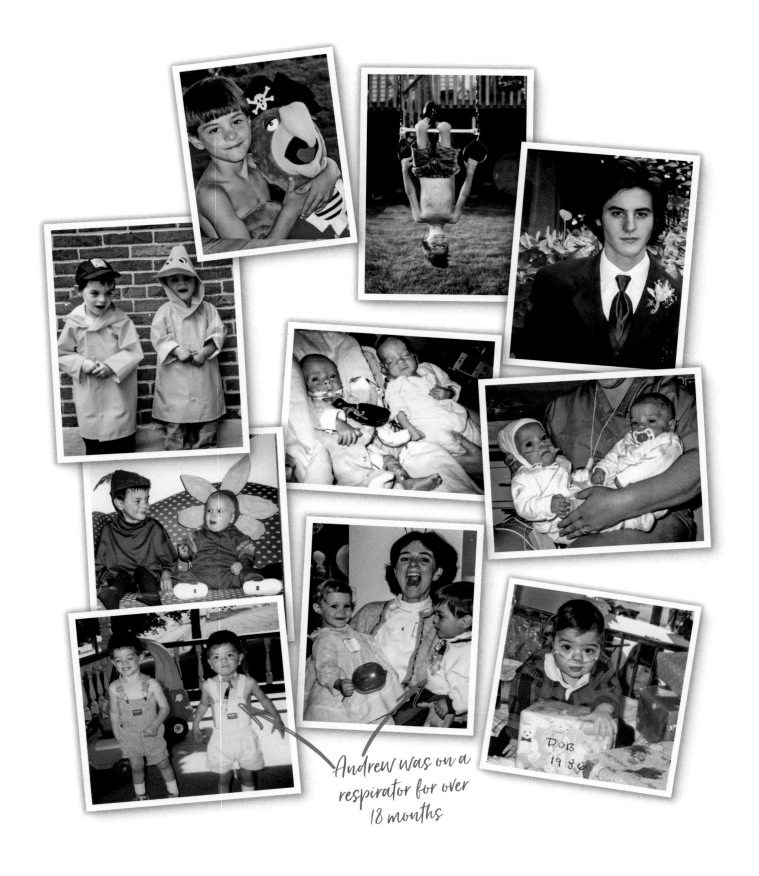

Andrew was on a respirator for over 18 months

DOB 1986

they got older, they played rugby. We tried our best to give them every chance to try any new things they were interested in.

Ryan earned a master's degree in Creative Writing from Trinity College, Dublin, Ireland. He played rugby, and was also on swim teams. He's very artistic, works as a chef in New York City, and writes and edits on the side. He plays the guitar with a small group, and occasionally plays in small venues in New York. He loves music and musicals, and often goes to concerts. He is getting married this year.

Andrew earned a liberal arts degree. He too played rugby and was on swim teams. He now works in construction, and plays the piano. Hallmark published one of his poems on a Halloween card.

I asked the boys if they have any memories of being in the hospital, the people, etc. Both said they do not. Probably for the best. The boys are very sensitive to individuals who have physical disabilities. Andrew is especially aware of others with tracheotomies, and often reaches out to them, showing them his trach scar.

5/31/2005

Dear Dr. Kaur,

We thought you would get a kick out of seeing Ryan. He is graduating soon and will be attending the University of Vermont. He wants to go to a good liberal arts school since he has so many interests. He is a fantastic artist and a great musician. He plays the guitar and is teaching himself to play the piano. He also loves to sing and dabble in acting. Anyway—I am sure he will find his way in college.

Andrew graduates next year and has been having a good time in high school. He is thinking of becoming a speech pathologist or a teacher. He loves medieval history. We'll see!

We hope you are well and not working too hard. I know that's next to impossible.

We send our love and thanks to you for everything you did for Ryan and Andrew when they were in your care.

Mark, Susan, Andrew, and Ryan

PS: The boys love their long hair!

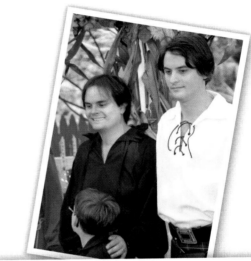

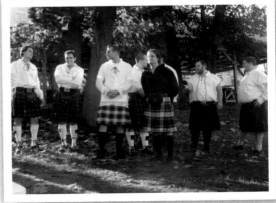

Intertwined: Two Peas in a Pod — Anna Kathryn and Cora

What a heartrending description of the trials and tribulations of your parents as well as both of you, little ones, as you came through every possible complication with gold stars.

I first met you, little Cora, when you were very sick and needed to take your first helicopter ride. Yet we thought of you as the "strong one," who would, with the strong faith of your family, come through every hurdle—and here we are, writing this testimonial today. Anna Kathryn, you gave us your share of trouble soon after birth, when you needed vigorous resuscitations in the NICU, as well as later, when you wished to trial "new endotracheal tubes."

I've always marveled at the strength and faith of your parents. When I was contemplating writing a book, I envisioned a great story of two little girls who required so many aspects of state-of-the-art technology, both prenatally as well as during the neonatal period—"mono-mono" or "mo-mo" twins—whose two physician parents, despite their professional demands, found the courage and strength for that long wait, a trying test of patience and faith, so that two little miracles could be home with their brothers and spend Halloween with the tiger and the pirate. What a lovely family photo!

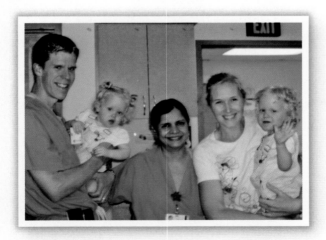

Two Little Angels

Just as close as peas in a pod,
Two little angels were conceived.
We call them mono-mono, gifts of God,
Arrived intertwined, too soon indeed.
Cora, dear, with a single lung,
Strong little warrior is she!
Enough to have a sonnet sung,
In praise of the Lord for thee.
Anna! Anna! Where art thou?
Your wayward heart makes the monitor ring.
Despite your pranks, you need a bow,
For all the joy that thou dost bring!
God bless!
—Manjeet Kaur

Anna Kathryn and Cora Hussar

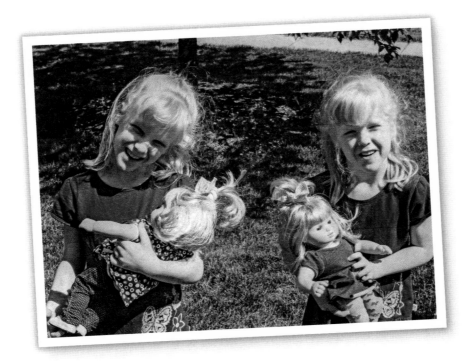

Parents:	Terra and Eric
Date of birth:	1/30/2009
Birth weight – Anna Kathryn:	2 pounds 6 ounces
Birth weight – Cora:	2 pounds 12 ounces
Medical conditions:	Preterm twins, Respiratory distress syndrome, Congenital hypoplasia of lung (in utero); Cora had spastic diplegia; Anna Kathryn had some mild hearing concerns.
Gestational age:	28 weeks
Hospitalization dates:	1/30/09–4/24/09

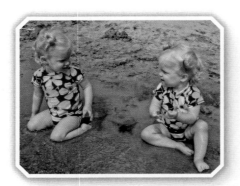
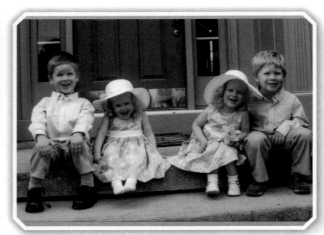
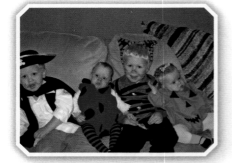
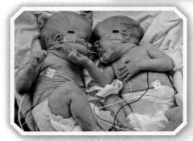
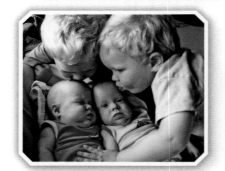
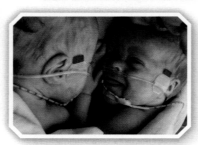
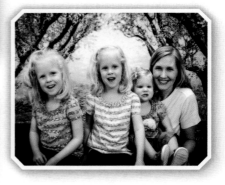
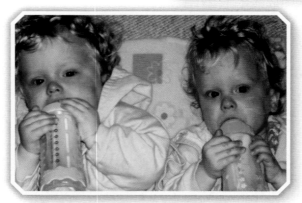
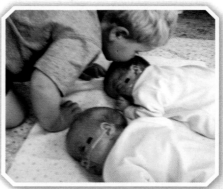

Terra and Eric's Story

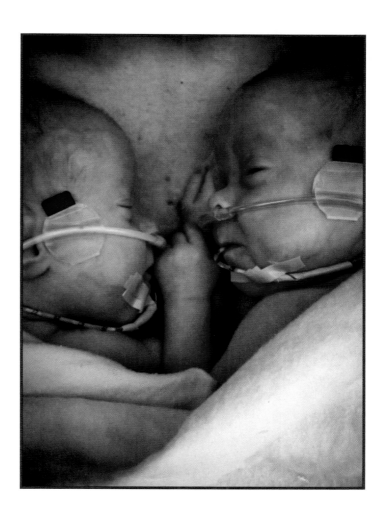

Our NICU journey began in November 2008. We waited eagerly for the ultrasound technician to tell us the gender of our unexpected twins. With one- and two-year-old sons at home, we were hoping for girls, and had already chosen one of the names.

We'd learned a few weeks earlier that I carried mono-mono twins, but we had no idea that their situation was rare and dangerous. The maternal fetal-medicine specialist didn't sugarcoat the news. Because our daughters shared the placenta and amniotic sac, this late split of the embryo translated into a 50 percent chance that one or both girls could die at any point.

Frozen in disbelief, I wept for the daughters I might never know in our pregnancy that we had not anticipated. A fight to save them was ensuing in Heaven and on Earth. We enlisted the prayers of everyone willing, and asked them to pray for the umbilical cords and for equal growth.

" Frozen in disbelief, I wept for the daughters I might never know.

We announced with tears to our family and friends what was to come: that our girls, who were not due until April 22, 2009, would be delivered at thirty-two weeks in late February, if not sooner. At Thanksgiving, we announced the girls' names to our families, as one of them is named after both of our living grandmothers. At Christmas I began aggressive monitoring at twenty-four-weeks gestation, with twice-weekly in-depth ultrasounds, watching for twin-twin transfusion and unusual or slowed umbilical-cord flow.

Birthday: At twenty-eight weeks I went in for another ultrasound and NST, but I needed a RhoGAM shot, which was scheduled for 1:00 p.m. on Friday, January 30, so I needed to move my usual morning MFM appointments to 2:00 p.m. When I arrived and the nurse put the monitor on me, she immediately started tracking my pulse. I still remember the look of concern, but not panic, on her face when she said that one baby's pulse rate was lower than mine. In a flash, I was moved to the exam room, and the doctor came in and started scanning the girls. He told me to call my husband, and said I was going downstairs for observation if her heart rate recovered, or for crash delivery if it didn't.

Everyone in the clinic seemed to be doing what he or she had been trained to do in an emergency. Phone calls were made, a wheelchair was secured, and the doctor himself pushed me straightaway to the pre-op holding area, the ultrasound technician chasing us the whole way. Once I was on the bed, they began again with continuous ultrasound, and the decision was made to do an emergency C-section. I couldn't have verbalized any thoughts or prayers in those hurried minutes, but firmly believe that there was One intervening on my behalf for my daughters' lives. My daughter was dying inside me, and though I couldn't feel it, the waiting in cautious optimism was ending.

It was time. In a gift of divine providence, my husband arrived (he'd been closer than usual to the hospital) in time to pray into my ear as I went under rapid-sequence general anesthesia.

A fight to save them was ensuing in Heaven and on Earth.

Delivery — Eric

Terra was under anesthesia in the OR as they started to operate. The doctors worked quickly and efficiently to bring the girls out. They handed each one to a waiting nurse, and offered me congratulations on the birth of my daughters. Congratulations that I feared at the time might have been premature. Both girls were intubated almost immediately after being put in the waiting isolettes in the OR and were attended to by a myriad of health providers. Cora seemed to be at least stable, and was being prepped for transfer to the NICU. Anna Kathryn, however, was in dire straits: Her pulse wasn't palpable, and she required

> " Everyone in the clinic seemed to be doing what he or she had been trained to do in an emergency.

chest compressions and epinephrine to restart her heart. It had been her low heartbeat that had initially caused concern for the MFM team when Terra came in. Eventually, Anna Kathryn also seemed to stabilize, and they readied her for the trip across the hall to the NICU as well. The doctor motioned for me to come over and showed me the umbilical cords. They had been braided in a way that had looked as if it was done intentionally and ended in a tight knot. I was grateful to God that Terra was where she needed to be when their situation became dangerous.

⌒

Terra

I awoke in the recovery room, and my husband confirmed that the girls had indeed survived. I don't remember much else. He didn't tell me about the events that occurred, just that the twins were alive and on ventilators. I have a vague memory of being wheeled into the NICU in my hospital bed, looking down two corridors where my daughters had been separated for the first time in their lives.

At 4:00 a.m., I met the NICU attending on overnight when he came to the room to tell us that our daughter, who we knew had only one lung, had developed a pneumothorax—a collapsed lung. This is a fairly common complication of mechanical ventilation following the use of surfactant, but most neonates have a second lung to compensate. Cora was made differently. They had discovered it in time to quickly insert a chest tube to decompress and drain the air, but she may have suffered some oxygen-delivery problems, and they'd do an echocardiogram and head ultrasound in the morning because other complications of intracranial bleeding or cardiac problems can sometimes follow.

By noon, Dr. Kaur, who had just met our girls, recommended Cora be helicoptered out to a tertiary children's hospital, based on the echo finding, which suggested early pulmonary hypertension—yet another potentially fatal complication. We hadn't even really seen our daughter, who at two and a half pounds was being prepped for a helicopter ride. No one had any smart phones yet, so we had no photos of the girls. The NICU had a Polaroid, and took a single snapshot of her isolette for me since I hadn't really visited her yet, and she was taking a risky helicopter ride (the changing pressure of air flight can cause recurrent collapse of the lung).

Once Cora was aboard, I watched the pilot and care flight team whisk her off. I still remember the sound of the helicopter takeoff. All the time, I was thinking, *What if she doesn't make it—and I never got to hold her, kiss her, and tell her, "I love you?"* I didn't want her to be there alone, so my husband drove there to meet the team and be with her in the other NICU.

"We spent five long weeks with twins in separate hospitals. Twice the fear, twice the travel, and all the while life went on at home.

It was now twenty-four hours after delivery, and Dr. Kaur turned her attention to twin A, whose respiratory disease was equally serious and required a great deal of ventilator support. I was still recovering from surgery, but eventually was able to visit Anna Kathryn (AK) in the NICU and start the long process of sitting, watching, waiting, and pumping. Though the girls' digestive tracts weren't ready for their mama's milk yet, the milk would be waiting for them.

The NICU staff was very generous and supportive of our predicament, and we spent five long weeks with twins in separate hospitals. Twice the fear, twice the travel, and all the while life went on at home. Eric worked, and I spent most days in between the two hospitals, watching my babies through their plastic cages hooked up to noisy monitors that signaled the sickness and struggles going on in their tiny bodies. Eventually we took a few photos and even a video.

The video is painful to watch, as it shows AK struggling to breathe and discolored from anemia and jaundice. Eric and I had Valentine's Day dinner at a restaurant close to one of the hospitals and then visited Cora afterward. It was a long, cold winter; many nights we took phone calls from the NICU about one daughter or the other having a new complication: a hernia, an infection, and several times Anna Kathryn self-extubated her breathing tube.

Eventually, Cora required surgery at an outside hospital in February. We were sitting with the cardiothoracic surgeon, signing the consent so that he could clip a tiny but crucial blood vessel inside her heart. It was then, while he was explaining the procedure, that she had extubated, and I heard her first soft cry.

Anna Kathryn had a more difficult course. One day, as I was doing kangaroo care with her, her color

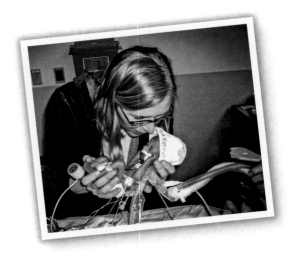
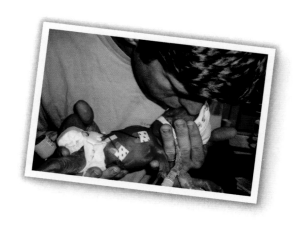

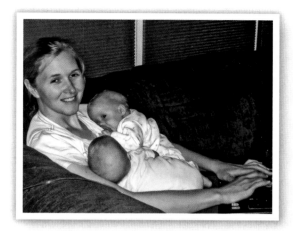

round and floppy. We brought our boys in and took our first family photo. It was quite an accomplishment with two toddlers and two girls on oxygen and monitors. I'll never forget that day—we had waited so long to all be together.

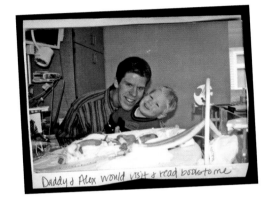

Daddy & Alex would visit & read books to me

turned gray and her monitor showed dropping saturations. The nurse took her from me, and I stood and watched her bag the blue baby, my smallest and most fragile one, limp and seemingly lifeless. She recovered, though, and spent forty-nine long days on a ventilator before transitioning to CPAP. In early March, Cora was well enough to return to the hospital of her birth, and we celebrated that she and her sister could be reunited.

The NICU was a strange and quiet place; our girls never really cried, and I don't remember hearing other babies cry much either. We brought our own music so as not to become too discouraged or distracted with the constant blipping and beeping of cardiac monitors. In the early days when touching/holding was not permitted, we often sang to the girls and played music. One day while driving to see Cora at the second hospital, I heard a song by Fernando Ortega that spoke of two friends walking a road together. I claimed it for my girls, and we sang it to

They were able to nurse eventually, and Easter was just around the corner. I remember that Easter because we visited them early in the morning, then drove to Philadelphia to be with family, and I felt a little guilty that we had left them behind on the most important holiday for Christians.

Spring was on its way; their health improved, and they were going to live. We transitioned from survival mode to preparation for discharge. I was able to hold both girls together, and we started taking more pictures and seeing the light in their eyes. Somewhere between the sleepless nights, tiny diaper changes, and bili lights, the girls grew. They started to look less frail and more like babies. They began to look at us, and AK seemed to always stick her tongue out. Even early on, Cora was so easygoing. For identical twins they were very different: AK, skinny and long; Cora,

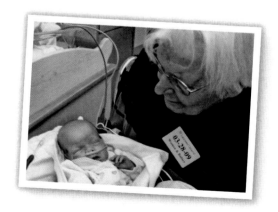

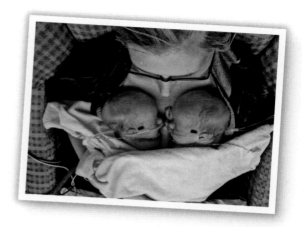

> " My most precious memories are when I was able to hold my girls together for kangaroo care for as long as I could stay …

them frequently: "Take heart, my friend, we'll go together."

After eleven to twelve weeks, we made the arrangements to go home and start the rest of our journey. We came home with two little girls just days before and after their original due date. Our Anna Kathryn came home on her great-grandmother's birthday—the one she was named after!

Here I sit, five years later, finally able to talk and write with only a few tears. We are so blessed to have seen our daughters survive, and we feel that the very Hand of God placed the team of doctors and nurses in the right places to care for us in so many ways. The girls are doing remarkably well. Anna Kathryn, despite being fully resuscitated, caught up and is enjoying most of the things her peers enjoy. Cora developed spastic diplegia, a mild form of cerebral

palsy, but shines like the noonday sun. She has a sweetness of spirit and is a tender and loving child. The sisters are best friends; we often find them curled into bed together, always sharing a hug or holding hands.

They bring us great joy, and though we knew we'd be at higher risk to have twins again, we added a fifth child to our family when the girls turned three. We wanted them to experience being the older siblings, and in January 2012, Eden Joy was welcomed and fought over by her four older siblings from day one.

Our lives are a bit crazy, but we wouldn't change a thing—except I'd love a full-time domestic specialist! It was all worth it: the fear, the anxiety, the pain, the tears, the almosts, and the could-have-beens, and we have no regrets. We recently met with a couple expecting their own mono-mono twins to encourage them in their journey and introduce them to our little miracle babies.

My most precious memories are when I was able to hold my girls together for kangaroo care for as long as I could stay and knowing that this was therapeutic for them. The most difficult time was every day having to say goodbye to them and leave them, always wondering if they would make it through the night.

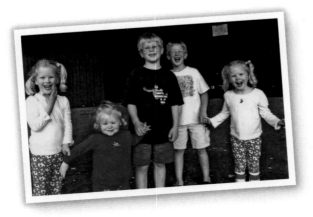

" Our faith is the beginning and end of the story—it is the Maker's story; He has given them to us to shepherd for a while.

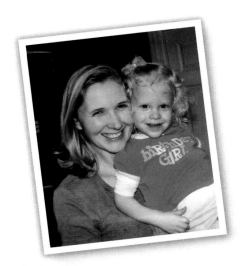

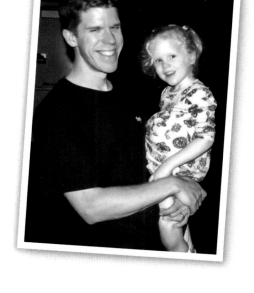

Our faith is the beginning and end of the story—it is the Maker's story; He has given them to us to shepherd for a while. I'm eager to see exactly what He has in store for these miracle girls. Already they know that they're a treasure and have a purpose. It was the support of our immediate family and local church family that carried us all those weeks. We believe God heard the prayers for our children and saved them.

The girls turned eight this year (2017), and are in first grade at school. They are growing, and will be tall for preemie twins (5'7" and 5'8" predicted).

They are loving reading and music. Cora has started English horseback riding and loves it. They jump on our trampoline and ride bikes down the street like everyone else. Now we have another sibling on the way via international adoption.

The adventure continues!

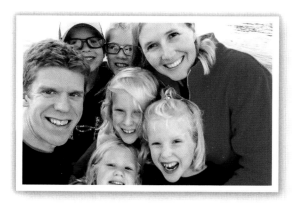

Born in "The Coolest Place in the World" — Amy and Emily

Lindsey, a "young Nightingale," called me one day to tell me about her sisters, who'd been in the NICU seventeen years ago, and to say she wished to share their story.

It's amazing how much she absorbed seventeen years ago, at the age of eight, obviously enough to last a lifetime.

She called the NICU (a scary place to children) "the coolest place in the world." What a compliment to our staff! She kept her promise to herself to become a nurse one day. We're privileged to have such a dedicated nurse in our NICU today. Thanks, Amy and Emily, for that inspiration!

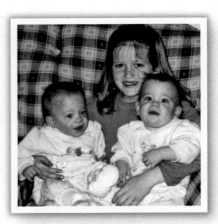

Amy, you've written such a lovely note. You're not only a talented singer but a superb writer as well, one who writes from the heart. I love to sing too, so maybe we can connect and make music someday. What fun that would be!

Sweet Emily, our athlete, a writer as well, who knows what you two sisters can compose? Good luck to both of you in all your future endeavors.

A Medley — A Marathon

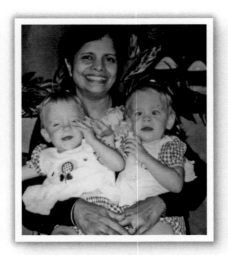

Seventeen years ago two pretty cherubs were born,
The light of many lives, numerous promises to adorn.
You gifted your sister with a dedication to heal,
To work in the "coolest" place in the world. What a steal!
Things happen for a reason, young Amy, you say,
How right you are ... you may be a singing star one day.
With medley and song, may you pleasure bring
To those in pain, a chiming breeze of spring!
And Emily, our athlete, a writer too,
May you make your mark in all you do.
With candor and diligence may you both excel in life,
You were destined to be special, may you win every strife!
—Manjeet Kaur

Amy and Emily Herr

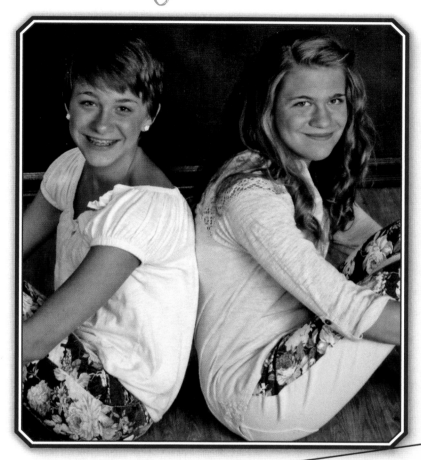

Parents:	Melinda and Dan
Date of birth:	3/10/1999
Birth weight– Amy:	2 pounds 12 ounces
Birth weight– Emily:	1 pound 12 ounces
Medical conditions:	Premature twins, respiratory distress syndrome; Amy: bowel volvulus
Gestational age:	30 weeks
Hospitalization dates:	3/10/1999–5/9/1999

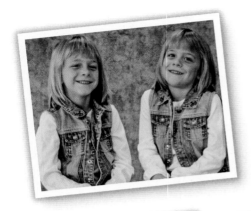
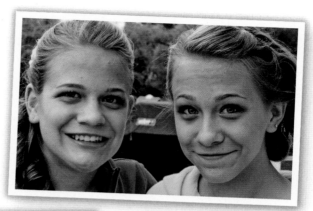
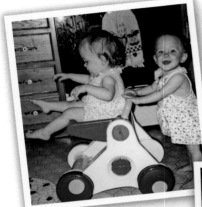
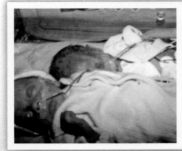
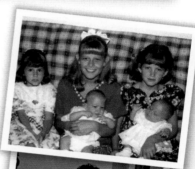
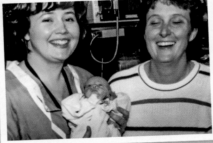
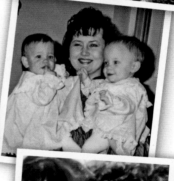
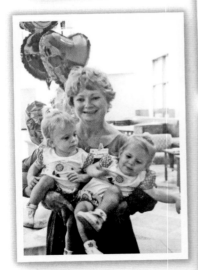
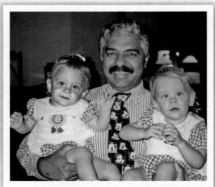
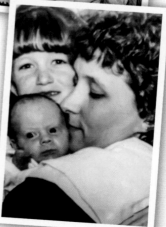

Melinda and Dan's Story

Our girls were born early due to placental insufficiency. We understood and were prepared, if there is such a thing, for the fact that we wouldn't be able to go past thirty-two weeks but deliver at thirty weeks. We weren't prepared for what a two-pound baby looks like. Both were on CPAP for only twelve hours, then room air within twenty-four hours—amazing.

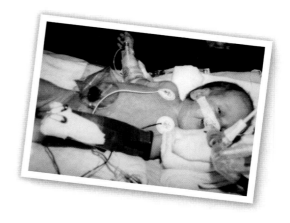

We felt at ease when both girls were at LGH. Amy got a volvulus (twisted bowel), which really wasn't due to prematurity. She almost died. When Amy was transferred at one month of age, our world became overwhelming. The hospital she was transferred to was so different from LGH: the facility, staff, and care so different. At LGH it felt like family, and when we left at night we had little fear, unlike when we left Amy. We knew from about five-months gestation that they would be in the NICU, and we were able to tour and ask questions, which helped.

We had three other girls at home: Stephanie, age eleven; Lindsey, age eight; and Danielle, age five. We have no family living nearby. We were grateful for the way visitation was set up, with a list of people who could visit when we weren't there. This definitely helped. (I think one parent must be present now.)

There are so many memories. I especially appreciated that when Dr. Kaur made rounds, she would always pick up and hold each twin for a few minutes, and all the nurses were so patient and kind. Our most difficult time, of course, was when Amy got deathly ill and the twins had to be separated, so for a month we had three children at home, one at LGH, and one an hour away. Amy needed to have a colostomy, which removed part of her intestine. She wasn't expected to survive.

> "We weren't prepared for what a two-pound baby looks like.

We're blessed with a wonderful, loving, and supportive church family. I'm not sure how we'd have made it without them.

Amy is now seventeen, and will be a senior in high school. She's an amazing singer, and hopes to pursue music and worship arts. Emily is also seventeen, and will be a senior. She was an accomplished runner till a broken femur and tibia put a halt to that.

We realize that we were extremely lucky. It was amazing to have twins who were two and three pounds not need any help with breathing. We were always told that things could change very quickly, but until Amy got sick it was smooth sailing—except that neither of them ever gained more than ten grams per day; it was discouraging when most other babies gained thirty grams or more each day.

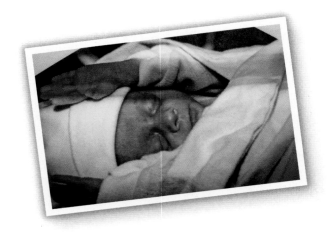

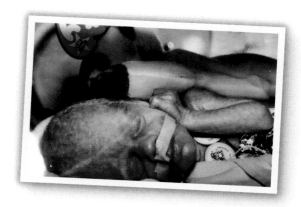

On Mother's Day, 1999, our twins were discharged from two separate hospitals. Emily weighed only three pounds ten ounces. Dr. Kaur wasn't there on that day, and I'm not sure she'd have let Emily go at that weight. I won't say we've had smooth sailing, and we do have some lingering effects that are most likely due to prematurity—eye issues, some coordination issues, and anxiety—but we're certainly not complaining and are so very thankful.

I'm a pediatric homecare nurse, and have cared for infants and children who are trached/vented and have many lifelong health issues, most due to prematurity (twenty-three–twenty-six-weekers), so I know

what could have been. I always tell people that it was likely the roughest time of our lives, but I wouldn't change anything (well, except for Amy's being transferred). It was a positive, eye-opening journey, and we have new friends because of it. Rhonda Urban was our primary nurse, and we will be forever grateful. I realize our journey was nowhere near as scary and up and down as many, and my heart aches for them, but if they're at LGH, they're in the best of hands. My hope is that someday LGH will be equipped to do surgery, so that no baby has to be transferred out and can experience the whole process with the best. Thank you.

> "I decided to believe that everything happens for a reason. I decided to tell myself that God spared my life so that I can praise Him and tell others about Him.

A Letter from Amy

I'll start by saying thank you for all you did to take care of me in the NICU. If having been a NICU preemie has taught me anything, I'd say I learned not only how valuable life is but also the importance of not giving up. As I got older, I remember looking at pictures of myself as a baby and asking my mom why I had all the tubes, a colostomy, and even a lazy eye. Mom eventually explained how I had a bowel obstruction and was going to die. Thanks to Rhonda Urban's urging, I had surgery in time to save my life. We call Rhonda our "NICU angel."

Anxiety, along with my lazy eye as a result of minor brain damage, can sometimes make learning in school difficult; however, my family has taught me that with a little faith and perseverance, I can get through any trial in life. One time when I was really discouraged and felt like giving up, my dad told me I couldn't. I asked him why. "Because you are a Herr, and the Herrs do not give up!"

So I kept going and discovered that I'm a talented singer. This discovery made me ponder the fact that I could have died but didn't. It's still hard for me to understand at times why God spared my life and gave me the gift of music. I decided to believe that everything happens for a reason. I decided to tell myself that God spared my life so that I can praise Him and tell others about Him. Singing not only gets me through tough times, bringing me pure joy and peace, but also helps me serve others. I'll be a senior in high school next fall and hope to pursue a career that involves working with young children and music. Dr. Kaur, I appreciate that you considered me as you work on your book. I wish you the best as you go forward in the future.

Lindsey's Story (Amy and Emily's Sister)

When the twins were born, Lindsey, then eight, would come into the NICU and hold and feed the twins. She told us then: "When I grow up I'm going to be a nurse, and I'm going to take care of these little babies."

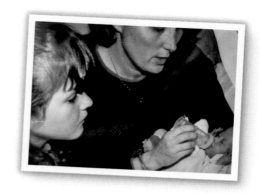

She never changed her mind. She went to LGH College of Nursing, graduated at age twenty, and worked at LGH on 4 West while getting her bachelor's degree. She applied to the   NICU at Women and Babies, and has been there since and loves it.

Amy Herr (twin A) and Emily Herr (twin B) were born on March 10, 1999, at thirty-weeks gestation. Amy weighed two pounds twelve ounces and was fourteen and a half inches long, and Emily weighed one pound twelve ounces and was fourteen inches long.

Both twins originally required CPAP for the first twelve hours but were weaned to room air by twenty-four hours after their birth. All was smooth sailing with the twins until they hit one month of age, when Amy was taken by ambulance to Polyclinic in Harrisburg (CHOP, Hershey, and DuPont were full) for a volvulus. Six inches of her intestine were removed, but she recovered quickly and hasn't had any issues since. Amy and Emily stayed in the NICU from March 10 until May 9, Mother's Day. Both came home weighing a little over three pounds.

My mother specifically remembers you and the loving care you provided to Amy, Emily, and our family. She said that of all the great doctors in the LGH NICU, you stood out from the rest. She'll always remember that it didn't matter if the twins were in their isolettes or being held by family; on your daily rounds you'd always ask to hold them. Mom said she could just tell how much you cared about your patients and your work.

When the twins were born, I was eight years old, and those little girls changed my life. I vividly remember the LGH NICU and all the time I spent there. I'll

> "I remember looking at my mom and asking, 'Mommy, are those real babies? They're too small to be real.'

never forget the two-minute "scrub in." I rubbed my poor little hands raw because I didn't want to bring any germs to my baby sisters.

I distinctly remember the first time I saw the twins. They were hooked up to so many tubes and wires and had on what I thought were sunglasses (for under the bili lights). I remember looking at my mom and asking, "Mommy, are those real babies? They're too small to be real." To this day I swear that the nurses in the NICU inspired me to become a NICU nurse myself. The NICU can be a very scary place for an eight-year-old, but every time I walked through that door, the nurses embraced my eagerness to learn: they let me help change diapers, they let me hold my baby sisters, they let me help with baths, and they let me help hold feeds for the NG tubes. I honestly thought the NICU was the coolest place in the world. It's a place where miracles take place every day, and I feel more than blessed to be a part of the same team that helped save my little sisters. I've worked in the WBH NICU for about two years now, and I can honestly say I have the best job in the world.

Amy and Emily are now seventeen and just got their driver's licenses (eek!). They're very involved at school and church. They live happy, healthy lives, and though they're "all grown up," they'll always be my babies!

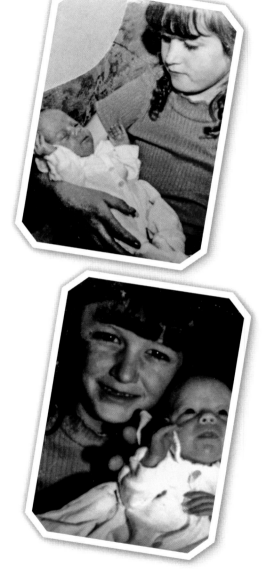

“ I've worked in the WBH NICU for about two years now, and I can honestly say I have the best job in the world.

Caring is Sharing—Alec and Taylor

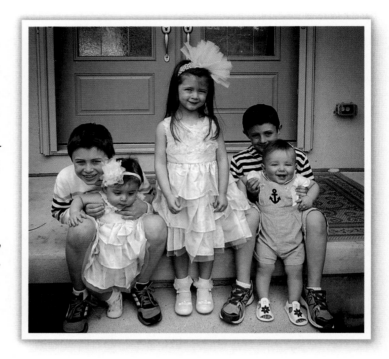

What a lovely recap of NICU stories of little ones who at thirty-one weeks were our "good gestation babies." In my career of more than three decades working with sick neonates, it was the only night I can recall when I intubated and put in a chest tube in each sibling within an hour!

"Togetherness" seems to be their code word and motto.

You both look adorable now, though, and fit in perfectly with your three siblings. God bless you and your family always!

Togetherness

A cute feisty duo, we happened to encounter,
Always so close, a sweet reminder.
Of togetherness, and camaraderie, of a law divine,
A unique sonnet, a genre, where all that is mine, is thine.
Sharing and enduring, both trivial and profound,
Alec needed a breathing tube, thus Taylor was bound.
Sweet kindered spirits, may you flourish and grow,
Fill your home with laughter, along with your loving trio.
—Manjeet Kaur

Alec and Taylor Medina

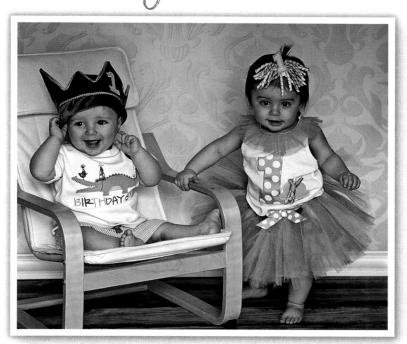

Parents:	Stacie and James
Date of birth:	5/1/2013
Birth weight – Alec:	3 pounds 11 ounces
Birth weight – Taylor:	3 pounds 5 ounces
Medical conditions:	Premature twins/respiratory distress, pneumothorax
Gestational age:	31 weeks
Hospitalization dates:	5/1/2013–6/7/2013

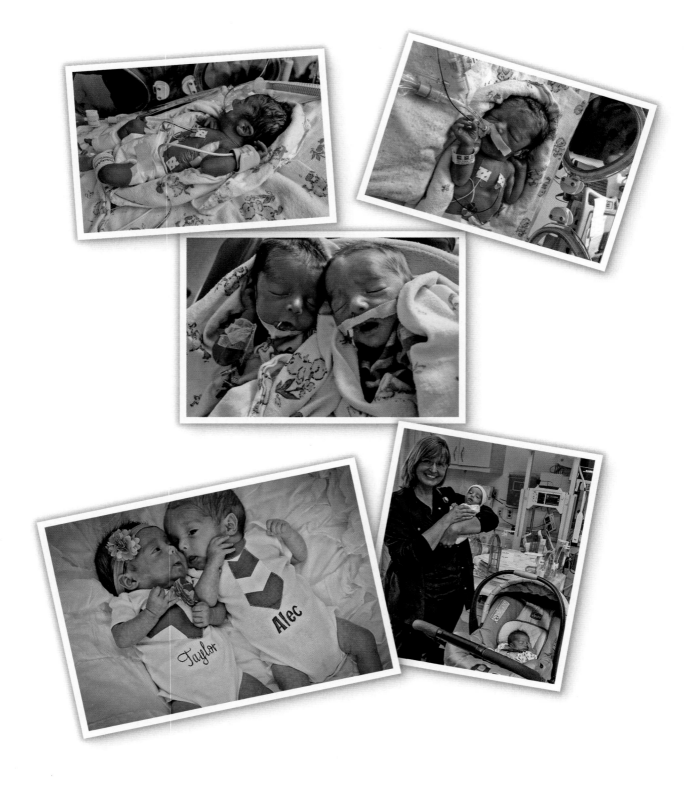

Stacie and James' Story

Delivery day was rushed. I'd had a headache for three days. Though my blood pressure was normal, my platelets were borderline low. On the third day of my headache I was seen in triage, where they admitted me and several hours later decided to take me for an emergency C-section due to my extremely low platelet count. The best words to describe our feelings at that time are "numb" and "anxious." We were worried about the twins' health, and since it was so rushed, I never had a chance to receive a steroid shot to mature their lungs. I was thirty-one weeks and two days along.

Our medical knowledge was both a help and a hindrance. I was a neonatal respiratory therapist before having children, and my husband is an ER physician. We knew everything that could go wrong, but we also knew how resilient preemies could be. It was my greatest fear to know that their lungs hadn't gotten the benefit of steroid shots, so I worried their respiratory status would decline rapidly.

My mother, mother-in-law, and sister-in-law were extremely helpful and supportive while the twins were in the NICU. On many occasions they took my older children, ages ten, eight, and two, to get them out of the house and keep them occupied. My children had quite a few sleepovers with their cousins at their aunt's house.

My most difficult moment was twenty-four hours after their birth. It was about 12:30 a.m., and I was visiting the NICU from my hospital room. I noticed that Alec looked as if he was struggling to breathe. He then turned blue. The nurse readjusted his CPAP mask, but that didn't help. Alec's heart rate plummeted, and his O2 saturation dropped into the fifties and forties. I was asked to leave the room while the NICU team rushed to work with him. From the hallway, I watched them try to resuscitate him and I broke down in tears. I was then asked to wait in my hospital room for an update on his condition. An hour later I received the call, yet heard unexpected news. A few minutes after Alec crashed, his sister did the very same. They both were put on ventilators. They both had left-sided pneumothoraces, and chest tubes were placed. On x-ray their lungs looked terrible. That was my most difficult night by far. Dr. Kaur said she would never forget the twins who did everything together! Crashed, chest tubes, ventilators, and then weaning from ventilators. They were truly kindred spirits.

> " The best words to describe our feelings at that time are 'numb' and 'anxious.'

"It was an extremely emotional moment for me when I was allowed to hold Alec for the first time.

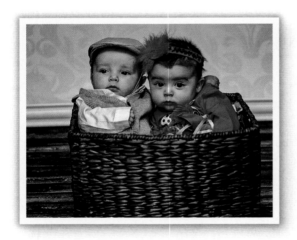

I have two very precious memories of the NICU: One was the day of my discharge after the C-section, when I was allowed to hold Alec for the first time. It was an extremely emotional moment for me. My other memory is of Mother's Day, when a very brave nurse moved mountains—those isolettes are very cumbersome—to allow me to hold both babies at the same time, even though they were connected to IVs and feeding tubes. I'll never forget how wonderful that was. She was so kind to do that for me.

We very often prayed for their recovery and healing, and our prayers were answered: they are currently a year old with absolutely no delays or restrictions and no residual effects from having been in the NICU.

We absolutely adored the team of nurses. Everyone was compassionate and understanding. Judy and Pam, their primary nurses, were amazing. They both went above and beyond to make the babies and me comfortable. I missed them terribly after discharge. The twins healed quickly in the NICU, and when all tests were normal they were discharged the first week in June. They did amazingly well at home, and grew into chubby, sweet, happy babies. Alec is such a lover-boy, and Taylor is the busiest little baby I've ever seen—she always has somewhere important to be!

Life at home with five kids was definitely an adjustment, but I wouldn't change any of it!

"I have a precious memory of Mother's Day, when a very brave nurse moved mountains to allow me to hold both babies at the same time, even though they were connected to IVs and feeding tubes.

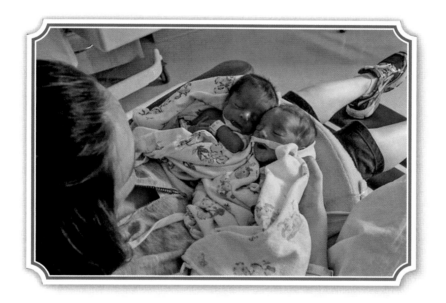

I'll never forget how wonderful that was. She was so kind to do that for me.

A Winsome Trio—Katie, Lindsay and Tiffany

These premature infants had a really rocky start and all the ups and downs expected of multiple births. They had many complications: pulmonary immaturity requiring ventilator support, pleural effusion requiring thoracentesis, intraventricular hemorrhages, sepsis, apnea, and renal issues. These three little angels went through a very rough time, but as we say, "They are the astounding newborns." We are delighted to see that our three little miracles are now lovely young women!

Your story truly embodies what I strongly believe: adversity brings you strength, strength brings you character, character brings you a firm destiny and an inner beauty—a beauty so visible in these charming portraits.

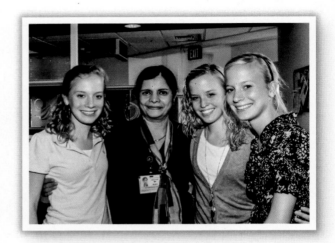

Three Lovely Maidens

Three little lilies, three little tarts,
Each sweeter than the other, despite a rocky start.
Athletic champions and honor scholars too,
Who would have guessed after so much ado?
As they conquered hurdles and hardships with grace,
Prayers reverberated, love and technology did race.
Our three precious babes—lovely young ladies today—
Katie, Lindsay, Tiffany, and sister Jamie, a special ray.
We are proud of your achievements, so much joy you have brought
To your family, friends, and the NICU lot.
May God bless you in all your future endeavors!
—Manjeet Kaur

Katie, Lindsay, and Tiffany Doughty

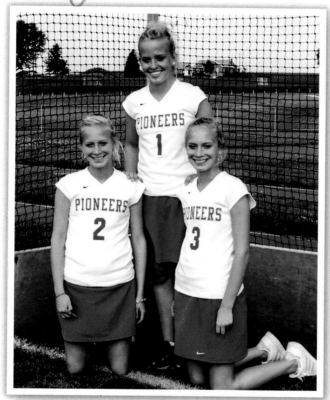

Parents:	Bev and Jim
Date of birth:	8/6/1991
Birth weight– Katie:	2 pounds 9 ounces
Birth weight – Lindsay:	1 pound 15 ounces
Birth weight – Tiffany:	1 pound 14 ounces
Medical conditions:	Prematurity, multiple gestation, respiratory distress syndrome, sepsis, intraventricular hemorrhage, apnea, bradycardia
Gestational age:	29 weeks
Hospitalization dates:	8/6/1991–10/18/1991

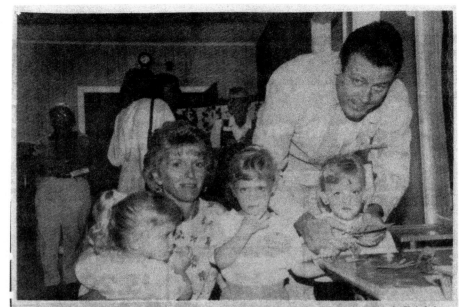

Bev and James Doughty are among the many area parents who have enrolled their children in the Great Beginnings Preschool held in the Strasburg Assembly of God Church. They are shown with 3 year old triplets (left to right) Tiffany, Lindsay and Katie.

"Great Beginnings Pre-School"

(continued from page 19)

to kindergarten. As they were invited to touch and explore, some were drawn by the playhouse, while others put together puzzles, examined "career" hats, donned dress up clothes, constructed block buildings or headed for the outdoor recreation areas, also arranged by Pastor Mark.

"We need a few more things," said Underhill, "like old jewelry, an area rug, and a photograph of each child to decorate our bulletin boards." Parents assisted their children as they traced a "helping hand" to pin on the boards, an invitation for everyone to get into the act and become involved in the success of the school.

With homemade cookies, balloons and baskets of flowers, the open house was a great beginning for everyone.

Three year old classes will be held on Tuesdays and Thursdays and four year olds will be held on Monday, Wednesdays and Fridays from 9 to 11:30 a.m. Julie Thiboldeaux is serving as registrar and can be reached at 687-0507.

" Our faith was tested many times but we always prayed, grasping the fact that we were blessed no matter what the next day brought us. We'd asked for these girls to be brought to us … for years, and God chose us for some reason.

Bev and Jim's Story

Our emotions around the time of delivery were very mixed. We were the parents of an already beautiful, active three-and-a-half-year-old to whom we devoted all of our time. Jamie was a very loving and intelligent little girl who always seemed mature for her age, and we had no doubt that she would be the greatest big sister anyone could ask for. We not only worried about the premature birth of our triplets but also how we'd handle doubling our family overnight, the medical problems they'd face, and all that we needed for one child, let alone four. Being on bed rest for the two weeks leading up to my emergency C-section only made it harder to give Jamie the appropriate attention. We feared finances as well. Jim was a social worker and worked long hours, but the pay didn't reflect the time he devoted, and now I'd need him here, too.

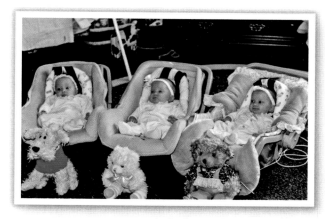

What helped us most was that our family and friends were close, and we had a great support network through them, our church, and our workplaces, which lessened our fear. What hurt the most was the fact that we could never simply run here or there as we had before. Loading up our family now took three of everything: three more people most of the time; nurses to carry the oxygen tanks, heart monitors, diaper bags, car seats, and whatever was needed for all the return visits to Hershey Medical Center, Lancaster General, the pediatrician, the specialists— you name it.

I joined the MOTC (Mother of Twins Club) and the Triplet Connection out of California once I knew I was having triplets. I read as much as I could to educate us on what we faced. The pictures of those little babies horrified me but also fully prepared me, because even though I tried to keep them growing in my womb, given the complications, I assumed it was inevitable they'd be born very premature and ill.

I knew that the NICU was prepared to give them the best care possible, which became an understatement as we grew close to the staff who saved our girls' lives at Hershey Medical and at Lancaster General Hospital. To this day we thank God for providing such caring, loving people for babies born like ours. It wasn't easy to leave for home each day, but we had a sense of peace knowing they would be okay—and they were!

> "My husband's most precious memory of the NICU was hearing the doctor at Hershey Medical Center say that they had a good chance of survival because they were all girls.

Having a three-year-old was a challenge while carrying the triplets. We tried to stay active with Jamie and make the most of the last months of our one-on-one time together. We prepared her by taking her to a sibling class, and we loved the expressions of the people when they asked how she felt about a new sister and she responded, "Good, but we're going to have 'free' of them!"

Jamie was our life for three and a half years, and it was important for us to continue to keep her involved with us and make her feel a part as well, since her world very soon would be turned upside down.

We hung a sign on the porch to anyone visiting: PLEASE ACKNOWLEDGE JAMIE, OUR 3½-YEAR-OLD, FIRST, AND THEN GO TO THE TRIPLETS. Whenever we were out, we were approached with oohs and aahs, and we made it a point to say, "This is their big sister, Jamie, who helps us so much!" Our family and friends treated Jamie like a queen; in fact, she's been to more places and done more than we have!

My husband's most precious memory of the NICU was hearing the doctor at Hershey Medical Center say that they had a good chance of survival because they were all girls. My most precious memory was the day we could take our first family photo. When they were stable enough, the girls were transported from Hershey Medical Center to Lancaster General's NICU via ambulance. That week we

> "My most precious memory was the day we could take our first family photo.

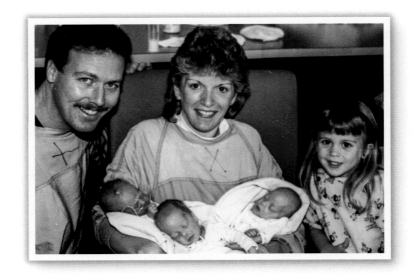

were able to get them out of their isolettes long enough for the family photo. It was beautiful, and made us finally feel a strong bond with our sickly infants. It was a small hurdle, but such a giant leap for us.

There's no doubt that we had many ups and downs through the course of Katie, Lindsay, and Tiffany's thirteen-week hospitalization. Our strong faith was really tested at the most difficult times, such as when we'd arrive ready to hold and love our babies and be told one or two weren't doing well, that we should just stroke and talk to them through the portholes of the isolette, as the staff had just gotten them settled and calmed from the many procedures they'd endured. Our tiniest miracle child, Tiffany, didn't have good veins for IVs, so they used the prominent one at the top of her head. It was awful to see a huge needle taped to her scalp in order to feed her. When they removed this needle several weeks later, she had developed a hematoma in that vein. It was engorged with blood and a huge bump remained on the top, which was there until it involuted at about age five.

Lindsay had difficulty feeding. She couldn't suck and breathe at the same time. This caused her to become cyanotic and need oxygen every time she was fed, which was very unnerving. Our worst time in the NICU was during Labor Day weekend. The girls were four weeks old, and we got an urgent call to come to the hospital immediately. Katie, the biggest at birth, had taken a turn for the worse, and there was nothing they could do for her. She was blown up with fluids, septic, and rapidly deteriorating. We called our family to watch Jamie and left in a hurry, not knowing what we'd face when we got there. We spoke with the doctor at Katie's bedside and Katie didn't even look like our precious daughter. Her veins were illuminated, her stomach immensely distended, and her little chest worked very hard to breathe. The chaplain met us, and we prayed and cried and hugged the doctor

who tried so desperately to save her. We visited our other two daughters as well, and they seemed stable, so we weren't sure what to do.

Torn, we left to go home with Jamie for a while and await the phone call, which didn't come till hours later, but it was a good call: they asked us to come back up, and to our amazement, our dear Katie had made a turnaround. A resident coming on duty had looked at her groin and thought that the catheter that was feeding her might have pierced her vein. Sure enough, that was what had happened, so all the fluids she was to be receiving were filling up her body cavity. The hospital staff did a thoracentesis and drained the cavity of fluid, and her condition was improving by the hour. We were so thankful to that intern, for he truly saved Katie's life.

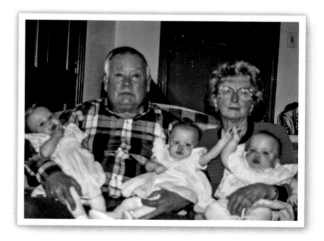

Another difficult time was, of course, when the girls were born. The medical staff had to be upfront with us about their condition, and tell us we had three critically ill babies. One had a grade III brain hemorrhage; the other two had grade II hemorrhages, which meant that only time would tell if they'd have cerebral palsy, be mentally challenged, or lack both fine and large motor skills. We were told that they had lung disease as a result of being born so prematurely. The smallest had hypertension due to her underdeveloped kidneys. All three were on ventilators, and eventually oxygen and apnea monitors. It was so overwhelming that we had to separate ourselves from emotions so we could care for them. This was how we dealt with all the problems, like knowing that we'd need round-the-clock nurses for at least the next year.

My husband and I were brought up in church-going households. He was Catholic and I Protestant, but we always went to church. That base helped us grow together as a married couple. Our faith was tested many times but we always prayed, grasping the fact that we were blessed no matter what the next day brought us. We'd asked for these girls to be brought to us as we struggled with miscarriages and infertility for years, and God chose us for some reason. We had the girls baptized by the hospital chaplain just in case anything happened. We knew it would be a journey and that the rewards would be here for us sooner than later. Though we've often been challenged financially, the rich blessings of so many memories of four daughters have taught us to appreciate the simple things and know that our life is what we make of it.

During elementary and junior-high schools the girls did really well in Girl Scouts, dance, softball,

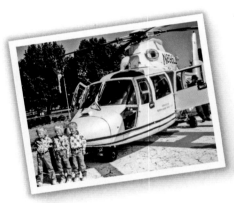

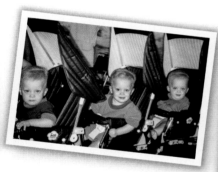

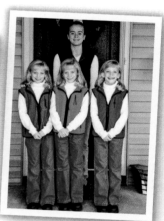

"The rich blessings of so many memories of four daughters have taught us to appreciate the simple things and know that our life is what we make of it.

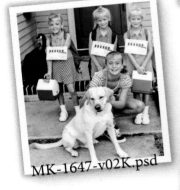

MK-1647-v02K.psd

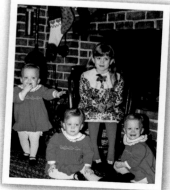

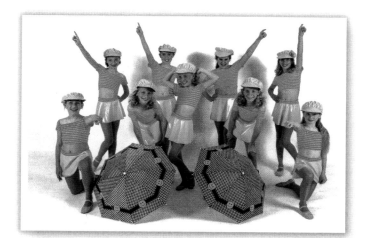

soccer, and many other activities. In high school they played field hockey. They never got caught up in cliques, and never had a lot of friends because they had each other. I believe that some, especially catty girls, were jealous of the triplets' relationship and that they didn't seem to need anyone else in their lives!

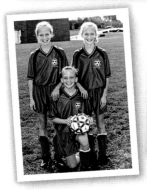
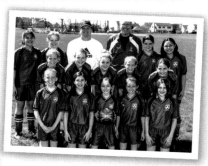
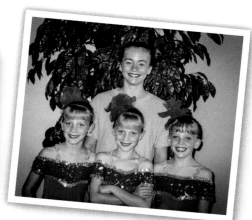

Even though they are very different—Katie is the mom of the other two, having been born first; Lindsay, the middle child, is easygoing; and Tiffany is the baby, since she was born last. They have a bond that's absolutely amazing! What else do you really need? This also includes their older sister, Jamie, who was their mentor and our third set of hands, and loved them just like a mom. They idolized everything she did, and strove to emulate her as an athlete and scholar.

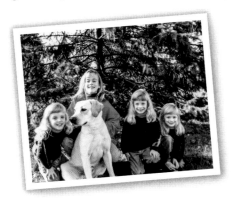
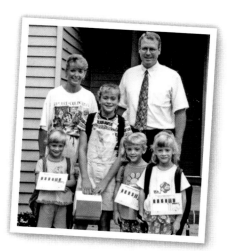

" My advice to everyone is enjoy the moment, little or big, simple or complex, because those preemies grow up in the blink of an eye, and after all the craziness you'll find yourself with filled hearts but empty homes.

The girls are seniors at Shippensburg University now. Katie and Tiffany have chosen the field of elementary education and wish to be teachers, while Lindsay has chosen social work. We are extremely proud of them. They have made dean's list all four years of college, have served as officers in clubs, and belong to an honor sorority. They didn't live together their freshman year, but after some negative experiences with roommates, they decided from sophomore year on that

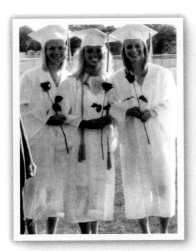

they'd be back together again. They're sisters, but are best friends too, and nothing is more satisfying for a mother and father to see. The girls have so much to give to others because people gave them so much at the beginning of their lives. To see where they've come in twenty-two years is unbelievable. If only we'd had a crystal ball to look into, how easy would our life have been? No worrying over the small stuff, like potty training three children at once or training three at once to ride a two-wheeler or training three at once to drive—and sending three away to college at once. God led us through each hurdle we faced, and when we look back it really wasn't as bad as we'd

anticipated. One just becomes stronger for the next obstacle.

In their earlier years, we wished their lives away, and now find ourselves wishing for more time to enjoy every minute with our daughters. They've brought so much joy into our hearts, and have touched so many people in our community. We, their older sister, their grandparents, aunts and uncles, friends, and neighbors will always feel their impact. On occasion, even total strangers ask, "How are your triplets doing?" We answer: "They're twenty-two years old and will graduate from college this May." We always get the same answer: "Oh my, that can't be!" All those years have flown way too fast, so my advice to everyone is enjoy the moment, little or big, simple or complex, because those preemies grow up in the blink of an eye, and after all the craziness you'll find yourself with filled hearts but empty homes.

Thanks for allowing us to share the story of our miracles, who changed our lives for the better. We're honored that God chose us and trusted that we could handle having three beautiful babies at once.

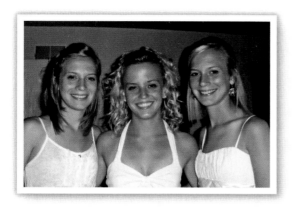

Katie Doughty's Comments

Thoughts of excitement and appreciation rushed into my head as I walked in to see Dr. Kaur. Our parents told us many stories of our first few months, but reuniting with one of the doctors who helped us when we were so helpless is indescribable. Dr. Kaur greeted us with open arms. Talking with her was like reconnecting with a friend I hadn't seen in years—genuine and natural.

Lindsay Doughty's Comments

Going back to Women and Babies NICU was a day I won't forget. It was really neat to be meeting the doctors, nurses, and other people who made a significant impact on our lives. When I look at baby pictures of the three of us, and hearing the stories of how sick we were as preemies, I feel forever grateful to all the people who helped my sisters and me become survivors. I'm also grateful for all the support they provided my family during our time at the NICU.

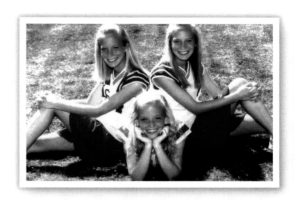

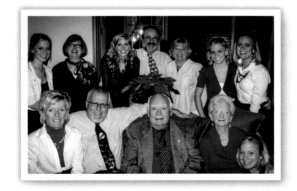

Tiffany Doughty's Comments

In the days leading up to the NICU reunion, I was anticipating the moment I'd be reunited with Dr. Kaur. As soon as my sisters and I walked into the NICU wing at Women and Babies Hospital, I felt right at home. Dr. Kaur embraced me with a warm smile and hug. It was an unforgettable feeling to meet one of the doctors who aided in my survival. Dr. Kaur is truly an inspirational woman, and I'm forever grateful for everything she's done for my family and me.

A Diverse Triple Medley
— Anjali, Alex and Andrew

*I*t's been two decades since our big surprise when your dad announced, "My wife is expecting triplets." It was a lovely prospect for our associate neonatologist to be having firsthand experience of expecting multiples, but we were anxious, too. Your mommy took great care of you and kept you in till thirty-six weeks. You boys were very considerate, to come in at the planned time and say, "Ladies first," allowing your sister to take the lead.

I took care of you, Anjali, and our colleague, Dr. Lebischak, took care of Alex, and then again I was there for Andrew. Things went well, and all three of you were placed in a row of beds among the "not-so-sick" infants.

I've had the privilege of remaining connected with you and your family over the years. You have done well in school, excelling in swimming, athletics, and ice hockey. I wish you all the best as you pursue your college careers—Anjali in psychology, Alex in biology, and Andrew in business. You were never three peas in a pod, but had diverse personalities to start with, so I'm certainly not surprised that you all have chosen different career paths.

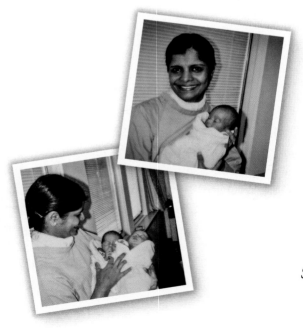

Triple Joy

Two decades ago, in an alluring spring,
Three little sweethearts did the April showers bring.
Anjali, a quiet sweet leader, led the trio,
As the rowdy duo followed in tow.
Alex and Andrew, you were a cute sight,
As your ultimate positions you sought to right.
You have brought oodles of joy, and much ado,
To your mom, dad, and Asha, your sweet sister, too.
Swimming and ice hockey are sports but a few,
That you've excelled in and studied anew.
As you spread your wings in a world so wide,
Seek truth and goodness, as towards success you stride.
God bless!
—Manjeet Kaur

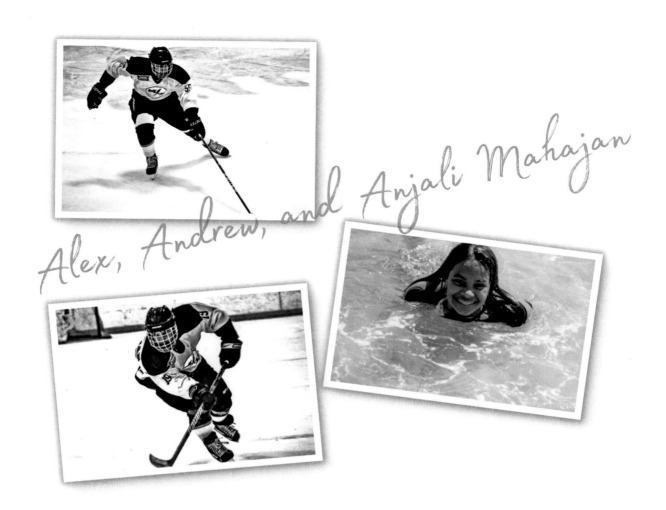

Alex, Andrew, and Anjali Mahajan

Parents:	Suzanne and Anand
Date of birth:	4/14/1995
Birth weight – Alex:	4 pounds 13 ounces
Birth weight – Andrew:	4 pounds 11 ounces
Birth weight – Anjali:	4 pounds 10 ounces
Medical conditions:	Prematurity, triplets
Gestational age:	36 weeks
Hospitalization dates:	4/14/1995–4/25/1995

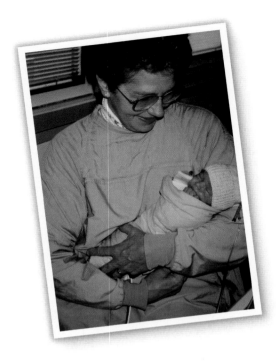
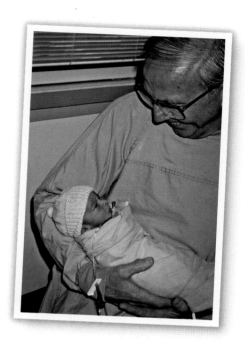
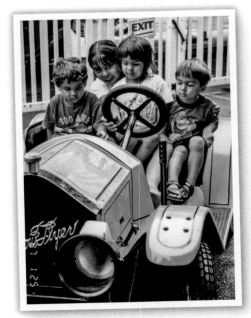
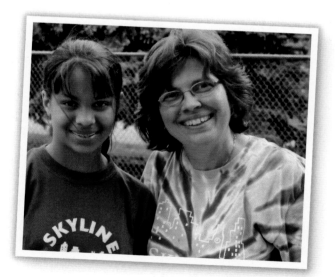

Suzanne and Anand's Story

All three of our babies were born healthy. What a blessing and what a joy that we had enough time and energy to care for and provide for all of them. Dad is a neonatologist, so we felt fully confident in the NICU. The babies received great care there, which was the answer to our many prayers.

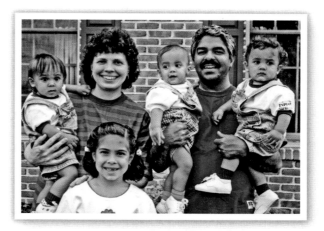

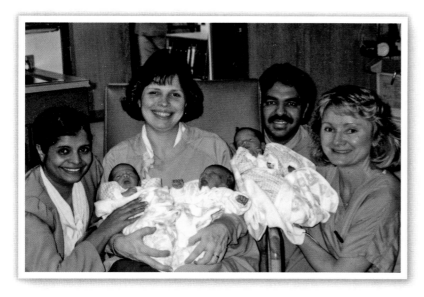

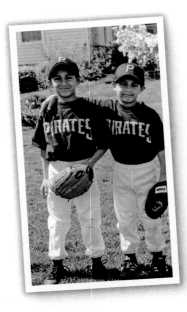

Andrew —"I love having
a brother to play with."

Alex —"We're always
there for each other."

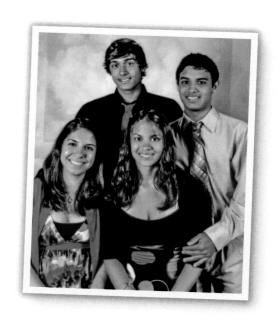

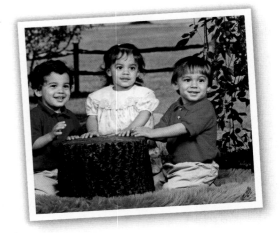

Anjali—"It's so much fun
to share a birthday."

Mom's mother helped care for the triplets' five-year-old sister. Our families were a great support, and friends helped too. Breastfeeding three babies was a challenge, but proved to be quite successful. Keeping a notebook handy to jot down important milestones was especially helpful while the triplets were under the age of two. They began to show more individualism and independence at three to four years old, though they loved to mirror each other.

They developed the typical sibling relationship—best friends one day, worst enemies another day. Each enjoyed having an older sibling and playmate as they grew up, and Asha was delighted to have a younger sister and two brothers.

All three have completed their sophomore years of college and will begin their junior years in the fall. Their bond can be seen clearly now that they're in college and are away from one another for brief intervals.

When, in a new class or club, each is asked separately, "Tell us something unique about yourself," the first statement is always "I'm a triplet!"

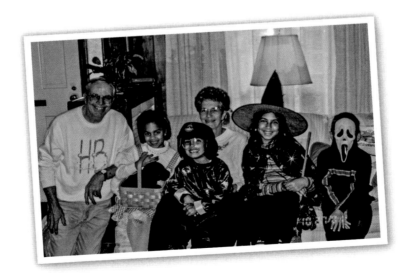

Little Footsteps — Mighty Imprints — Adam

As I write your story, the years roll back to when I first met your parents. Like others before them, your mom and dad were very anxious. Being highly educated, they were well informed, even though the early 1990s was the pre-Internet era—if we can imagine such a time today!

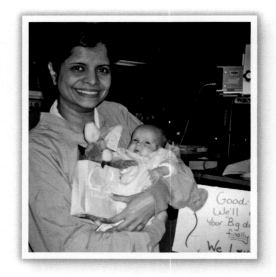

The next four months were the usual roller-coaster ride we often talk about. Our NICU family connection, however, continued after your discharge. I remember photos, reunions, and you and your family at our house at Christmas parties. In the rather relaxed HIPAA privacy protocol of those days, we proudly displayed our NICU Grads' photos, sent by each family, on our bulletin board. That was a great boon to other little ones' parents, who delighted in seeing such testimonials—especially about our preemies—and often spoke of the comfort it brought them.

Over the years, Adam, I've been in touch with your mom, received updates, and have seen you at NICU reunions or seen photos from time to time, celebrating the achievements of both you and your sister, Sarah. You can't imagine the immense pleasure it gives us all, and speaking for myself, it's been a special privilege to follow my little NICU godchildren through their life journeys.

A Son of Lancaster

If I close my eyes I see to this day,
Your mom and dad in the NICU bay.
Anxious, yet pleasant, absorbing the ambience anew,
Of alarms, beeps, and wires surrounding you.
Yet amidst all the clamor, Adam, you did pursue,
The tumultuous ride and came sailing through.
Now a graduate of Agricultural Mechanics—a true son of the soil,
May you achieve every ambition and grow in every way as you toil.
—Manjeet Kaur

Adam Mumman

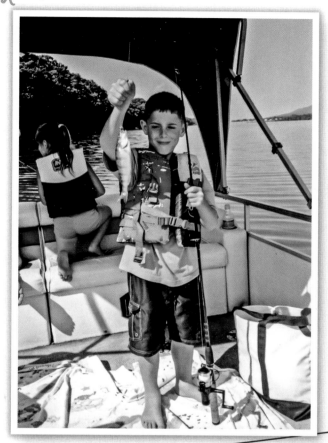

Parents: Sheri and Arlen
Date of birth: 11/9/1992
Birth weight: 1 pound 12 ounces
Medical conditions: Prematurity/respiratory
                            distress syndrome, apnea, and
                            bradycardia
Gestational age: 25 weeks
Hospitalization dates: 11/9/1992–3/9/1993

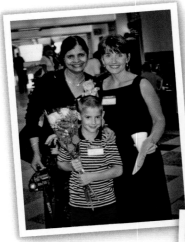

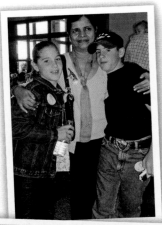

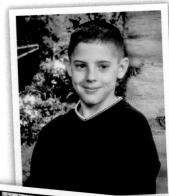

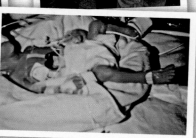

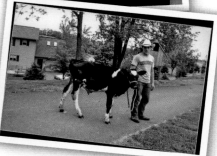

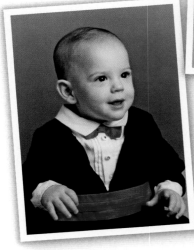

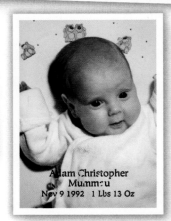

Adam Christopher
Mummau
Nov 9 1992   1 Lbs 13 Oz

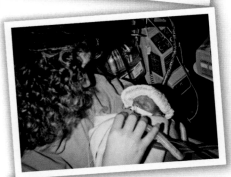

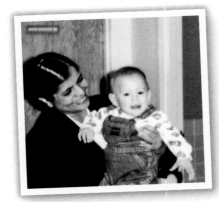

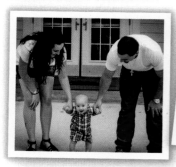

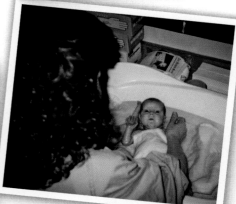

Sheri and Arlen's Story

Around the time of Adam's delivery, there was a maelstrom of emotions: we felt confused, frightened, sad, guilty, helpless, and woefully unprepared. The initial moments were all a blur; however, the excellent care from the doctors and nurses, the facility, and the education and information that they provided helped alleviate our fears.

My inability, as Adam's mother, to help him, hurt me deeply. I was sad that I couldn't be with him, but was relieved to know that he was at a place where excellent doctors and nurses could give him the specialized care his medical condition required.

We had little family support, and were pretty much on our own. I think most folks really have no clue as to what takes place in terms of baby care or the parents' emotions.

▷ My most precious memory of the NICU is the *Footsteps* book, especially the nurses' notes.

▷ Adam opened his eyes for the first time, November 14, 1992.

▷ Mom held him the first time, November 27, 1992.

▷ Breastfed him for the first time, January 22, 1993.

▷ Reached three pounds, January 26, 1993.

▷ First tub bath, January 28, 1993.

▷ Adam could breathe without the ventilator, January 8, 1993.

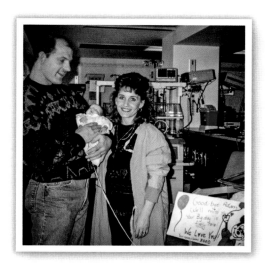

" There was a maelstrom of emotions: we felt confused, frightened, sad, guilty, helpless, and woefully unprepared.

> "I sat wondering if my son would live or die. I didn't know what to do, and I felt helpless, so I prayed and prayed that if only my son were allowed to live, I'd never ask anything of God again.
>
> God answered my prayers, and I've been faithful to my promise.

My most difficult times there were when Adam needed to be re-intubated when his oxygen-saturation levels dropped, and when blood gasses were done, requiring lots of needles and IVs—the one in his head bothered me the most! It was also tough when they gave us the statistical data on babies born Adam's size and what we might expect, but our faith and prayers uplifted us, since we, his parents, were so helpless otherwise.

Born at twenty-five-weeks gestation, Adam weighed just one pound twelve ounces and was thirteen and a quarter inches long. My pregnancy was stressful, as I'd experienced some bleeding. I was sick all weekend, and on Sunday evening, November 9, 1992, I went to St. Joseph Hospital in Lancaster, where I delivered my first child at 8:02 p.m.

When I arrived at the hospital, the women who checked me in were making popcorn, and I feared that I was going to have my baby before they finished the check-in process. On completion of the check-in, I was transferred to my room. Shortly after that, the doctors and nurses gave me some medication. Unfortunately, it was unsuccessful in stopping my contractions. I was then quickly taken to a delivery room, where Dr. Lebischak attended the delivery of our tiny baby boy, Adam Christopher Mummau—AKA Baby Boy Mummau—as labeled on his isolette in the NICU. (Ironically, I'd actually known Dr. Lebischak several years prior, as I taught her in an adult-education computer course.) As soon as I was wheeled into the delivery room, my water broke and Adam was born. He seemed to shoot from my womb into the arms of the delivery nurse. How tiny and dark he was—he looked like a bird that had fallen out of its nest. He made a little squealing noise because he couldn't cry, as his lungs were too weak.

He was too sick for me to hold him, but I was relieved to see that the nurses and the doctor were trying so diligently to help him. We were informed that once he was stable, he'd be transported to the NICU at LGH. I got a quick glimpse of him and was barely able to kiss his tiny hand prior to his departure. His first ride was in an ambulance, where only medical staff accompanied him. Adam's daddy drove to LGH to be with him and talk to his doctors, but I wasn't allowed to leave.

“The NICU became our home
every day for the next four months.

Being unable to go to the NICU with my husband and newborn was one of the worst nights of my life. Each time the telephone rang or a nurse came into the room, I was terrified of what news I'd hear. I sat wondering if my son would live or die. I didn't know what to do, and I felt helpless, so I prayed and prayed that if only my son were allowed to live, I'd never ask anything of God again. God answered my prayers, and I've been faithful to my promise.

The next morning, when I was discharged, Arlen and I went directly to the NICU to see Adam. He was very sick, but we were more hopeful, as he'd lived through the night. We saw this as his first big step toward survival. We knew we had a long journey ahead of us, but we felt comfort and strength in knowing that extremely knowledgeable and skilled doctors and nurses were caring for Adam. We knew that they were doing all they could to help him and us through our difficult journey, and we trusted them to guide us through it, regardless of the outcome.

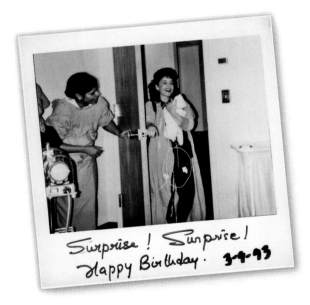

The NICU became our home every day for the next four months (i.e., Thanksgiving, Christmas, New Year's), as Adam remained there until his discharge on March 9, 1993— my thirtieth birthday.

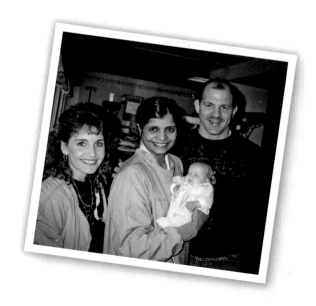

> "Adam truly is our miracle, and we're so thankful to everyone who took care of him in the NICU. … We are truly blessed.

My memories of this time are good ones, overall. Setbacks occurred, but what I remember the most are the good events. I remember the first time I saw Adam in the NICU, when his eyes opened a few days after he was born, and when I arrived at the NICU and was greeted by a sign on his isolette announcing that he had finally reached three pounds.

I recall the first time I held him with all his blankets, hat, tubes, etc., when I was able to breastfeed him instead of pumping milk into a bottle, which would later be fed to him through his tube, and when he finally got promoted to the "other side," where I could bathe him. I remember, too, when he was finally able to breathe on his own without a ventilator that supplied oxygen to his tiny lungs. But what I remember most, and for which I'm most thankful, is the excellent care he received in the NICU under the direction of Dr. Manjeet Kaur. The manner in which his doctors and nurses interacted and treated both Adam and us was amazing, and we'll be forever grateful.

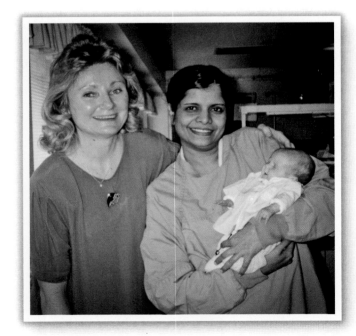

My best keepsake, which I'll treasure forever, is his *Footsteps* book. The detailed memories recorded in it are priceless, especially the note written at the end by his nurse Sandy:

Adam,

You're a very special boy. I really enjoyed taking care of you and watching you grow. I'm happy to see you go home, but sad because I'll miss you and your family. Stay healthy, Adam, and give Mommy, Daddy, and Jordan a hug for me every once in a while.

I love you,

XO, Nurse Sandy

Thanks to Sandy and Vicky; Drs. Manjeet Kaur, Carol Lebischak, and Anand Mahajan; and all of the nursing staff, Adam is a strong, healthy, happy young man who celebrated his twenty-second birthday in November.

In April 2014, he graduated from Montana State University-Northern with an associate degree in Agricultural Mechanics and Diesel Technology. A varsity member of the Montana State University Northern Rodeo Team, he enjoys hunting, fishing, horseback riding, and weightlifting. He and his wife plan to live in Montana, and they have a brand-new son, Stetson Luke Mummau.

I believe that much of who Adam is today can be attributed to his birth experience. Since his first breath, he's been a strong, independent, adventurous, and loving person. He's content with who he is and happy for what he has. He's patient and forgiving and has a high tolerance for pain. He's loyal to his friends and family, and his needs are small. Adam has taught me more about life than anyone else has: At a time when I felt weak, he taught me to be strong. As I watched him fight so hard to live, he reminded me to be patient and to have faith. He has taught me to see the glass half full and to be thankful for what I have. We witnessed many situations during Adam's stay in the NICU, and not all parents were as fortunate as we were. We got to take our baby home, and we don't take this blessing for granted. Adam truly is our miracle, and we're so thankful to everyone who took care of him in the NICU. Without them, and the grace of God, we wouldn't have our son and our grandson today. We are truly blessed.

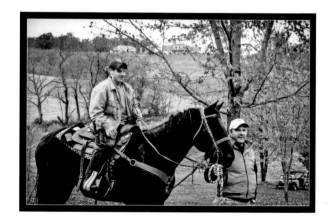

“Adam has taught me more about life than anyone else has:

At a time when I felt weak, he taught me to be strong. As I watched him fight so hard to live, he reminded me to be patient and to have faith. He has taught me to see the glass half full and to be thankful for what I have.

To Heal the World — Sarah

You, Sarah, were a relatively easy child. Your mom and dad were familiar with the NICU, and of course you were born at thirty-two weeks, which makes a great difference, i.e., fewer medical problems and a shorter NICU course.

When your mom called me regarding your high-school project and said that you wished to spend time shadowing me and learning more about the NICU, and that you wanted to become a neonatologist, I considered it a tribute to our NICU. This was certainly positive feedback about your family's medical experiences. I was happy and proud to introduce you as "one of my NICU graduates" whom I was helping realize her dream. Wouldn't it be wonderful if you became a neonatologist and worked at the same NICU where you and your brother were born? I might not be there that day, but my blessings will always be with you. I still have the framed photo you gave me at the completion of your project.

God bless you, my child! May you fulfill your dream!

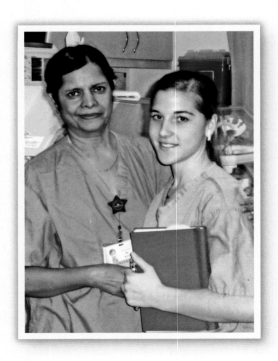

A Dream to Heal

A lovely little babe was born one September,
To visit the NICU, her brother's haven a past November.
A pretty rose, now a winsome young girl,
With thoughtful ways, a bright future to unfurl.
With passions and faith, a dream for tomorrow,
To help the ailing, to rid them of sorrow.
Your dreams, dear Sarah, do pursue,
Unique joy and fulfillment on this path await you.
Make this dream a labor of love so bold,
Color it with compassion and make kindness your stronghold.
—Manjeet Kaur

Sarah Mummau

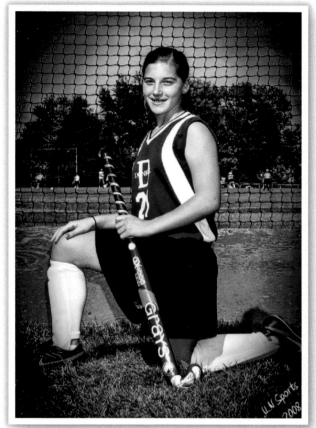

Parents:	Sheri and Arlen
Date of birth:	9/9/1994
Birth weight:	4 pounds 0 ounces
Medical conditions:	Prematurity, apnea, GE reflux
Gestational age:	32 weeks
Hospitalization dates:	9/9/1994–9/27/1994

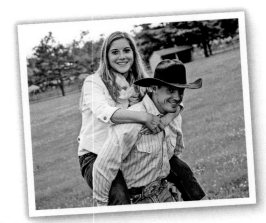

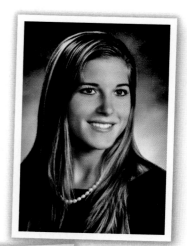

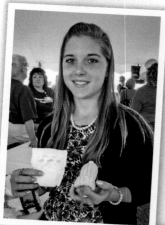

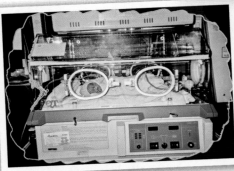

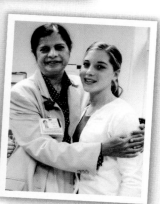

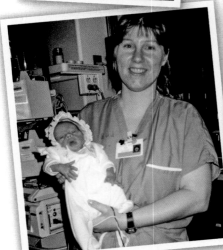

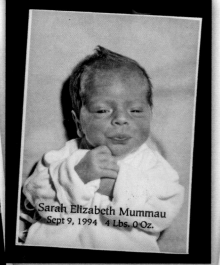

Sarah Elizabeth Mummau
Sept 9, 1994   4 Lbs. 0 Oz.

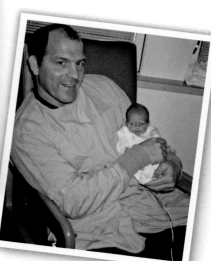

Sheri and Arlen's Story

At the time of Sarah's delivery, we both felt excited about having another child. The morning after I gave birth to Sarah, an obstetrician told me that I shouldn't have any more children. This caused me great anxiety, but our previous premature birth experience and the caring staff at the NICU were a great help in reducing our fears.

My most precious memory of the NICU is of being able to take care of Sarah's needs: holding, feeding, and bathing her.

It was difficult to manage the care of our older child while having a newborn in the NICU, **but our faith, which is an important part of our daily lives, sustains us through the highest and lowest times of our lives.**

I gave birth to my tiny baby girl, Sarah Elizabeth, twenty-one months after the birth of her micro-preemie brother, Adam. Having had a previous premature infant, mine was a high-risk pregnancy and was monitored closely. Being a teacher, I was off work during most of my second trimester, which was when I gave birth to Sarah's premature brother, but with the advent of the new school year, I returned to work in early September.

On the evening of Thursday, September 8, 1994, my husband, Arlen, and I had just finished our last prenatal class. I was feeling a lot of pressure as we were leaving, and shortly after our arrival home, my water broke. Thus, we left for Lancaster General less than twenty-four hours after our receiving a certificate of completion for the Expectant Parents' Class. The doctor delivered Sarah at 2:28 a.m. on Friday, September 9. Sarah was born at thirty-two-weeks gestation, weighed four pounds, and measured seventeen and three-quarter inches long. She had dark brown hair, and she was precious!

Our new baby spent the next eighteen days in the NICU under the care of Drs. Manjeet Kaur, Carol Lebischak, and Anand Mahajan; Nurse Sandy Riese; and the rest of the wonderful nursing staff. Sarah spent her days growing bigger and stronger. She received breast milk through her tube, and was eventually breastfed.

In addition to caring for her older brother, Arlen and I visited Sarah each day until her homecoming. During NICU visits, we enjoyed helping care for her, changing her diapers, and giving her a bath. In addition, we helped dress and feed her, and enjoyed talking and reading to her. Finally, on Tuesday, September 27, Sarah was discharged, and we brought our little girl home to meet her big brother, Adam.

Upon discharge, Sarah, like her brother, was adorned with an oxygen monitor. Its job was to observe Sarah's breathing and alert us in the event that she was too tired to breathe. A few weeks after her arrival home, I noticed that her breathing was becoming more labored each time she breastfed. I wasn't extremely alarmed, as I knew from previous experience that this is common for preemies; however, she didn't

> " My most precious memory of the NICU is of being able to take care of Sarah's needs: holding, feeding, and bathing her.

respond to my attempts to stimulate her during feeding. As her monitor continued to beep, indicating that her oxygen level was low, I became increasingly concerned. Sarah's normally pink lips were showing purple, so I called her pediatrician to schedule an appointment. Finally, Sarah was so unresponsive that I called her doctor and said we'd be arriving as soon as I could drive to the office. Upon Sarah's arrival, the medical staff quickly intubated her. Once stabilized, she was transported via ambulance to the hospital for further observation. After many tests Sarah was diagnosed with a silent reflux, was put on the prescription drug Reglan, and was discharged to return home once again.

At age nineteen, Sarah still has a sensitive stomach, but is otherwise very strong and healthy. She's an intelligent young woman who has scored "Advanced" on all standardized tests, achieved all A's in her elementary- and high-school career, and earned a score of five out of five on multiple advanced-placement exams. In elementary school, Sarah was diagnosed with dyslexia, so she must work harder and longer than many of her peers to achieve her goals. Nonetheless, she sets her goals high and works exceedingly hard. We're enormously blessed, as our daughter is an extremely motivated, morally conscious young woman—it was just like Sarah to make sure that she wasn't born prior to our receiving our Expectant Parents' Certificate!

Sarah continues to inspire everyone around her as she strives for excellence in all she pursues. She has always been a wonderful big sister and outstanding role model. She graduated in the top five of her high-school class, despite a rigorous schedule; was an officer for the National Honor Society and Student Council, a member of the Key Club, and a starter on the Donegal Field Hockey team.

Sarah's goal is to become a Neonatologist. She is now a premed student, at the University of Pittsburgh, one of the best premed programs in the nation. In addition, Sarah earned a four-year Air Force Reserve Officer Training Corp (AFROTC) scholarship. These highly sought, extremely competitive scholarships are awarded to students who demonstrate the ability to endure rigorous schedules and display excellent leadership qualities. Through the AFROTC program, Sarah is required to rise early, work hard physically and intellectually, and continue to meet specific grade requirements—despite the intense coursework required of premed students—in return for the financial benefits the program provides for its cadets.

Sarah aspires to help care for premature infants. It's an understatement to say that she has a long road ahead and will need a tremendous amount of support to achieve her goals. Her fate, however, is in God's hands, and we trust that He will continue to guide her as He has since her birth. We couldn't be prouder to have Sarah as our daughter, but more importantly, we're proud of the person she is. Despite her fragile beginning in the Lancaster General NICU, we're confident that, with God's grace and the support of her family and friends, Sarah will improve the lives of others and leave her fingerprint on our world and future generations.

> " I wasn't extremely alarmed, as I knew from previous experience that this is common for preemies.

Sarah's Story

Life is precious, and every newborn, regardless of gender, race, culture, or IQ is a miracle and a gift from God. It's astonishing when one takes time to think about all the knowledge and care a mother must put in during her pregnancy to help her baby undergo a healthy development while in the womb. The mother can only do her part, however, while biology and genetics are left to take care of the rest of the baby's development.

My fascination with neonatology began with the NICU graduates' party held by Lancaster General's Women and Babies Hospital. Attending the event was a yearly occurrence, something my siblings and I looked forward to each year, but it wasn't till late elementary school that I noticed the common theme among its attendees: we were all preemies or infants who had been ill and needed the highly specialized care the NICU staff provides for newborns. A light went on in my head, and I realized that my sister attended the event because she was a family member, and my friends didn't attend because they weren't NICU graduates. My brother and I were special!

I began to ask my mom about why Adam and I had required additional care. Also, I began to notice in some of our baby photos that my brother was very small, and his veins protruded more than those of other babies. In most of my baby photos, a box always sat next to me; I later learned that this was a ventilator, which helped me to breathe. These weren't the things my mom mentioned when she talked about neonatology. Instead, she talked about all the nurses and doctors who helped her little miracles survive. She told stories about how the nurses would make signs to go in our isolettes, and how caring and sensitive the doctors were about my parents' feelings and educated them on taking care of a NICU infant.

I decided in high school that I wanted to learn more about neonatology and the work of a neonatologist.

Dr. Kaur graciously took me under her wing and allowed me to shadow her in the NICU. During this time my love of neonatology grew even greater. I witnessed firsthand the great patience and understanding required of a neonatologist, one that can only be fueled by a passion. Dr. Kaur is the prototype of a neonatologist.

Today, heading into my sophomore year of college, I aspire to be a neonatologist. I hope one day I'll be able to demonstrate the same selfless kindness and love that Dr. Kaur did to my family and many other NICU families. I can't think of any better way to contribute to society. Were it not for the dedicated staff at Lancaster General's Women and Babies Hospital, my parents wouldn't have a son, and my sister and I wouldn't have had the opportunity to share our childhood with our older brother and look up to him as a role model. When I think of neonatology, I think of everything I value: life, selflessness, caring, families, children, passion, and, no doubt, faith.

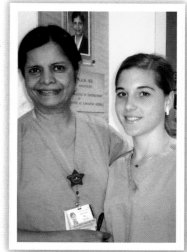

The Warrior and The Star

Ryan, I remember your stay in the NICU so vividly, perhaps more so since it engendered a continued connection with your mom. After your birth, your mom told me about choosing your name, and informed me that Wyatt (your middle name) meant "brave warrior." *How appropriate,* I thought. You sure gave us some scares, but our brave little warrior marched on, facing all the upheavals, and continues to do so.

It's been a great pleasure to know such a delightful family. I'm so glad you made it to the wedding of my son, Arun, now a pediatrician himself. The memory of dancing with a NICU graduate whom I cared for brings tears of joy, as I think about the frail little one in the NICU and the strong, handsome young man you are now.

Only recently I was at your wedding to the lovely daughter of our wonderful head nurse. A glorious day, a great celebration.

Such poignant memories!

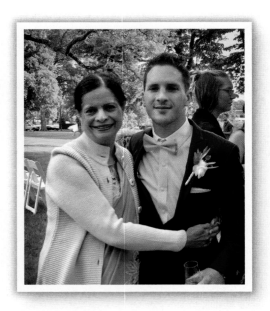

A Wyatt Story

A little baby, a frantic mom,
As nature did intervene on that morn,
A scrawny little soldier, did we greet,
Who had a cry real soft, yet so sweet.
As tubes he encountered, monitors and vents too,
He marched bravely on, without much ado!
A little king! A warrior in his glory!
That is our Ryan Wyatt's story!
An inspiration to your mom, we do surmise,
A new role to this nightingale, a new enterprise.
We love your achievements in medicine too
And rejoice for your upcoming nuptials, we do!
—Manjeet Kaur

— Ryan Wyatt and Alex

What a lovely little bundle you were, almost a year after your brother's birth. When I went to your mom's room, she said, "Oh, I'm not worried, Dr. Kaur. I know you'll take care of him." It was a very different feeling from the one before when Ryan was born. You had your little problems, but did well. After two children in the NICU, your mom decided she wanted to go into the nursing profession and take care of babies. What a wonderful salute to the nursing staff of the NICU. Becky now works in the nursery at WBH, and she's a great nurse. It's always such a pleasure to run into her at work and ask about Ryan Wyatt and Alex!

Alexander's Cove

A year after your brother's birth, Becky decided to renew
Her love for the NICU, the WBH rue.
She thus begot a little ethereal star,
Who from his brother was never far.
Hark! Within the year, the art of technology grew,
Very soon by divine grace, under the azure hue,
Alex, you were on your way home, bless you!
Let's celebrate your school and work evermore,
As the mazes of life you do explore.
Your mom is special, and serves to this day,
With dedicated love, keeping maladies at bay.
Ever remembering her two angels
—Gorgeous young men today!
—Manjeet Kaur

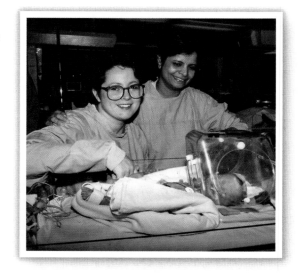

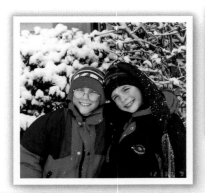
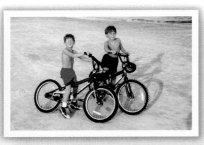
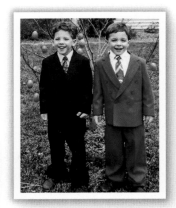
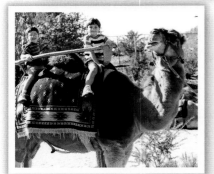
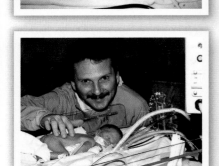
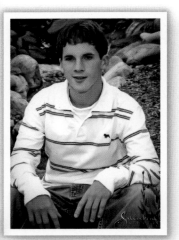
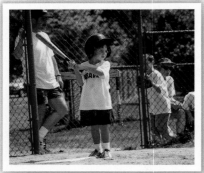
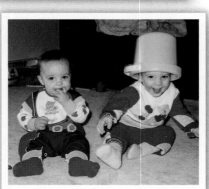
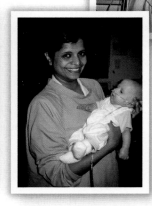

Ryan Wyatt and Alex de Lorraine

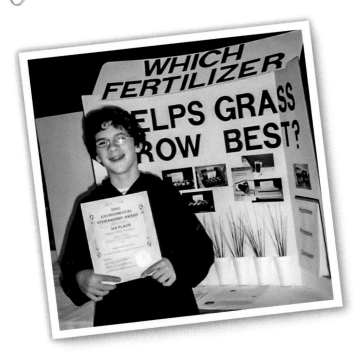

Parents:	Becky and Claude
Year of birth:	Ryan (1989); Alex (1990)
Birth weight – Ryan:	3 pounds 2 ounces
Birth weight – Alex:	4 pounds 12 ounces
Medical conditions:	Prematurity/Respiratory distress syndrome
Gestational age:	Ryan - 30 weeks; Alex - 32 weeks

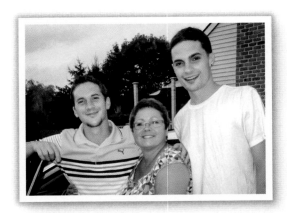

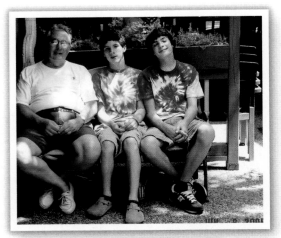

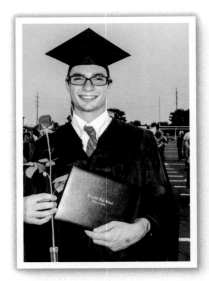

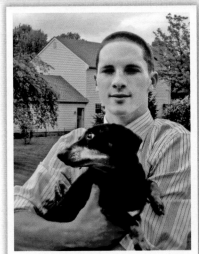

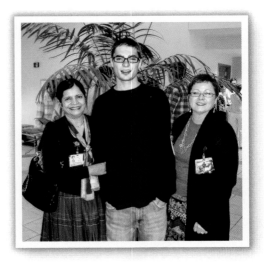

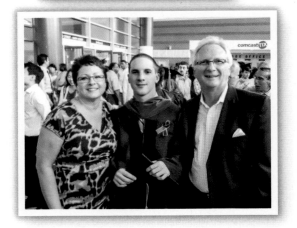

Becky and Claude's Story

My husband, Claude, and I first met Dr. Kaur in the delivery room at Lancaster General in 1989. I was about to deliver our son, and I was only thirty weeks pregnant. I was scared to death. We had lost our first son when I was six months pregnant, from what was misdiagnosed as appendicitis requiring emergency surgery. As it turned out, I had a degenerating tumor on my uterus that was eliciting the same symptoms as appendicitis. Our son was unable to survive the anesthesia, and is in the safe and loving hands of God now and watching over us.

I was monitored very closely during this pregnancy, and considered high risk. Much to our fear I went into labor at thirty weeks. I lay in the delivery room, terrified of losing another son. Dr. Kaur was on call in the NICU that night, and she was a blessing to us all. She arrived right before Ryan was delivered. They whisked him off to the NICU immediately. I was in a panic, hyperventilating and crying, worried about our three-pound two-ounce baby. Dr. Kaur was very calming, reassuring me that they would take very good care of him and I'd be able to see him shortly. They needed to get him stabilized and hooked up to monitors and a respirator to help him breathe, all of which was very foreign to Claude and me.

> "I was about to deliver our son, and I was only thirty weeks pregnant. I was scared to death.

> "I was blessed to be able to hold the life that was given to me, created out of the love of my husband and blessed by God.

"The first time I went [to the NICU] it was overwhelming.

The room was big, with maybe eight baby stations, each with monitors and machines, some of them sounding alarms.

I was terrified and worried about Ryan.

Claude got to see Ryan first, as I wasn't able to go to the NICU right away. The first time I went, it was overwhelming. The room was big, with maybe eight baby stations, each with monitors and machines, some of them sounding alarms. I was terrified and worried about Ryan.

When I first saw Ryan's little body, I cried and thanked God he was still with us. He had so many tubes and lines and monitors on him, and all I wanted to do was hold my baby. Unfortunately, that couldn't happen. Dr. Kaur was right there with me and told me what was going on with Ryan and what he needed. She explained that we could not stress his fragile body, and his need for oxygen, and the use of a machine to help him breathe. I wasn't able to hold him at this point, but could hold his hand and talk to him. I cherished every moment I could spend with him. On the eighth day of Ryan's life, I was able to actually hold him. I was afraid I'd hurt him. He was still intubated and hooked up to monitors, and all the equipment weighed more than his little body, but to hold him, if only for a few minutes, was the most amazing experience. I was blessed to be able to hold the life that was given to me, created out of the love of my husband and blessed by God.

Since Ryan was only thirty-weeks gestation, we'd thought we had ten more weeks to come up with a name for him, and we were now faced with the dilemma of what his name would be. Claude and I hadn't even begun to think of names. We started with the idea of one that would represent the strength he needed to pull through the fight ahead of him. Eventually, we chose Ryan Wyatt, which means king and brave warrior. We called him "little king–little warrior." We felt this name was very appropriate for the uphill battle he was undergoing. Dr. Kaur especially liked Wyatt, and teased us many times by calling him Wyatt Ryan. To this day, she still likes to call him Wyatt when she talks to him.

"Claude and I hadn't even begun to think of names.

The nurses who took care of Ryan were very caring, and spent time helping me understand what all the equipment was doing and why. It was comforting to know Ryan was being well taken care of by these wonderful nurses and doctors. Over the two and a half months Ryan was in the NICU I considered them my family. The day Ryan was finally able to go home, on monitors and oxygen, was incredible, but it was frightening because Claude and I were now on our own, just our family to watch over him. He was coming home on monitors and oxygen. Would we be up to the task? Thanking the staff for all the love and support they'd showed our son and all of us during this very scary time never seemed enough. We'd have never gotten through this time without them; they helped us feel competent when we left that we could handle whatever came. We were put to the test as soon as we walked in the door and laid Ryan down. Alarms started going off, and Ryan stopped breathing for a couple of seconds. Very calmly, I stimulated him; he remembered to breathe, and we were good to go. I thought, *Yeah, I can do this!*

Alex

Surprisingly enough, I was back in the hospital thirteen months later having our second son, Alex, who was only thirty-two-weeks gestation and weighing in at four pounds twelve ounces. This was a totally new and different experience. Dr. Kaur showed up in my hospital room again and, instead of being in a panic and hyperventilating, she brought a very calming feeling to me. I knew all was well when Dr. Kaur arrived. I could have this baby now, and everything will be fine. This baby is in great hands and will be loved and cared for like one of her own.

You might think Claude and I would've learned our lesson with Ryan being born early, and picked a name early in this pregnancy. I guess we'd hoped to carry full term, so again we had a baby with no name for a couple of days. We chose Alexander Christian, defender of mankind and follower of Christ, which we thought appropriate for the challenges ahead. His battle was a little different from his brother's. The year between their births had brought great advances in medicine and technology. Alex was given a new drug called surfactant, which helps the lungs mature. This is something that the body produces naturally, but can't produce enough this early. Alex was weaned off O_2 in the first week, where Ryan was on it for six months.

Walking into the NICU to see Alex for the first time was like coming home after a long trip, and I had no fear of all the equipment. I was much calmer and able to absorb the situation with better understanding. Alex did have some hurdles to overcome, such as jaundice, but I viewed it as a new learning experience instead of being a terrified new mother.

During the five months in the NICU with my two boys, I felt this was something I would like to do myself. When the boys were both in school, I went back to school to become a nurse. My months in the NICU, and the compassion and caring I experienced there, are why I am a nurse today.

When I started working as a nurse I was hired at Women and Babies Hospital, not in the NICU but in Couplet Care, working with postpartum moms and families. I enjoy having families whose babies are in the NICU, as I can relate to their situation and help them through their fears. While working, I'd see Dr. Kaur, who always asked about Ryan and Alex. I love her and think she's a remarkable doctor and caring person.

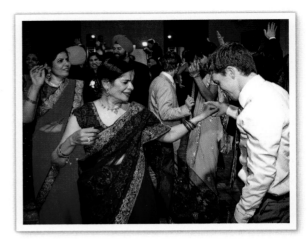

Twenty-six years later, Ryan happened to attend the wedding with us of one of Dr. Kaur's sons. It was so good to see Ryan and Dr. Kaur dance together, knowing she helped save his life and was there for him from the start.

Claude

After losing our first child, experiencing the births of Ryan and Alex was a blessing. The premature arrival of our first son, Ryan, was one of the happiest moments of our lives. Being premature brought on additional challenges and required persistence, faith, and reliance on Dr. Kaur and the medical expertise provided to us.

For the next three months, Becky and I visited the hospital daily to be near Ryan and let him feel our presence. Being born at three pounds two ounces, Ryan needed twenty-four-hour maintenance. Seeing him attached to all the monitors indicated the critical care he required. Ryan improved day by day, and after three months he was ready to be taken home. After his release from the hospital, Becky's family played an important role in Ryan's day-to-day care. Becky's grandmother, Nanny, drove from York to Lancaster

daily to help Becky. Her parents would come to the house in the evenings after work to help. We were so blessed and thankful to have family in the area to help us care for Ryan. As he matured, we noticed that he had a lazy eye, so we took him to Hershey Medical Center and started a program to correct his eye alignment. Ryan also had a condition called "rapid heart rate." No one knew when it would strike, and when it did, we'd have to turn him upside down until his too-rapid heartbeat slowed.

Ryan grew into a healthy person. He graduated from Hempfield High School in 2007, and was accepted by the University of Sciences in Philadelphia College of Pharmacy program, from which he graduated as a Doctor of Pharmacy in 2013. Looking back, Ryan has overcome many challenges, and has worked hard to be the person he is today. His survival all began with early intervention from Dr. Kaur and her staff, Becky's family, and our belief in God watching over Ryan.

Alexander Christian was born thirteen months after Ryan Wyatt. Alex, too, was born premature at four pounds twelve ounces. Though he weighed more at birth than Ryan, Alex had many medical challenges to overcome. Thanks to Dr. Kaur and her staff, Alex was released from the hospital after two months. Having two babies at home just thirteen months apart was like having twins. Becky had her hands full taking care of them. The daily support from her family was instrumental in Ryan and Alex getting the care they needed. The boys grew up together as best friends and playmates. Having them so close in age became an advantage in school-bus schedules, sports schedules, and various family activities. Alex excelled in a variety of sports. He graduated from Hempfield High School in 2009, was accepted at Shippensburg University, and is currently employed at Armstrong in Lancaster.

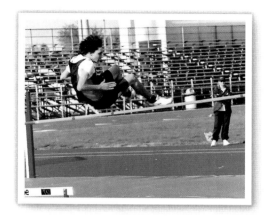

We took vacations together as an extended family with Becky's parents. It was important to Becky and me that Ryan and Alex have a solid relationship with their grandparents. To this day, the boys stay in frequent touch with them. Becky and I are blessed to have two great young adults who overcame premature birth. We're grateful to Dr. Kaur and her staff, our family, and our faith in God for helping us.

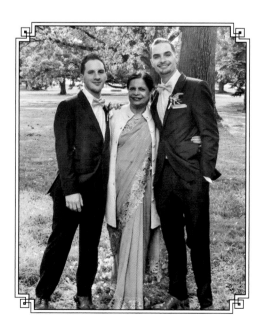

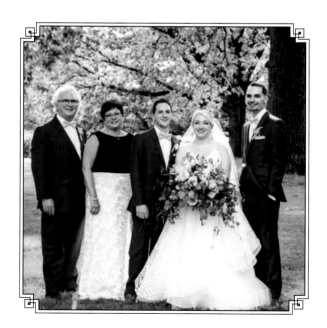

A "Big Cherub" — Bobby

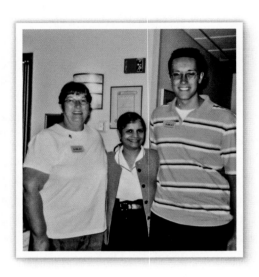

A Story of What Wasn't and Then Was

A sweet large cherub mama bore,
Long awaited in the days of yore.
A tough start! A rough gale
Awaited Bobby in this tale.
Who could predict in this time of woe,
Which way and how the winds would blow?
Yet this valiant soldier swept
All perils away when we met.
In a few weeks, with His blessings, to our delight,
You went home that winter, warm and bright.
A future musician, an athlete, a professor-to-be,
Who knew then, what the cards held for thee!
—Manjeet Kaur

*I*t is amazing, when facts of a few months ago have been forgotten, how I can actually replay events from years back on "my brain, my video" so vividly. I remember marveling at your size, Bobby, when you were transported to St. Joseph Hospital (now Lancaster Regional). At nearly twelve pounds, you were by far one of the largest babies that I had cared for, but unfortunately you were pretty sick with neonatal seizures amongst other things.

You were a big baby with meconium aspiration and seizures that were difficult to control initially. Besides using phenobarbital and Dilantin, which still remain the first-line treatment, I had to use a paraldehyde drip, a strong-smelling medication (not used much today), before the seizures could be controlled.

Your family was delightful to work with, though they were very anxious. It's such a joy to remain connected with families—every Christmas I received a card with a photo of "big little Bobby," a little older and a little taller. I remember your photos: as a toddler, school photos, one with a trumpet, another on a boat at a beach, and of course the favorite amusement park where you worked.

Another memory that definitely stands out—when I was buying my first laptop computer many years ago, I was approached by a polite, gentle, tall youth who seemed so familiar that I asked, "Are you Bobby Sharpe?" And of course you were! You were working part time at Circuit City. The acquisition of that computer was so special, sold to me by my NICU graduate, and I still have that laptop to this day.

Then you found a beautiful young woman, and we got a photo of your wedding and one of a cute little daughter. Thanks, Helen, for keeping me posted over the years. When we talk, it's not as physician and patient but as friends. What lovely memories.

Robert (Bob) Sharpe

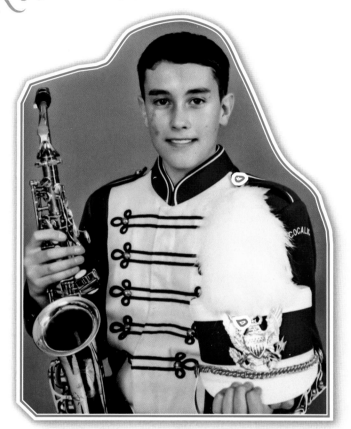

Parents:	Helen and George
Date of birth:	1/2/1985
Birth weight:	11 pounds 12 ounces
Medical conditions:	Meconium aspiration, neonatal seizures
Gestational age:	42 weeks
Hospitalization dates:	1/2/1985–1/14/1985

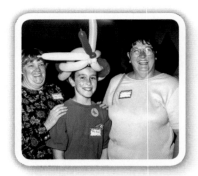

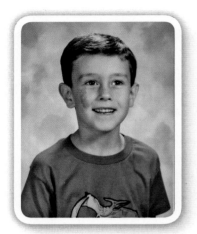

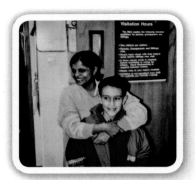

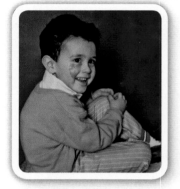

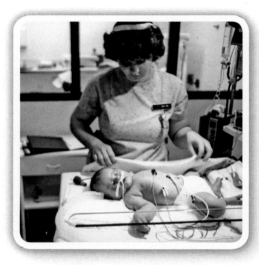

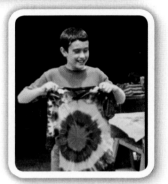

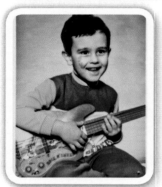

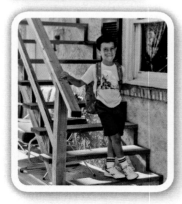

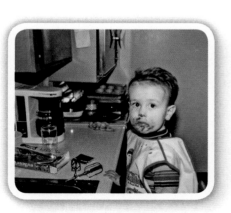

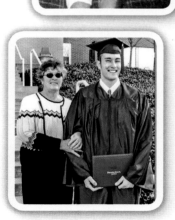

Helen and George's Story

How to put twenty-nine years on paper? When Bobby was born, we were happy beyond belief, though I wasn't certain whether I'd be a good mom, and my husband, George, was concerned about our ages. When we found out how sick Bobby was, it helped to know that a NICU had opened in Lancaster—otherwise they'd have transported him to Hershey. Nonetheless, after having waited nineteen years for a pregnancy, we were very worried about the possibility of losing our precious one, and were very fortunate to have the emotional support of our family.

After five years of marriage, we had tests done to find out why I hadn't gotten pregnant. Fourteen years later, never suspecting that a pregnancy could happen, I thought my nausea was due to flu. When I realized that wasn't the case, after getting over the initial shock, then happiness, worry, and other emotions took over.

I gained quite a lot of weight, but other than that the pregnancy was great. I was told our baby would be big. We never imagined he'd be eleven pounds twelve ounces, twenty-five inches long, and so beautiful.

I gave birth at St. Joseph Hospital. Bobby was very sick. Thank God, the new neonatal unit had opened at Lancaster General. They rushed him there, and I never got to see our son until four days later, which was also my first time to hold him in my arms. When I was released from St. Joe's, I could see and hold him. He looked at me with a little smile, as though to say, "Where have you been?" That's my fondest memory of the NICU. While in St. Joseph Hospital, Dr. Kaur sent me daily pictures of my sweet baby.

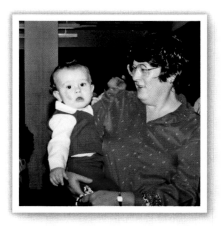

MK-2204-V01K.psd

> " We were very worried about the possibility of losing our precious one, and were very fortunate to have the emotional support of our family.

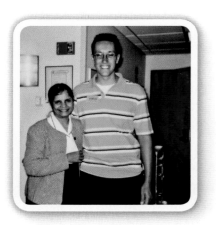
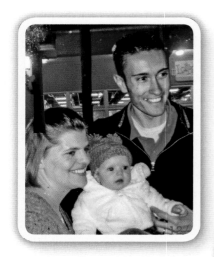
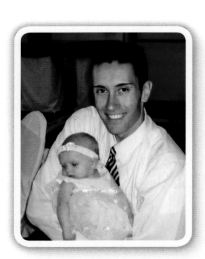
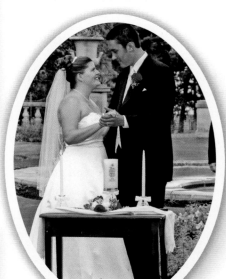
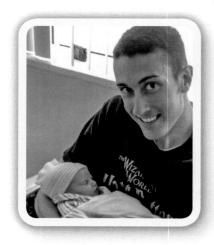
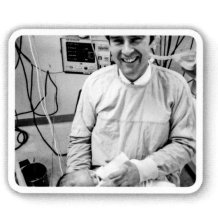
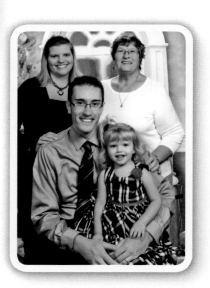

When I held him in my arms I was so happy I couldn't stop crying tears of joy. Bobby remained in the hospital for twelve days. It was hard to leave Bobby there and go home without him each day, even though we knew he was in good hands. Our trust in the Lord helped preserve our sanity. He then came home with a monitor that detected when he'd stop breathing. Despite his health problems, he grew to be a healthy, happy little boy who loved to hang out with his dad and play with his friends. Also, he loved swimming, picnics, boating, playing in the snow, and acting out movies he'd seen.

We had many happy and sad times, but the hardest was when George passed away. Bobby was only ten years old.

> *When I held him in my arms I was so happy I couldn't stop crying tears of joy.*

During Bobby's school years he tried soccer, basketball, football, choir (both church and school), playing saxophone, band (orchestral and marching), and computers. His interest always came back to music. He was in chorus and band, and in his junior/senior high-school years became a drum major, winning Best Drum Major at competition, and still plays the saxophone. At age fourteen he went to work for Dutch Wonderland, and his love for amusement parks continues to this day.

Bobby graduated from high school in 2003, went on to college, and graduated in 2006. While working at Dutch Wonderland he met his soulmate; they married in June 2006, and then moved to Florida, where Bobby worked at a Florida theme park. In 2010 he obtained a master's degree (the first in our family).

In June 2011, the birth of their first child, a beautiful daughter, added more sunshine to our lives. Also that year, Bobby began a journey of health and fitness. He lost seventy pounds with the P90X and Insanity workouts and now helps to inspire others. Bobby and Cristen now have another girl.

In 2012 he became a Professor of Business Ethics at University of Phoenix.

In 2014 Bobby participated in his first Spartan Race and, in April 2014, his second endurance race. I'm such a proud mom, and I know his dad would feel the same. I'll never forget George's face when I told him, "Yes, I'm pregnant," and how he beamed with the birth of our son—worried about Bobby's health, but a proud papa!

> *Our trust in the Lord helped preserve our sanity.*

Building the NICU He Was Born In — Ross

Ross, it was a wonderful surprise to meet you in the NICU a couple of years back. You introduced yourself and told me that your mother had asked you to look me up as I had taken care of you in the NICU many years ago. I was really gratified with that warm hug.

It certainly is one of the best parts of our profession as neonatologists—seeing these tiny, sick helpless infants grow into, as per potential, strong, intelligent, and talented young men and women. You were there for construction of the addition to the family wing of our neonatal intensive care unit at Women and Babies Hospital (WBH). What an irony—helping to build a wing in the same NICU you had been born in. Though we had moved from Lancaster General Hospital (LGH) on the sixth floor (where you were born) to WBH, the parent facility remained the same. The hospital staff were very excited, and the administration actually had us take a photograph together, which they posted in the LGH magazine as well as in the NICU.

You had been one of our very sick NICU babies, being sent for ECMO (extracorporeal membrane oxygenation), which back then was done only in limited facilities, and it seemed that, in some cases, the only way to oxygenate the lungs with persistent pulmonary hypertension was to bypass them. You were a feisty one, though, and up for a lot of bigger things. It warms my heart to see you now with your hockey stick while playing ice hockey. I remember the invitation your mom sent me for your wedding; she was planning to surprise you. Congratulations on your achievements and I hope you continue to have a fabulous life. Remember, when you come to any hardships in life, how you crossed so many hurdles in the NICU and that you are strong!

God bless.

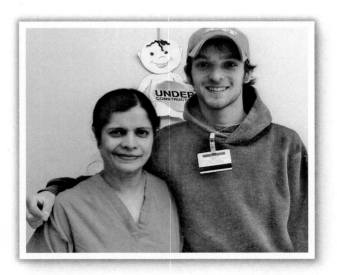

NICU to Ice Hockey

Years have gone by, yet memories remain strong,
Of a day when something went wrong.
A dream, a mist, a tangible song,
A story of a babe, 'tis hard to believe.
Destined for every skill to achieve
A play of hockey or a NICU tapestry to weave.
You have surpassed all hurdles, Ross,
As a brand-new dad, may you always toss
Every impediment, at every hill you cross.
—Manjeet Kaur

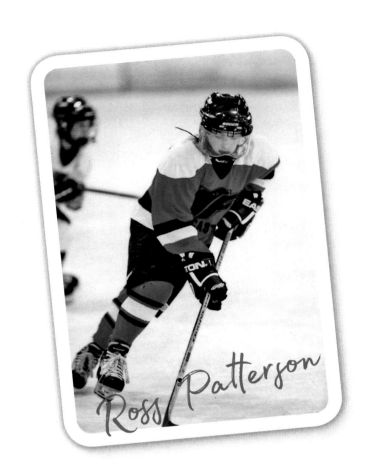

Ross Patterson

Parents:	Sue and Ron
Date of birth:	10/26/1987
Medical conditions:	Amniotic fluid aspiration, persistent pulmonary hypertension, pneumothorax
Gestational age:	40 weeks

> " What an irony—helping to build a wing in the same NICU you had been born in.

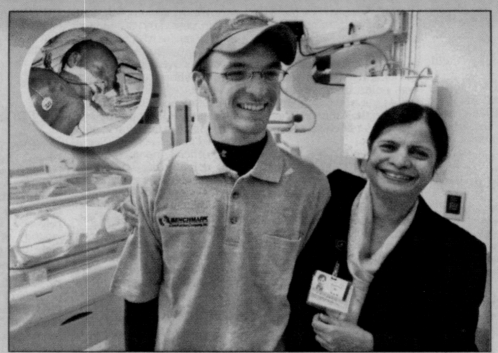

LANCASTER, PA, NEW ERA   FRIDAY, FEBRUARY 20, 2009

Carpenter has special bond to Women & Babies expansion

MARTY HEISEY / NEW ERA

Ross Patterson worked on the Lancaster General Women & Babies Hospital addition. Patterson was cared for in the neonatal intensive care unit at Lancaster General as a baby (inset), by Dr. Manjeet Kaur (right).

Refer page 53 for the full story

Sue and Ron's Story

Our son Ross was born on October 26th in 1987. After his cesarean delivery he developed persistent fetal circulation, which was caused by him possibly aspirating fluid. The attending nurses moved quickly to provide Ross with the appropriate care that he needed without alarming me and my wife Sue. We did realize that he needed care and would be put into the NICU. Sue and I were all too familiar with the NICU at Lancaster General Hospital, as they had saved our daughter Leslie and provided great care for her just three years earlier.

Although we knew Ross was having difficulty with his breathing we didn't realize the severity of the condition until later the next day. Sue was informed that his condition was poor. This news was devastating and caught us somewhat by surprise. I personally was trying not to come unraveled, having been through a similar situation with Leslie. Many questions raced through my mind as I drove to the hospital: How did we not realize that he was this sick? Did his condition worsen suddenly, or was it that critical all along? How do they treat this? The most important question I had was how bad was he, and would he survive?

My father was with me when we arrived at the NICU early that evening. Sue was unable to leave her bed having had surgery the day before and was relying on the doctors and nurses to keep her informed. She had been sedated after the surgery, and was feeling disconnected from Ross and everything that was taking place.

We first met with a resident doctor who tried to answer those important questions. The nurse who was on duty in the NICU that evening was a friend of ours. She was a calming presence and told us that Dr. Kaur would be able to fill us in on everything we needed to know. Dr. Kaur was very straightforward with explaining how grave Ross' condition was. This

"Dr. Kaur was very straightforward with explaining how grave Ross' condition was. This was very helpful to me. It enabled me to grasp how serious things were, and that there was a definitive plan to try to save him.

> **I now knew that we all were in another battle for life.**

was very helpful to me. It enabled me to grasp how serious things were, and that there was a definitive plan to try to save him. She told us his lungs were basically clogged with fluid and were unable to oxygenate the blood. Dr. Kaur then said Ross would need to be flown by helicopter to Georgetown University Hospital in Washington, DC to receive treatment on a relatively new machine called ECMO. The machine receives blood from one of the carotid arteries and oxygenates the blood. By bypassing the lungs during the process the lungs are given a chance to clear and heal.

I now knew that we all were in another battle for life. Ross was very sick and needed to be flown to Washington. There was another hurdle that evening: The weather was bad. Thunderstorms and high winds prevented any chance of a helicopter flight happening that night. All we could do was wait overnight and hope the weather cleared the next morning.

When morning came the skies were clear and a medical crew was dispatched from Georgetown to pick Ross up and take him back via helicopter. Sue was wheeled down to the NICU to watch Dr. Kaur and the nurses prepare Ross for his journey. This gave her some time to love him and nurture him.

Sue and I along with my father watched the helicopter arrive, and the crew came in and helped with preparation and consulted with Dr. Kaur. Suddenly there were alarms going off and the staff was rushing all around Ross' incubator. His lung had collapsed. Dr. Kaur quickly inserted a tube into his lung and saved him. The staff then was able to finish preparing Ross for the trip, and we all said goodbye as they wheeled him to the helicopter.

> **The chopper lifted off the pad. At that moment I felt alone and uncertain—uncertain and worried that I may not ever see my son again.**

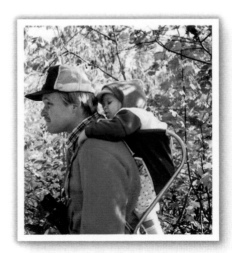

It was a beautiful late October morning as I stood near the helicopter pad outside the hospital. Tears filled my eyes as the chopper lifted off the pad and started to disappear around the corner of the building. At that moment I felt alone and uncertain—uncertain and worried that I may not ever see my son again.

My mother volunteered to accompany me to Georgetown and stay for a few days. Our daughter Leslie would be home with Sue's grandmother. Sue again was confined to Lancaster General, not being able to travel so soon after surgery.

Ross spent the next four days at Georgetown University Hospital. On the third day Sue was cleared to travel and my uncle drove her down to us. By the time she had arrived Ross had been sedated to help him rest and possibly recover faster. He was inactive since his arrival. When Sue walked over to him and started talking to him, he started to blow little air bubbles out beside his ventilator. That was one of the most touching moments I have ever witnessed. The bond between mother and child is amazing.

Miraculously, his lungs cleared up without the help of the ECMO. He was flown back to Lancaster General where he received excellent care from Dr. Kaur and her staff. They became like our extended family and shared in the joy of his continued improvement until he was sent home.

He certainly made up for the first month of inactivity in his life. As a toddler he was always on the go, didn't like to sleep, and kept us on our toes. He eventually played ice hockey for fifteen years and is an avid outdoorsman.

Now Ross is twenty-six years old. In 2011 he married his wife Melissa and they have a one-year-old son, Skyler. I know Ross doesn't remember any of what happened back then. We have told him that he had a lot of people praying for him, and those prayers were answered when he was blessed with the care of so many good doctors and nurses.

Thank you, Dr. Kaur!

> " *He had a lot of people praying for him, and those prayers were answered.*

2/24/2017

Born to Lofty Goals — Miles

This is a story about a strong young man who was born with "low platelets." Platelets are small cells in the blood that help with clotting, so one doesn't want them to get too low or there may be bleeding issues. Miles needed repeated platelet transfusions. We sent some special tests to Philadelphia, as they weren't done in Lancaster back in the 1980s.

I remember photos of Miles that his mom and dad sent, playing all kinds of contact sports, such as soccer. Many years later, I saw Miles—now an exceptionally tall young man—at our twenty-five-year NICU reunion, and his was one of the stories included in the newspaper's feature article about the event. It's been wonderful to connect with this lovely family.

Thanks for keeping in touch all these years. Good luck and God bless!

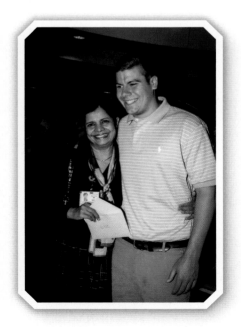

Salutations to a Captain

A winsome infant I was asked to greet,
His name was Miles, with platelets low,
Who would know that in two decades we'd meet?
A tall handsome man, always on the go,
A writer with a lofty goal, and a special song,
Keep that special zeal in life, every enterprise strong.
A soccer champion, a true sportsman, and a kind heart too,
Keep it up, Captain Harriger, salutations to you!
Our NICU kids are special, we say, both in actions and in name,
We hope to see your wish fulfilled as you make it to the Hall of Fame.
God bless.

—Manjeet Kaur

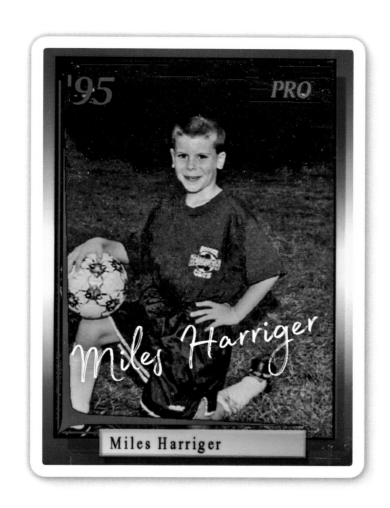

'95   PRO

Miles Harriger

Miles Harriger

Parents:	Julie and Joe
Date of birth:	1/18/1988
Medical conditions:	Thrombocytopenia (low platelets)
Gestational age:	Term
Hospitalization:	1988

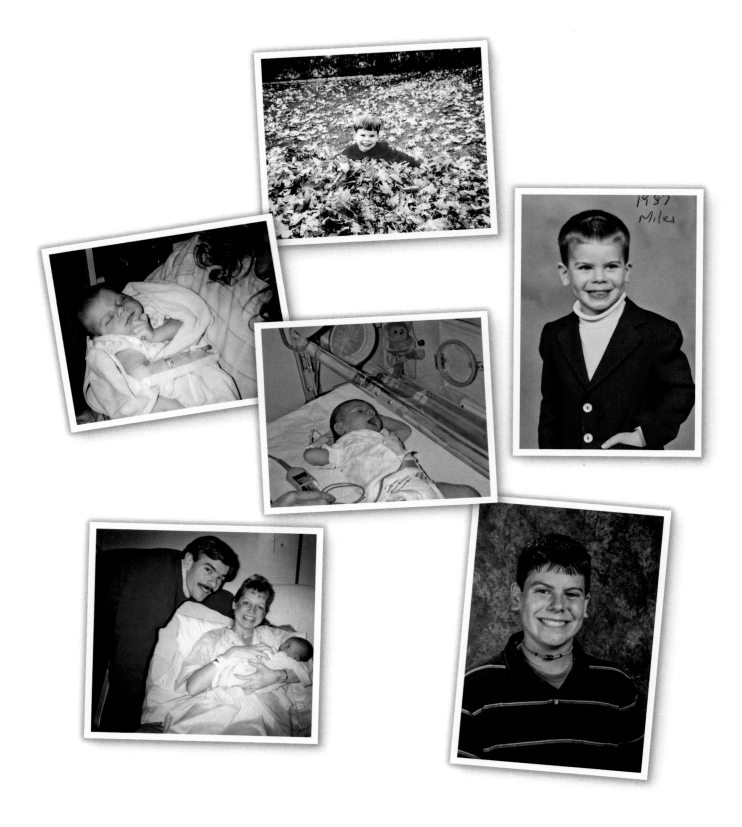

1987
Miles

Julie and Joe's Story

Miles was our first child. We were extremely excited to bring him into this world and have him be a part of our life journey. We received tremendous support from Dr. Kaur's team. The staff was empathetic, and our family and friends visited the hospital and called daily. I don't think I fully realized the value of that support until I got older. I cannot imagine going through such a difficult time alone.

We were very worried when we got word that Miles was being transferred to LGH from Regional (formerly known as St. Joseph Hospital). We were told the ride would be delicate, and that they needed to avoid bumpy roads: due to his low platelets, Miles could easily bruise, causing further complications. That was scary! It broke our hearts to know that he was going into the NICU and that we weren't going to leave the hospital with him. We didn't know how long he'd be there, and the uncertainty of his outcome compounded our fears.

> "It broke our hearts to know that he was going into the NICU and that we weren't going to leave the hospital with him.

Miles has no siblings, so we had no other children to care for. Julie and I were each other's rock. The situation was out of our control, and our lives grew stronger as those three weeks helped deepen our faith and our appreciation of LGH.

Julie: When I called the NICU early one morning, the nurses were drawing blood from Miles' heel, which was done multiple times daily. He was kicking and screaming, and I thought he was saying, "I am done with this and I'm going home." A few days later, he was released. That was my happiest memory of the NICU.

Joe: One of my most precious memories was seeing Julie sleeping with Miles and never leaving his side.

There was a twenty-four-hour period when Miles was most vulnerable. We were aware that he needed to make progress or suffer a major setback. That was extremely tough, but we never lost faith even in the most difficult times. Dr. Kaur's diagnosis was positive, and the staff did their job exceptionally well, monitoring Miles' platelet count and making certain they did everything possible to keep it moving in the right direction.

Miles has had no platelet-related health problems since his release from the hospital in 1988. His hobbies include soccer, basketball, and working out. He graduated from Hempfield High School in 2006 and Shippensburg University in 2010. While attending Shippensburg, he captained the men's soccer team to a PSAC championship for only the second time since 1975 and their first ever NCAA tournament bid. He received numerous awards, including Daktronics All American Status. He is employed in Baltimore, Maryland, and is a healthy six-foot one-inch man who hasn't had any serious health issues since the day he was released from LGH.

Note from Miles

To Dr. Manjeet Kaur,

I received your letter, and would be honored to help you with your book.

Writing comes pretty easy to me, but when you're writing to the person who saved your life it's hard to put into words how appreciative you truly are. I'm glad you reached out. Staying in touch with you has meant more and more to me over the years. It's important to remember the sacrifice that my parents, family, the NICU staff, and you made to keep me alive when I was a newborn.

I'd like to tell you a story of my biggest achievement. My college soccer career at Shippensburg University was rough. We were the worst team in the PSAC Conference every season. In my junior year we finished 1-15-4, which was not only the worst in the PSAC but also the worst in the history of the school. As team captain, I understood that things needed to change. Off the field, we started by improving our academics, focusing on better grades, more study-hall hours, and enforcing the no-drinking rules. We then moved onto the field with a week of conditioning before our preseason, dedicating time to watching film and longer practices. After coming off the worst season ever, in my senior year we started 2-5, then won thirteen

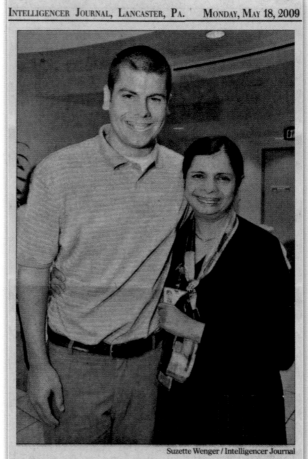

INTELLIGENCER JOURNAL, LANCASTER, PA.   MONDAY, MAY 18, 2009

Suzette Wenger / Intelligencer Journal

Dr. Manjeet Kaur, a neonatologist, stands with Miles Harringer, who as a baby was a patient at Lancaster General Hospital's Neonatal Intensive Care Unit, during a 25th anniversary celebration of the NICU.

> " When you're writing to the person who saved your life it's hard to put into words how appreciative you truly are.

games straight to win the first PSAC Championship since 1975. We won in a PK (penalty kick) shootout!

We received our school's first-ever bid to Nationals. I got the honors of All-American, First Team All PSAC, and the Academic Momentum Award for improving my GPA every semester. I hope someday to be inducted into the Hall of Fame. It was a good feeling to help change the culture of a program and impact the lives of so many teammates.

I've lived in Baltimore for the past three years. I work for an emergency notification company called Alertus Technologies. I help colleges and universities with plans to save lives. It feels good to work in an industry like yours. In my spare time I work out with a personal trainer. I keep active in sports leagues like soccer and kickball. Most importantly, I'm extremely

healthy. I picked up good eating habits from my mother.

I have a great relationship with my parents, whose support is the reason I'm so successful and happy today! You have impacted our family so much and it's something we'll always hold special. In my opinion, you are the reason we're so close—a reminder that we have to live every day to the fullest.

It was great to see you at the twenty-fifth NICU Reunion. If you need anything else from me, please let me know. I hope to see you again soon.

Sincerely,

Miles Harriger

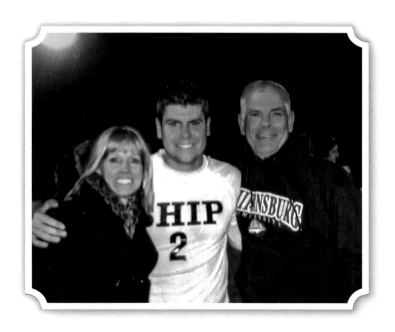

NICU Babies Having Babies — Chelsea

*C*helsea, you and your family have been wonderful in staying connected. You had a relatively benign course in the NICU. Obviously, you enjoy the medical field, coming back to work in the same hospital where you were born. The support and love of your family over the years have been great. They have kept me updated, and I remember you coming to our twenty-fifth reunion.

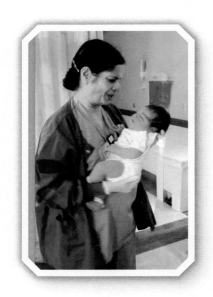

Then I met you again at the birth of your baby. I really enjoyed being at the birth of a NICU grad's baby. Events such as this are a special bonus of being in this field of medicine, and holding your little one was such a unique experience.

The Cycle of Life

Amazing is the cycle of life,
Babies having babies, of happiness and strife.
What lovely stories, what lovely tales
Beautiful sonnets, few awesome gales.
Of Life, of beauty, of rhetoric vales,
From the scenes of connection, a continuity hails.
Continue the work of healing in your specialty, too,
Remain connected, Chelsea, may God bless you!
—Manjeet Kaur

Chelsea Grove Workman

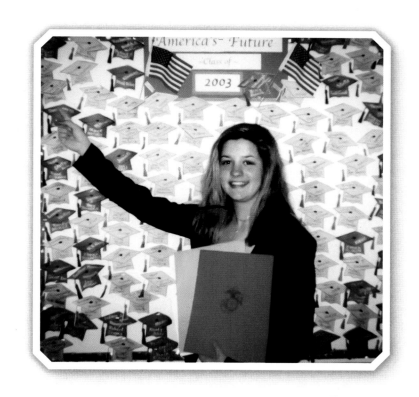

Parents:	Charlene and Michael
Date of birth:	9/25/1984
Birth weight:	8 pounds 12 ounces
Medical conditions:	Pneumonia
Gestational age:	Term

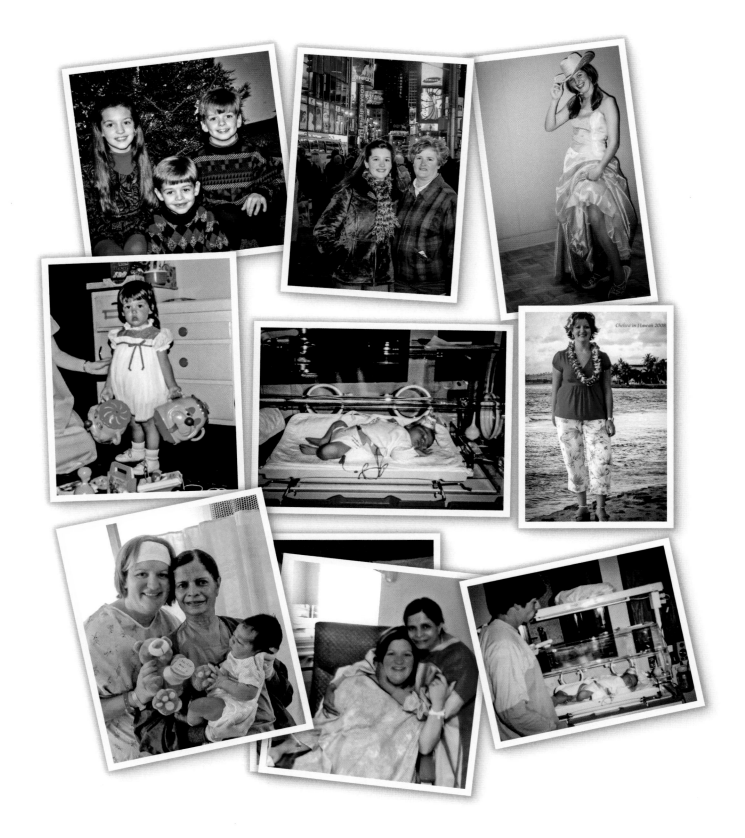

Chelsea in Hawaii 2008

Charlene and Michael's Story

Chelsea Lynd Grove was born on September 25, 1984, at Lancaster General Hospital. She weighed eight pounds twelve ounces and was twenty-one and a half inches long. After her birth, Chelsea was taken to the NICU and was placed under the care of Dr. Manjeet Kaur. This was surprising to us, because we thought all NICU babies were tiny and premature, and Chelsea was certainly not in this category.

Chelsea was our firstborn, and this was a brand-new experience. Eventually we learned that due to Charlene's long labor, Chelsea was born with bacteria around her eyes, nose, and mouth, thus requiring special care that only a NICU could provide. Fortunately for Chelsea, as well as for us, the NICU had just opened in the beginning of September 1984. This expedited Chelsea's care and made it easier for our family to participate.

All kinds of emotions arise when having your first child. The anticipation of having a healthy baby was foremost in our minds. We looked forward to the joy and pride that come with having a child to cherish and foster. Chelsea was also the first grandchild and great-grandchild on her father's side, and her grandparents and great-grandparents anxiously awaited her arrival, so it was a large extended family.

Our experience with the NICU was both hopeful and scary. We were most grateful that our little girl didn't have to be transported to another facility.

Charlene had fallen down twice the week prior to Chelsea's birth and had sustained a broken tailbone, which would've made it very difficult for her to travel back and forth to see Chelsea in another hospital. Charlene was allowed to stay at Lancaster General as long as Chelsea needed to stay in the NICU.

> " Our experience with the NICU was both hopeful and scary.

Chelsea had to stay there for seven days. Because she was jaundiced, she was placed in an incubator, and she was also hooked to an IV for administration of antibiotics to clear up the bacterial condition. It was first put in her foot, but after a few days it was placed in her head. This was unpleasant, because Chelsea was born with a beautiful head of dark hair and they had to shave it, first on the side near her temple, and eventually on the other side too.

Seeing all the apparatus needed for babies to have a chance at life was the most difficult thing. There was that fear of the unknown. We just expected beautiful babies and warm, fuzzy blankets everywhere.

"There was that fear of the unknown.

We just expected beautiful babies and warm, fuzzy blankets everywhere.

While our situation was difficult for us, the experience with the NICU was very enlightening. At around the same time as our daughter, twins were born who weighed a little over a pound each. They were so small and hooked up to far more lifelines than Chelsea was. It was unbelievable that they could survive, but we've learned that they both did!

"Family support is crucial during any new birth, especially when a child has medical needs.

Family support is crucial during any new birth, especially when a child has medical needs. We were most fortunate in having abundant family support and encouragement. Our faith also played a major role in our lives. We prayed for our daughter's health and healing. We prayed for wisdom for the doctors to make the best decisions while caring for our child. We prayed that the equipment needed for her care would not fail. We prayed that the skills the entire staff needed to run the NICU would suffice in such a new unit.

Due to cold symptoms, Chelsea had three back-to-back visits to the doctor, and one return to the hospital for dehydration. With that re-admission to the hospital, we made many more decisions about her continuing care, and we believe this was what changed the course of Chelsea's health for the rest of her life as well as that of her two brothers to come.

Chelsea's childhood was normal and healthy. She was a very good student, and participated in athletics. While in elementary school, Chelsea learned to play T-ball and then softball. Her favorite position was catcher. She also learned how to play the flute. In junior high, Chelsea tried the cross-country team and then track, where she also ran the long-distance events. She continued to play the flute, joined show choir, and continued to play softball with the local athletic association too.

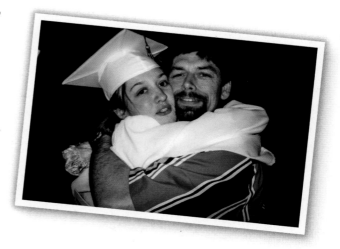

> *Our faith also played a major role in our lives, and we were most fortunate in having abundant family support and encouragement.*

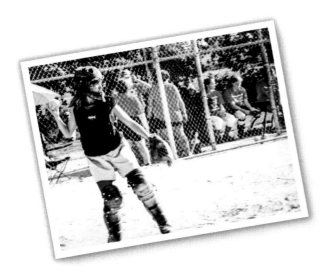

Chelsea also did well in high school, where she was a member of the Music Club, and the girls' softball and basketball teams. As part of the Music Club, Chelsea played flute in the concert band and marching band. She sang in the choir, and learned to play the piccolo and eventually the bassoon for orchestra. An outstanding scholar, Chelsea was inducted into the National Honor Society. She received varsity letters in both softball and basketball, and was named Female Athlete of her graduating class.

Within two weeks of starting kindergarten, Chelsea had decided that she wanted to be a teacher. She was always a very helpful older sister to her two younger brothers, Michael and Seth. She also loved helping with other little children, whether at church or in our neighborhood. Chelsea started babysitting the neighbor children when she was twelve.

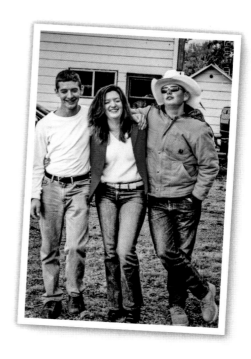

While in high school, Chelsea took a child development class, which was a key factor in leading her to her career as a Certified Surgical Technologist. The child development class required a visit to a NICU at a local hospital in Harrisburg, Pennsylvania. After visiting there with her class, Chelsea was so inspired that she wanted to become a NICU nurse. Her next step was a health-careers course at the local Lancaster County Career and Technology Center during her senior year in high school.

Chelsea was a healthy child growing up, but she did have a couple of medical setbacks. During the summer between her junior and senior years of high school, Chelsea's nose was broken during a church-league softball game. She finished playing the game after a brief break. The doctor recommended surgery, but only after Chelsea was done playing softball for the season. Chelsea's nose was straightened, but that was only the beginning of what was to come. After examining her nose, the doctor—an ear, nose, and throat specialist—found a lump in Chelsea's neck. It was an enlarged thyroid gland, and he told her that once her nose was healed he would take care of it.

Chelsea had surgery over Christmas break 2002. This may have seemed like terrible timing to most, but Chelsea had perfect attendance in high school and didn't want to ruin her record. After surgery, Chelsea was diagnosed with thyroid cancer on December 31. This was devastating for our beautiful young lady. Surgery had left a scar on her neck, and a second surgery was going to interfere with her perfect attendance. She went through weight loss, radioactive iodine treatment, and a full body scan. We were amazed at her resilience and strength through all of it. Chelsea graduated from high school with honors in June 2003. After a checkup in the spring of 2013, we can report that she has been cancer free for ten years. We are blessed.

After high-school graduation, Chelsea entered a two-year program to get her Associate Degree in Nursing. We later learned, however, that the school she attended was not accredited at the time. In January 2006, she became a Patient-Care Assistant at Lancaster General, where she found that she really enjoyed the personal interactions with people.

That spring, Chelsea applied to the same school to take the Surgical Technology Program, and was thrilled to learn that the school was now a certified college. Thinking that this program would lead to an actual associate degree, she could then move to another college to complete her nursing degree. Well, Chelsea loved the surgical tech program so much that, after getting her degree in August 2007, she took a position at LGH. This job truly fit her like a glove. In December 2007, Chelsea passed her certification exam, becoming a Certified Surgical Technologist. Ever since, she has been employed at the same hospital where she started her somewhat fragile life.

> " Ever since, she has been employed at the same hospital where she started her somewhat fragile life.

On family vacations, Chelsea has traveled all over the United States, visiting every continental state by the time she graduated from high school, which was her personal goal. She has been on a mission trip to Jordan and vacationed in Hawaii with her cousin Trista. Chelsea continues to play slow-pitch softball in a local church league, and has served in the church nursery for many years. She also enjoys watching NASCAR, football, and baseball, and likes country music and line dancing.

In 2008, Chelsea bought her first new car, a Ford Mustang. In 2009, she purchased her first home. Chelsea traded in her first Mustang to get a brand-new one in 2013, this time with the "pony package." Her favorite number is thirteen, and on July 13, 2013, Chelsea was married to Jesse at 1300 hours. They had their first child in July 2014.

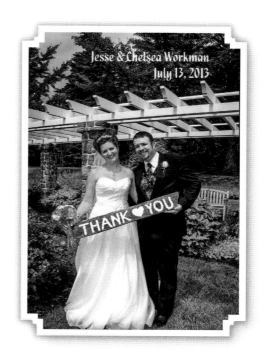

We're so proud of our daughter and her achievements. Our wish for any family who experiences that unexpected circumstance and finds their baby in the NICU is to know that there's unending hope for all newborns that find their way into a NICU today. May you take comfort from our daughter's story, and find blessings in life's small miracles. We will always be grateful to Dr. Kaur and the staff who took care of our daughter. Thank you and best wishes to all!

Here's to the NICU, which is celebrating thirty years with Lancaster General. We are glad you came!

> "Our wish for any family who experiences that unexpected circumstance and finds their baby in the NICU is to know that there's unending hope for all newborns that find their way into a NICU today. May you take comfort from our daughter's story, and find blessings in life's small miracles.

A Pale, Little Narcissus — Little Mandy

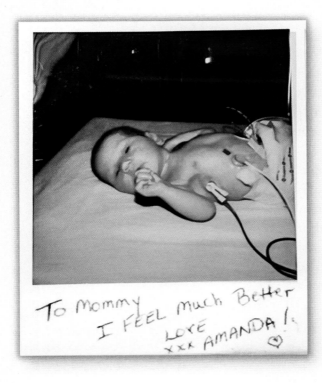

To Mommy I FEEL much Better LOVE xxx AMANDA !

*I*t was great to recapture the story of your birth with your family, Amanda; a family of one baby with severe anemia and one who required an exchange transfusion. It didn't end there though, as your daughter was in the NICU as well. You certainly are a NICU family in the truest sense.

I often tell the residents that it's most rewarding to treat a baby with severe anemia like yours. With optimal support and treatment, complete recovery occurs within days. Thus the "Kool-Aid blood" baby was soon ready to go home.

Good luck with your young ones!

Kool-Aid Mandy

A heartwarming story of a lovely young lady,
A Kool-Aid blood baby, a very pale Mandy.
Now a mother herself, able to relate
To her own little progeny, her saga of fate,
How precious blood was pumped into that lily so white,
Had only fair Narcissus had the ethereal fluid to right,
The ancient Greek legend would be sung differently too,
Had the god Apollo healed his floral crew!
The cycle of life goes on, behold
As the saga of Mandy's little angel now unfolds.
—Manjeet Kaur

258

Amanda Miller

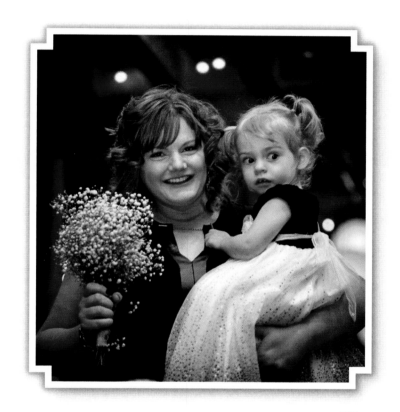

Parents:	Theresa and Steve
Date of birth:	7/11/1986
Birth weight:	6 pounds 4 ounces
Medical conditions:	Severe anemia
Gestational age:	39 weeks
Hospitalization dates:	7/11/1986–7/17/1986

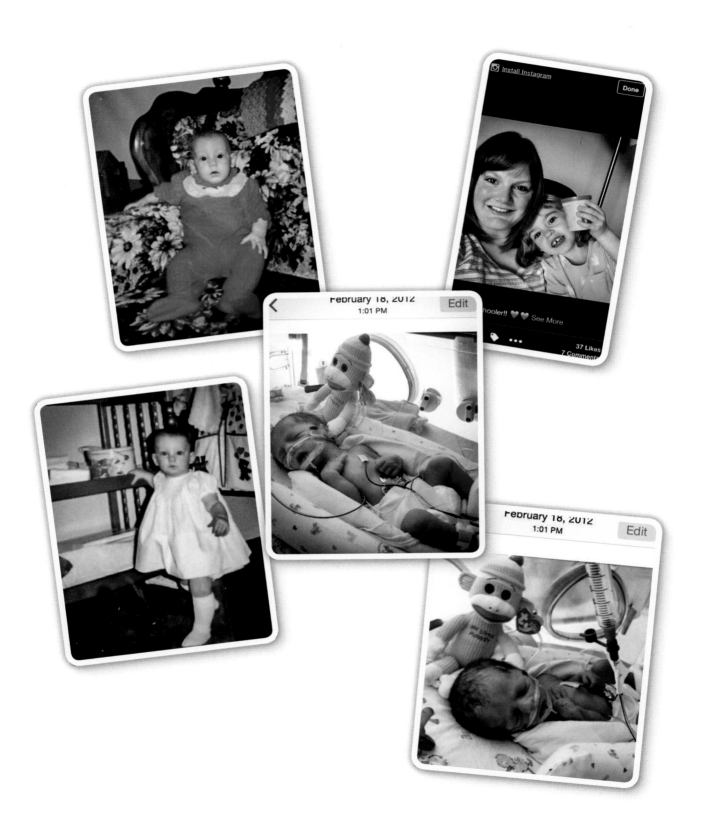

February 18, 2012
1:01 PM   Edit

February 18, 2012
1:01 PM   Edit

Install Instagram   Done

37 Likes
7 Comments

Theresa and Steve's Story

My wife and I were expecting our first child in the summer of 1986. It was Friday, July 11th, and Theresa was in labor at the former St. Joseph Hospital. Everything was going smoothly, and all signs pointed toward a normal, natural delivery. Being old-fashioned, we chose not to learn the gender beforehand. Like all new parents, our only concern was that he or she be born healthy.

Early that afternoon, the obstetrician saw something on the monitor that he didn't like. Shortly thereafter, Theresa was wheeled into the OR for an emergency C-section. When our daughter, Amanda Marie, was lifted from the womb, she was pale and lifeless. The doctor and nurses tried to reassure us by saying that she had all her fingers and toes; however, we sensed something was wrong. St. Joseph didn't have a neonatal unit at that time, so after Theresa was allowed to briefly touch our firstborn, Mandy was transferred by ambulance to Lancaster General. We had our share of anxiety and fear, but it was reassuring to know she was going to an excellent facility where she'd be well cared for by NICU physicians.

Because of her severe anemia, hospital personnel nicknamed Mandy "the orange Kool-Aid blood baby." Multiple transfusions were required to save her life. The blood supply was low at the time, so frozen units had to be quickly thawed. I spent the next several days traveling between hospitals to visit my wife and daughter. Our prayers were answered, and after a weeklong stay in the NICU, Mandy was able to go home without any long-term effects.

> " When our daughter was lifted from the womb, she was pale and lifeless.

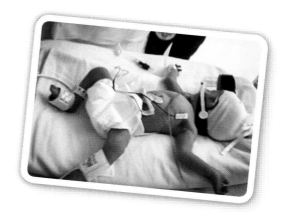

" Today, Mandy is a perfectly healthy thirty-year-old with three children of her own.

We had a second occasion to use the services of LGH NICU and physicians when my wife was pregnant with our son Matthew. Theresa had an amniocentesis every week for six weeks to monitor the baby's bilirubin levels, and because his levels were too high, Matthew was born at thirty-seven weeks. This resulted in his having to receive a blood exchange, also performed by a LGH NICU physician at St. Joseph, which was the first one performed at that hospital. Having used their services seven years earlier, we had full trust and faith in the NICU physicians. They were very thorough and always took the time to answer our questions.

There is another twist to this story; when Mandy was pregnant with her first child, her husband was serving in the United States Army and was stationed at Fort Hood, Texas. In mid-February 2012, they drove home to Lancaster County for a baby shower, arriving in the early-morning hours. Mandy's due date wasn't till April, and she anticipated giving birth at an army hospital in Texas. Later that evening, she developed a severe headache and vomiting, and her husband, Todd, and I took her to Lancaster General. The doctors recognized the symptoms of preeclampsia (a serious pregnancy condition marked by high blood pressure), and Mandy was transported by ambulance to Women and Babies Hospital. Out of concern for the health of the mother as well as the baby, Samantha was delivered by C-section nine weeks premature. She weighed just three pounds, and spent the next five weeks in the NICU at WBH. My wife and I visited our granddaughter there many times, and have high praise for the doctors and nurses. We felt very fortunate to have such a top-notch facility just minutes from our home.

In the hallway outside the NICU is a plaque recognizing Dr. Manjeet Kaur for her contributions to neonatology. Dr. Kaur was in charge of the NICU at Lancaster General some twenty-nine years prior, and my wife and I credit her with saving Mandy's life.

Today, in 2017, Mandy is a perfectly healthy thirty-year-old with three children of her own: Samantha, age five; Christopher, age four; and Sadie, born this past January and four months old.

Benevolent Bliss

My boat is drifting in mundane waters,
Onwards towards the whirlpool of oblivion.
Take me ashore to thy kingdom O' Lord!
Grant me the strength, perception and virtue,
To recognize that light, the benevolent bliss,
That can only shine through you!
When the covenant I meet and keep O' Lord!
—Manjeet Kaur

Born to Heal — Rebecca

Rebecca, my child, your story grew in importance as you yourself became part of the medical profession, a nurse, and from all the input I've received, a super RN, as our expectations of a NICU graduate would be.

Your NICU course was a relatively benign one compared to some, being post-term with meconium, but the NICU family connection has remained strong. I've seen you at reunions and met your parents off and on. The last meeting was at our twenty-five-year NICU reunion where you were featured in the paper as well.

It was a proud moment to see my NICU godchild graduate as an RN. Thanks, Mr. and Mrs. Sauder, for keeping me updated about her progress over the years. What a coincidence that one of the first people you met was an Indian doctor, and your husband, Aashish, is from India as well—a lovely universal connection!

Congratulations, Rebecca—you're a great role model for our future NICU Grads.

God bless!

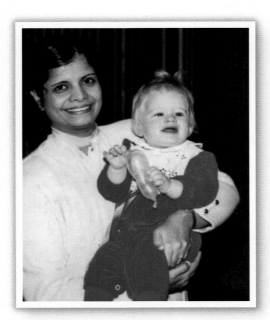

To a Lady with a Lamp

The true art of healing
Is the nature of nurturing.
The sweetness of caring
Makes pain worth bearing.
When the battles get rough
And the day is tough.
Remember, Rebecca,
Rolling hills are easy, mountain peaks are steep,
The brooks can frolic, but the ocean is deep.
Climb that mountain, sail that ocean
Bearing gifts of patience and a freight of compassion.
But lastly, unconditional love brings solace
A true gift, a spiritual grace!
—Manjeet Kaur

Rebecca Sauder

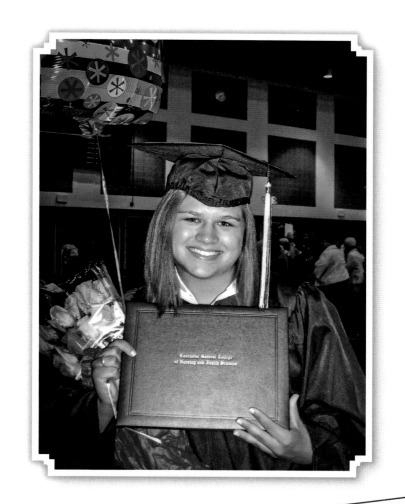

Parents:	Twila and Don
Date of birth:	1/16/1989
Birth weight:	6 pounds 0 ounces
Medical conditions:	Meconium staining/pneumothorax; Apgar scores: 1 at birth, 7 at 3 minutes
Gestational age:	42 weeks
Hospitalization dates:	1/16/1989–1/24/1989

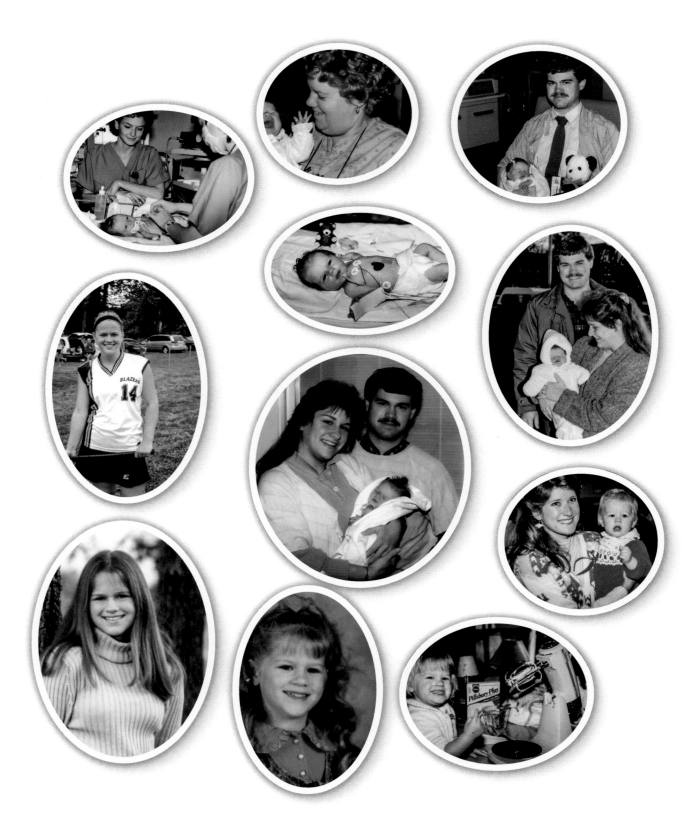

Twila and Don's Story

Our baby was sixteen days late, and we were so eager for her arrival. When, during labor, her heart rate dropped and they took me stat for C-section, we were somewhat afraid, but so thankful that everyone moved so fast. Dr. Kaur's sweet, kind way of relating helped, as did good communication and the gentle care of the nurses. Rebecca was taken to the NICU right away, and were it not for their care, we probably wouldn't have our Rebecca. Also, we felt strongly supported by grandparents and family praying for Rebecca's safe delivery and healing. We're very thankful to everyone.

Our most difficult time in the NICU was when we heard that Rebecca's oxygen was at the highest level and wasn't stabilizing, and could see our dear little one but couldn't hold her. My favorite memory is of when we were finally able to hold Rebecca for the first time at two days of age.

Our family and our church family played a huge role in praying for Rebecca and us. The first time my parents came in, they laid their hands over Becca and prayed for healing and God's peace. That gave us hope.

"We felt strongly supported by grandparents and family praying for Rebecca's safe delivery and healing. We're very thankful to everyone.

INTELLIGENCER JOURNAL, Lancaster, Pa., Monday, May 18, 2009

Marking a 'miracle'

Lancaster General's Neonatal Intensive Care Unit celebrates its 25th anniversary

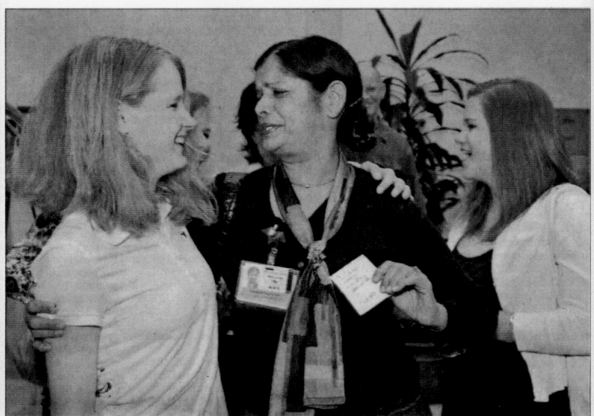

Suzette Wegner / Intelligencer Journal

Dr. Manjeet Kaur, who founded Lancaster General Hospital's Neonatal Intensive Care Unit in 1984, speaks Sunday with 13-year-old Jacqueline Hynes of Lancaster, a NICU graduate, during a 25th anniversary celebration at Women & Babies Hospital. At right is Rebecca Sauder, 20, of Mount Joy, also a NICU graduate and a recent nursing school graduate.

Twila's Story

As I look back twenty-five years, I remember that our Rebecca Lynn Sauder's due date was January 1, 1989. This baby was to be the first grandchild on both sides of the family, and everyone was thinking she might be born around Christmas. But Christmas came and went, and so did New Year's Day. We were eager for this birth. Being a week late, I'd wake up most mornings feeling sad that I hadn't gone into labor the night before.

On January 14th, when Becca was two weeks overdue, contractions began around 10:00 p.m. and were regular for several hours. We called the doctor, who told us to come in. We got to the hospital around 3:45 a.m. on the fifteenth. I was so glad to be going to have our baby! To my disappointment I wasn't even dilated any more than I was at the doctor's visit a few days ago. I had more contractions, was in the hospital for a few more hours, and then the contractions all but stopped. They did a non-stress test, and the doctor came in and told us that the baby appeared to be healthy and that we should head home till labor intensified. I was in tears as we left around 9:30 a.m. We were so discouraged. I slept a few hours and then woke to more contractions, which got stronger that evening; we waited till we knew they weren't letting up.

We went to the hospital that night and they monitored the baby and me as my labor intensified. Our baby's heart rate changed more than was normal with each contraction. I was dilating some, but not progressing as they would have liked. The doctor decided to break my water, and when he did they discovered meconium in the fluid, which meant Rebecca had had her first bowel movement in utero. She was showing signs of distress with each contraction, and around 11:50 p.m. the doctor said, "Prepare her for a stat C-section."

I remember everyone quickly unhooking me from stuff in the room and then rushing the whole bed and me to the OR. They told my husband, Don, to wait outside. He waved to me, and I was soon unconscious. The team moved very quickly, and at midnight Rebecca Lynn Sauder was born; she weighed six pounds and was nineteen and a half inches long. Her Apgar score at birth was one at one minute, but within three minutes it was a seven, thanks to the quick, efficient work of the doctors and nurses. As an LPN I know the seriousness of such a low Apgar score.

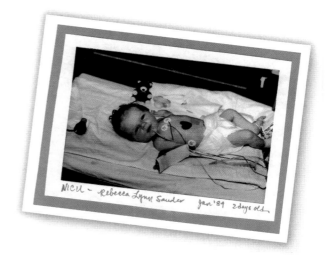

NICU ~ Rebecca Lynn Sauder Jan '89 2 days old

As I came out of the anesthesia in recovery, I heard the nurses talking about a baby girl and Don's voice saying, "Rebecca Lynn." *We had a little girl,* I thought, but wasn't "with it" enough to speak right away. I'd sensed during my pregnancy we were having a boy, so it was a surprise to hear girl. "How is she?" I was finally able to ask. Don said, "She has a lot of dark hair, and I got to see them working with her for a while. She's in good hands in the NICU and is on oxygen."

"So many people are praying for her and that's why she's doing so wonderfully.

Even though Becca needed special care, I felt an overwhelming sense of peace. I was eager to see her, but needed to wait till I was out of the recovery room. I remember them wheeling me to see her; she was so beautiful, perfect round face with a head full of dark hair. I so wanted to hold her, but she needed to be in the isolette with tubes and monitors. The nurses reassured us they'd care for her and we could call any time. Having just had surgery, I needed to get to my room and rest. I remember thinking, *God is so good. We have our dear little Rebecca, and she's in good hands.*

This is some of what I wrote in my journal during the days after Rebecca was born:

January 17, 9:45 p.m.: Lord, I just love Rebecca so much! Don and I had a beautiful time with her this eve. Les and Pam came, and Rich and Bonnie too. We visited awhile with them and they got to see Rebecca from the doorway. So many people are praying for her and that's why she's doing so wonderfully. Her oxygen level is down to 42 percent—and to think yesterday she was on 100 percent. Don and I sat and talked and stroked her from 8:30–9:30 this eve, and we laid hands on her and prayed for her. She is in your hands, Lord. Thanks for guiding the hands of the nurses as they care for her. You have done great things, whereof we are glad!

January 18, 8:45 p.m.: This evening we held our beautiful daughter for the first time … such a beautiful experience! Tears of joy.

January 20: I awoke at 5:10 this morning, pumped my milk, and thought, *I should just take it over to Rebecca and see her.* I'm so glad I did; I got to change her diaper and then hold her for an hour and a half! She was awake, and I fed her nasogastric tube (a tube placed from her nose to her stomach for feeds) and then sang her to sleep. It felt so wonderful! Becca's off oxygen, and her saturation level was ninety-four and above the whole time I held her. Thank you, Lord, for the wonderful way you are caring for her.

Looking back, I remember how well the nurses showed me how to care for Rebecca and always explained what they were doing. Dr. Kaur, with her sweet, gentle voice when talking about Becca, made us feel secure in knowing she was in the best of care. I remember how hard it was to leave her at the hospital when I was discharged to go home. I was glad I was healing well, but wanted our baby home too. I was so glad for the nurses who told us to call anytime. I called in the next morning after we had gotten home and wrote this in my journal:

"I so wanted to hold her, but she needed to be in the isolette with tubes and monitors.

Sunday a.m.: I am so happy—I just called in to check on Rebecca and was so encouraged. Marian is her nurse again; I'm glad. She said Becca likes to eat every three hours instead of every four. They ran out of my breast milk again and gave her formula, which she spit up. I'm so glad she handles my milk best. Today she starts her twelve-hour pneumogram test at 3:00, and if her heart monitor doesn't go off and her breathing doesn't stop for more than twenty seconds, she'll be able to come home without a monitor. Rebecca is wonderful, Lord. We are so blessed. Our prayer is that you'll be near her during this test and she'll have a perfect score. Thanks, Jesus. We love you.

Rebecca came home January 24 at eight days old. What a happy day! She did need to wear a monitor, and we got adjusted to making sure it was hooked up correctly. She did pretty well with it. It went off a few times, but often when we didn't connect it properly. After a few weeks she no longer needed her monitor. Praise to God.

Rebecca has been a healthy, happy child and full of joy in life. She began walking at eight and a half months, and would walk under the table.

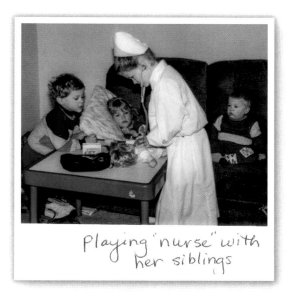

Playing "nurse" with her siblings

Rebecca was eighteen months old when her sister, Melissa Joy, joined our family. They are good friends to this day. Rebecca also has two brothers who were born by the time she was six: Jason Daniel when she had just turned four, and Jonathan David when she was in kindergarten.

Rebecca went to Kraybill Mennonite School from kindergarten through eighth grade. In middle school she enjoyed playing soccer, basketball, and field hockey. In high school at Lancaster Mennonite she played varsity field hockey all four years. She was chosen the Rotary Club's Student of the Month during her junior year.

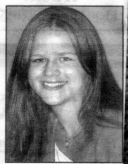

Rotary Club Honors Sauder

Rebecca Sauder was chosen as Student of the Month in March for Lancaster Mennonite High School by the Paradise Rotary Club.

Rebecca, daughter of Don and Twila Sauder of Mount Joy, is a junior at Lancaster Mennonite High School. Rebecca is a member of the National Honor Society and PALS (Peer Assistance Leaders). She is on the varsity field hockey team and was named a first team All-Star Player.

Rebecca sings in Campus Chorale at her school and helps lead the weekly Bible study. Rebecca is co-president of her church youth group at East Petersburg Mennonite Church, where she also teaches Children's Church and sings on a worship team. Rebecca was honored at the Paradise Rotary Club monthly lunch meeting in March.

Rebecca Sauder

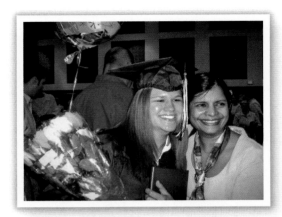

Rebecca went to Lancaster College of Nursing and graduated in 2009. Dr. Kaur and her husband even came to Rebecca's nursing-school graduation! She's been working at LGH as a Registered Nurse since then.

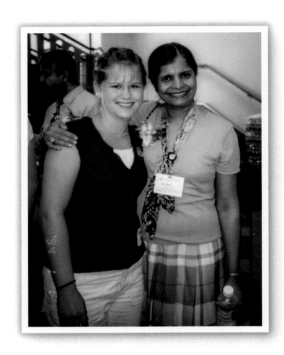

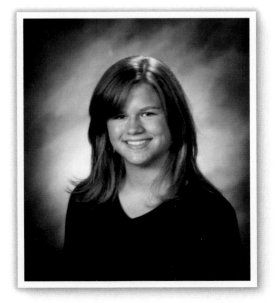

She's also a Junior Girl Leader at her East Petersburg Mennonite Church. Rebecca loves life and shines Jesus' love and light to all she meets. Many people have told her she is a wonderful nurse.

We are so grateful to God for the wonderful care of the nurses and all the staff at LGH, and especially the NICU staff who helped Rebecca as a newborn. It was so important we were where the best medical care was available, or Rebecca might not have survived. I can't imagine life without her. She is such a delight to her family and those who know her. Jesus' love radiates through her life!

Rebecca married Aashish in 2014. She is currently working as an infection control nurse at Lancaster General.

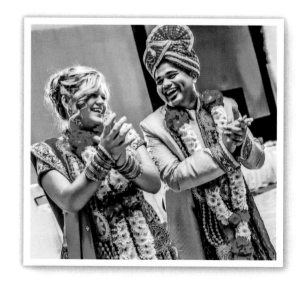

A Mother's Lament — A Farewell

Can one ever forget,
That tender gift,
An interlude so brief?
A cherub so sweet,
That gentle kiss,
Of lips so pale,
Frail tiny arms …
Unable to face the gale.
Anger and anguish,
A sheer pain so deep,
Helpless to part, yet powerless to keep.
Unable to unfurl
That bud so bold!
Had a sacred covenant with the Lord to uphold!
Those tiny feet trudge a path forlorn,
Through a milky way
To a starry morn.
Little Flora, you shall now adorn,
A heavenly abode, an angel reborn.
Thy gentle touch! Thy memories I'll keep,
Of a brief interlude, so precious, so sweet
An encounter so short, yet so sublime
Tiny footprints on the sand of time,
Adieu, my little angel, adieu, adieu, adieu!

—Manjeet Kaur

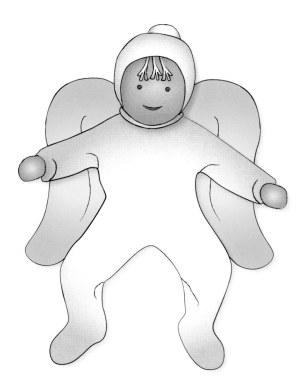

The glory of life is real, but the memories of the tiny buds that could not bloom certainly remain very precious. Many a time, we need to bow to the inevitable, knowing that there is nothing more medical technology can do. We sit teary-eyed with families, holding their hands at this difficult time.

Walking alongside family members with empathy and love brings about not only some ease in acceptance of the inevitable of this brief interlude but also helps to create memories that can be lovingly remembered over the years.

In the following pages, Mary Ann Wolpert and Carolanne Hauck have written beautifully about their experiences providing fantastic support for bereaved families.

Miracles of the Heart

A NICU Nurse's Reflections on the Death of an Infant

Miracles happen every day in the NICU. It's a blessed place to work and care for others. The tiniest, most premature babies survive, and some of the sickest receive treatments or surgeries that make them well.

Being a NICU nurse is the best job in the world; it's the happiest place on earth to practice nursing. It can also be the saddest, most heart-wrenching place to work, because sometimes the hoped-for miracle doesn't happen and a sick or too-small baby dies.

Within a very short time, tiny, precious babies, so fresh from heaven, arrive in this world, both elating and breaking the hearts of those who love them so much. To have seen, held, and hoped for the life of an infant and then give it up to death is a journey of deepest emotion. It seems a paradox of life.

Sometimes people ask me, especially in difficult situations with infants or loved ones, "How can you do what you do? How can you work in a NICU where there's so much loss and pain every day?" For some reason that only God knows, which is sowed deep in my core, my answer is "How can I not?" It's what I was born for, and is what so many of my devoted NICU colleagues were born for. It's a sisterhood and brotherhood of taking care of the tiny ones, the fragile ones, the most vulnerable. It's not a calling for the fainthearted, but at the same time it demands the softest of hearts and a true willingness to be open to, and molded by, the mysteries of life and death.

That statement, however, is a philosophical one, and not at all what the reality of losing an infant looks like in the everyday life of the NICU. If I could sum up the guiding words for all of us who must bear witness to the pain parents experience when their beloved, longed-for baby dies, it is

"Sacred Time, Sacred Space."

"Sometimes people ask me, 'How can you do what you do? How can you work in a NICU where there's so much loss and pain every day?" … My answer is "How can I not? It's what I was born for.'

Amidst all the medical mayhem, we nurses are called to help families keep their footing in the present and seek some higher ground in their grief journey. We're called to meet families where they are at, and respect their culture and beliefs, while recognizing the universal human emotions that unite us all. I have had the humbling experience of walking this journey with many families over many years.

I think of so many families that I've led through the experience of saying both hello and goodbye to their babies. I can tell you about each one. What our NICU team does for families in the hospital has a commonality, but each one is a unique and individual story. Each experience, as important and precious as the next, has changed me in profound and unforeseen ways.

"It's not a calling for the fainthearted … it demands the softest of hearts and a true willingness to be open to, and molded by, the mysteries of life and death.

*I*t' s been ten years since I cared for one tiny and beautiful infant girl who was born around twenty-five weeks, which is very early. She was quite sick with an infection, and she also suffered a severe brain hemorrhage. Her parents were devastated by the prognosis for their new little daughter, which was death or severe lifelong mental and physical disabilities.

The doctors met with her parents to explain how nothing more could be done for their baby. That discussion led to the decision to provide comfort care for the tiny baby, eventually discontinuing the life-sustaining measures. Because of the baby's critical condition, her mother had never been able to hold her. She longed to hold her baby before she passed; a plan was made that the family would gather on a certain day to say goodbye, and at that time all of the machines would be removed.

I cared for this baby and her family on the day this was scheduled. I remember the exact spot in the NICU where her incubator was. I remember helping her mother dress her daughter in the NICU. We had a beautiful handmade smocked dress and hat, with tiny booties to dress her in, so her mother could cradle her.

We dressed her gently, with all the tubes and IVs still running. Carefully, we wrapped the baby in a soft handmade blanket, and I lifted the baby into her mother's arms. Her husband and sons were with her. The baby girl looked so sweet.

~

In that moment everything changed. The baby's mother could not allow the machines to be turned off. She wanted the medical team instead to continue all the life-sustaining care the baby was getting. She shared with me her hope for a miracle, if only she just waited a little longer.

A mother myself, I knew intuitively what she must have been going through and why she couldn't turn off the machines that day. At the moment that I placed the baby in her arms, the baby was no longer the object of a medical decision-making process but her own little girl, real and alive, and she wanted her to live with all her heart and soul. Medically, I knew that the baby's outcome wouldn't change, but emotionally, I knew the mother needed more time and I supported her. After I left her with her baby girl, I spoke to the neonatologist and explained all that had transpired.

~

"She shared with me her hope for a miracle, if only she just waited a little longer.

Before leaving the hospital at the end of my shift that night, I stopped by to check on the family. The mother asked me if I thought the baby seemed better in any way. It was in my hands to talk to her honestly and gently. I sat down on her bed while her little boys slept in a nearby stroller. We talked about the next day and the day after that, and slowly, painfully, the reality settled in, that those extra days of waiting for a miracle would not heal the damage the baby's brain hemorrhage had caused. The mother began to understand what she needed to do to love her little girl in the brief time she was given with her.

> " The mother began to understand what she needed to do to love her little girl in the brief time she was given with her.

After the weekend, on Monday morning, the medical team wondered why "the plan" had changed; essentially, why was the baby still alive on the ventilator? A part of me reacted with some anger, fueled by the compassion I felt when I saw this mother hold her sweetly dressed daughter and bond with her as only a mother can. I explained that the mother needed a little more time to have her baby alive, so that she could seal in her heart the memories of holding her and knowing her a little before she died.

The baby girl passed away in her mother's arms early that week. I attended her funeral service a few days later. Dressed in a tiny dress sewn and hand embroidered by her maternal grandmother, this tiny baby had clearly drawn her family into a circle of love and mourning during her brief life.

> " Dressed in a tiny dress sewn and hand embroidered by her maternal grandmother, this tiny baby had clearly drawn her family into a circle of love and mourning during her brief life.

Every year since, around the anniversary of her baby's life, this mother comes to see me or contacts me with photos of her growing family. I've come to think of it as a remembrance of the gift of time and heartfelt recognition of her little baby girl as a precious member of the family. She continues to thank me for something I didn't even know I'd given her. A bond was formed during our time together. I was one of few who knew and remembered what her baby looked like, in the tiny clothes and blankets that made her a "real baby," for her mother to snuggle and hold.

Ten years later, this baby girl still lives in her mother's heart, forever tiny as she was, but also imagined as the growing ten-year-old she might have been today. This baby also lives in my heart, this tiny patient of mine who changed me in profound and unforeseen ways. It is a sacred trust when a family who has lost a child allows you to take part in their journey of mourning, a journey that lasts a lifetime.

> " She continues to thank me for something I didn't even know I'd given her.

It's important as a professional to understand mourning as the lifelong work of living meaningfully after significant loss. Losing a child is recognized almost universally as the most difficult of losses. Those of us who are privileged to walk alongside, and tend to the hearts of, those facing such loss have ourselves been educated by families as to what they need most.

I'm just one of many nurses who've become more intimately involved over the years of my nursing life, finding ways to meet the needs of grieving families. I've worked with other nurses and our hospital chaplain to form our hospital Bereavement Team, a committed team of professionals who meet monthly to ensure that everything that can be done is being done as effectively as possible. Our focus, and the most important aspect of our work, is the coordinated care that's delivered daily, as nurses, doctors, chaplains, patient-care assistants, and all hospital team members interact with a family whose baby has died.

Our team's mission starts with education and providing avenues of hope and healing as families journey through their loss. Most significantly, we want families to know that we recognize their babies as special persons, irreplaceable and worthy of time and attention to all that is unique about their brief lives. We do as much as possible to create memories and give families time with their infants and each other during their hospital stay.

Part of the Bereavement Team's role is to coordinate donations of infant clothing: hand-embroidered dresses and nightgowns, crocheted and knitted blankets, and the tiniest of booties and hats, which are

"We do as much as possible to create memories and give families time with their infants and each other during their hospital stay.

made by community groups and individuals who know about our hospital's service mission.

Infants are lovingly dressed in these special outfits, and photographs are taken—respectful, beautiful photographs that reflect the essence of each baby, held in the loving arms of family members. A single photo of tiny feet or a little hand wrapped around a father's finger tells the story of lifelong attachment and the miracle of an infant's development, even at the earliest stages of life. Footprints and handprints are made. A lock of hair is saved. Hand and foot impressions are molded in soft clay.

A child conceived is a member of a family forever. When, during the mother's hospitalization, that baby is lost, it's imperative that all caregivers involved are sensitive to the nature of this experience. The hardest thing to integrate into practice is the reality that when miscarriage, stillbirth, or neonatal death occurs,

it is inevitable. The nature of nursing and medicine in general is to treat or cure, and by accepting the reality of the NICU we must also accept that, sometimes, to treat or cure is not possible.

The healing of a parent's broken heart after losing a baby takes a long time. Our hospital team is connected to community support groups for bereaved families. We give parents information and encouragement to look for the activities or resources that will help them move through their grief in a healthy way.

Miracles do happen every day in the NICU. Miracles of the heart occur when bereaved families are touched by compassion and empathy, by kindness and caring. Each little life has taught me to embrace each moment in love as a nurse and as a person.

—Mary Ann Wolpert, RNC-NIC,
NICU Representative/Bereavement Team
NICU Staff Nurses Clinical Ladder IV

"He has been a trouper, fighting hard for so long, so maybe it's time to let him go.

Blessings of the Heart (Chaplain)

For ten years, I have been privileged to walk alongside the NICU staff as they cared for hundreds of families and their precious babies. It was easy for me to understand why, despite the sad moments, nurses and physicians continued their work in the NICU.

One of the most memorable moments was when I accompanied a young couple whose twin sons were born at twenty-five weeks. We prayed together and held vigil at the bedside. I watched this young couple parent their twins as best as they could. I watched loving nurses and physicians gently caress the babies. Conversations were never rushed, truth was spoken, and hugs were all around.

I sat at the bedside with the parents when the nurse shared the news that the one baby was failing fast. The father became somewhat angry in his grief and said, "Are you telling me to give up? Are you giving up?"

The nurse put her arm around the father and quietly said, "No, I would never give up hope. My faith tells me to hold on to hope. As your baby's nurse, though, I am charged with telling you what your baby's body is saying. At this time, your baby's body is getting tired."

I saw the father immediately relax, and tears began to fall down his cheeks. He shook his head yes, and said, "He has been a trouper, fighting hard for so long, so maybe it's time to let him go."

I can only describe those moments as sacred. The nurse allowed the father to express his grief, and at the same time she joined him in his sorrow and gently shared the reality of his baby's precarious situation.

Another time that stays with my heart is when I worked with one of our neonatal palliative care families. As the mother held her baby boy, surrounded by family and staff, he died quietly in her arms. It was a peaceful death. The baby knew only love. The mother shared what it was like when she found out she was pregnant and how excited she and her husband were to have their first baby. There was laughter and tears. All the while the baby was passed around and lovingly held by all present.

Once the mother and father had said their goodbyes and everyone left, the nurse practitioner and I worked to prepare the baby's body for his final resting place. We bathed him and dressed him in a beautiful little outfit chosen by his parents for his burial. We took many photographs, as is our practice, and at one point the physician stopped by and asked if we needed any help with anything. We thanked him and told him we were just about finished. He came over to the bassinet and gently rubbed his thumb along the baby's cheek. It was very touching for me to see that kind of love expressed. I will never forget the time with the family or the way that doctor said goodbye to the baby.

I will forever be grateful to the families, nurses, and physicians who invited me to accompany them on so many sacred journeys. A NICU nurse once told me that her heart is filled with tiny footprints of all the babies she cared for. Looking back, I know exactly what she meant.

—Carolanne B. Hauck, MA,
BCC (Board Certified Chaplain)

NICU Staff Reflections

In the following pages, some of our staff relate their experiences during the early years of the NICU at Lancaster General Hospital.

~

Lynn Balmer, RN — "The Pre-NICU Era"

When I started at the hospital in 1973, I was assigned to the Newborn Nursery/Preemie Nursery. In the preemie nursery, they cared for sick and slightly premature newborns. The capacity of the preemie nursery was ten infants, usually staffed with one Registered Nurse and a nurse's aide. If it was really busy, the staffing might also include a Licensed Practical Nurse.

We had one cardio/respiratory monitor for the whole unit—a very large Hewlett-Packard monitor on wheels, so we could push it from patient to patient if need be.

Every baby was kept NPO (nothing by mouth) for at least the first twelve hours of life. Once the doctor OK'd feeding them, they would all be fed on the 9-12-3-6 schedule, which means that all babies were fed at the same time, around the clock.

Nurses were not allowed to start IVs on the babies. That was the duty of a doctor or a resident. If a child needed an IV antibiotic, the nurse had to call the on-call resident, and he would give it. Many times, the nurse would have to explain to the resident how to administer the medication after she had drawn it up for him to give.

There were very few NICUs at that time. When we had a really ill infant whom we couldn't take care of in our unit, we would transport the infant via ambulance to a hospital in Philadelphia. I remember a very ill infant who couldn't breathe on his own and needed transfer to a higher level of care. The problem was that there was a severe snowstorm on the East Coast and nothing was moving. The doctors and nurses took turns "bagging" the baby for over twenty-four hours, till the weather cleared enough to allow travel. They took one-hour shifts caring for an infant, who was finally transferred to a hospital in Philadelphia and continued to recover there.

[Lynn worked in the NICU from its inception in 1984 until her retirement in 2014.]

⇒

"When we had a really ill infant we couldn't take care of in our unit, we would transport the infant via ambulance to a hospital in Philadelphia.

Judy Coble, RN — *"A Pioneer"*

The director of nursing at Lancaster General Hospital (LGH) hired me in January 1965, and I started work in the Newborn Nursery. After two years there, I transferred to the Premature Nursery, or "Preemie Nursery," as it was usually called. Our patients were the babies born preterm and term infants who were too ill to be admitted to the well-baby nursery, as they had congenital anomalies, cardiac defects, or respiratory distress. Our infants were managed by staff pediatricians and cared for by RNs, LPNs, and nurse's aides. An infant who was too ill to be cared for in our Preemie Nursery was transported in an incubator by ambulance, with one of our nurses and possibly a resident, to either St. Christopher's Hospital or Children's Hospital of Philadelphia (CHOP, as it was called). This was before Hershey Medical Center existed.

Fast-forward to 1984 and we were told that LGH had hired a Neonatologist for our Preemie Nursery.

That was Dr. Manjeet Kaur, and what a delight she was. Then the nurses were informed that we were going to open a Neonatal Intensive Care Nursery, and if we wanted to work in the NICU we'd have to reapply for our jobs. We had to go through an interview process, and if selected we'd have special training.

The chosen RNs took classes taught by a NICU nurse clinician from the Medical College of Philadelphia (MCP) and by Dr. Kaur. After that, we each had a week of training at MCP. I was really excited when I came back to LGH from my training in the NICU at MCP. I remember going to Kmart to buy a cart. I felt that if we were going to be a NICU, we'd be starting a lot of IVs, and I thought it would be helpful to have a cart in which to store all the needed supplies so we could easily move them where needed. I bought a white vinyl-coated wire cart on wheels. I doubt it lasted a year before it fell apart.

[Judy worked in the NICU from 1965 until her retirement in 2001.]

"I remember going to Kmart to buy a cart. I felt that if we were going to be a NICU, we'd be starting a lot of IVs, and I thought it would be helpful to have a cart in which to store all the needed supplies.

Brenda Sollenberger, RN —"Compassionate Care"

I've worked in the NICU for over thirty years, since it was established in 1984, and I've seen it advance from a tiny "preemie nursery" to what it is now—an eminent, twenty-nine-bed, level-4 NICU.

I was nine months pregnant when I met Dr. Kaur. One of my first memories is how she and I laughed together at the first C-section we attended. There was very little space allotted to us in the room, and with my large belly and the cumbersome box that held our supplies, Dr. Kaur and I walked very gingerly through that delivery!

Through the programs that she established, we learned the skills to provide care for the smallest of patients. Even though it often meant working around the clock, 24/7 in the early days, babies were able to remain with their families at LGH, preventing the stress of transportation to a care center many miles away.

What I admire and wish to emulate most is Dr. Kaur's compassion and connection to families. She has hugged families as well as shed tears with them. She has sat by the bedsides of critically ill patients. She always takes time to educate and update and answer questions, and when the patient is discharged, her compassion continues.

Even decades after a tiny patient has been discharged, she receives invitations to, and attends, their graduations, Eagle Scout ceremonies, weddings, and family celebrations, and she is always receiving updates, photos, and cards.

Another fond memory began in 1984, when the local TV station filmed a news segment about our new NICU, and interviewed the mother of our first NICU baby as she held her newborn daughter. Recently, that baby girl, now grown up and a mother herself, held her own newborn daughter in our NICU. Those three decades have flown by so quickly!

I would like to share with my colleagues who've never had the privilege to work with Dr. Kaur some of the core values I learned through her mentoring: Never lose sight of the reason we are in a caring profession. We'll have bad days and stressful days, and go through some personal trying times, but remember, kindness and compassion can make all the difference in someone's life. We may only be with a patient or the family for a short time, but the memory we leave with them will last forever.

I cherish the years I have worked with Dr. Kaur. I learned so much, not only about science and medicine but also about compassion, kindness, and dedication. My fond memories of working with Dr. Kaur will last a lifetime.

[Brenda has worked in the NICU since 1984, and continues to the present day.]

❝ Kindness and compassion can make all the difference in someone's life. We may only be with a patient or the family for a short time, but the memory we leave with them will last forever.

Beth Yeingst, RN — *"Aeonian Connection"*

> "We practiced primary-care nursing in the NICU, which resulted in tight bonds of trust between nurses and families, as parents could leave knowing that the nurse taking care of their baby really knew the child and them; knew how to hold their baby like mom did; and knew the best way to comfort their child.

I began work in the NICU in 1986 at age twenty-one, at that time the youngest nurse working there. Dr. Kaur was our only Neonatologist at the time, and I honestly don't know when she ever had the time to sleep. She always greeted the day with enthusiasm despite her tough schedule. Her dedication and compassion were, and are, unparalleled.

Though our census in 1986 was nowhere near what the NICU census is today, and extremely critical babies requiring surgery or ECMO sometimes had to be sent to other facilities, the babies who entered the doors of the Lancaster General Hospital NICU were received by extremely skilled hands and a woman/physician with more knowledge and heart than I'd ever before had the pleasure of seeing or working with. In fact, when I left the NICU in 2004, I was asked at my next job interview whom I considered to be my mentor, and through tears and a smile, I immediately said, "Dr. Kaur, because she has taught me so much about neonatal nursing and has constantly demonstrated how to not lose touch with the baby as well as the family behind the tubes and monitors."

As a team, we would try to make having a baby in the NICU as "normal" as it could be, allowing parents to participate in their baby's care as early as possible. In the 1980s, many of our babies were with us until they were ready for discharge. Home care for babies and step-down facilities were not available as they are today. One baby, named Zach, was with us for eleven months. I remember sitting him in his highchair to feed him his baby food, tucking him in for naps, and taking him for a walk around the hospital block when we were at last able to get a portable ventilator for him. I'll always remember his bright eyes (behind sunglasses, of course) as he could finally have sunlight and fresh air on his face.

> "As a team, we would try to make having a baby in the NICU as 'normal' as it could be, allowing parents to participate in their baby's care as early as possible.

I was fortunate to be able to ride along with him in the ambulance when he got to go home.

We practiced primary-care nursing in the NICU, which resulted in tight bonds of trust between nurses and families, as parents could leave knowing that the nurse taking care of their baby really knew the child and them; knew how to hold their baby like Mom did; and knew the best way to comfort their child. I had the pleasure of being primary-care nurse to two twenty-eight-week twins named Andrew and Ryan Huntley. That bond has never been severed, as I still keep in touch with them today, thirty-plus years later. I was privileged to attend Andrew's wedding, and was excited to have been invited to Ryan's. There were days when we worried whether Andrew (Twin "B") would survive. I remember getting those phone calls from Susan and Mark, the twins' parents, after Andrew was discharged, saying, "Beth, Andrew is being admitted again; we're on our way in." Andrew had a trach until he was a little past two, and he had many respiratory issues. Now he's a handsome married man, and I'm blessed to have been involved in the care of these two amazing young men.

We NICU nurses often celebrated with parents and grieved with them as well. Sometimes a baby would be born with obviously different features, and I remember nurses and physicians sometimes pondering what the possible genetic defect could be. Dr.

Kaur would often walk up, take one look, and say, "Oh, I believe that this baby has this," whereupon we'd consult the reference book and she'd be right. Her knowledge never ceases to astound me.

I remember Dr. Kaur's office walls being literally papered with photos of "her babies," because she always treated every one of these precious babies as if they were her own. She often gave them endearing nicknames, sometimes referring to the weather on the day they were born. I recall one baby she nicknamed "Snowflake," as he was born during a snowstorm. Every year we held a NICU reunion, and Dr. Kaur never forgot a face or a name, even though the little faces looking up at her looked nothing like that micro-preemie she had first met.

Technology was constantly changing in the NICU. I remember going on transports and suctioning babies using DeLee suction, which was basically a chamber that had a straw that went in your mouth and a tube that went into the baby's mouth, allowing you to suck the fluids into a connected trap. It wasn't long before portable suction units were in place and we no longer had to use the DeLee. Before today's flight teams, the NICU nurses, physicians, and pulmonary staff did air transports. Sometimes we flew via small private jets from Lancaster Airport, and once we even flew in a National Guard helicopter.

Anand Mahajan, MD, FAAP (Neonatologist) — *"Technology as an Art"*

> "Our outcome for babies in the community continues to improve. Extreme premature babies have survived with good results. Parents have brought their bundles of joy back to the NICU to show us their wonderful progress.

After finishing my Neonatal-Perinatal fellowship in 1988 at Georgetown University Hospital, I joined a private practice of Neonatology in Oklahoma City. In 1989, after our daughter, Asha, was born, my wife and I wanted to relocate so that we would be close to my in-laws, who lived in Reading, Pennsylvania. After a discussion with my colleague, Dr. Gross, I contacted Dr. Manjeet Kaur (Chief of Neonatology at Lancaster General Hospital) who, in 1989, offered me a position as a Neonatologist at Lancaster General. Dr. Kaur had started the Neonatal Intensive Care Unit at LGH in 1984, and I was very excited to work with her and Dr. Lebischak.

Dr. Kaur had worked countless hours to establish the NICU, and I was amazed to see her dedication, personal sacrifice, and commitment to teamwork. Even though I was trained with all new technology, Dr. Kaur has taught me compassionate care, and she has been a mentor to me at different levels of care. Our outcome for babies in the community continues to improve. Extreme premature babies have survived with good results. Parents have brought their bundles of joy back to the NICU to show us their wonderful progress. This has all been a very rewarding experience to the NICU team and me.

When we found out that my wife, Suzanne, was pregnant with triplets, Dr. Kaur helped us tremendously, comforting us and reassuring us that our delivery would be a smooth one.

Dr. Kaur, Dr. Lebischak, and the NICU team gave them excellent care, and Anjali, Alexander, and Andrew were born by C-section at thirty-six weeks on April 14, 1995—they gave me the role of Dad! Dr. Kaur continues to be an advocate for our children. We really appreciate her involvement and thank her from the bottom of our hearts.

"It wasn't the machines that made the NICU so special—it was the passion that we all shared to give every infant in our care the very best chance of life, and his or her parents the blessing of taking their child home.

Sherry Smith, RN — *"Teamwork"*

I remember how excited and nervous we nurses felt in 1984 when Dr. Kaur came to start a NICU at LGH. Everyone attended classes that she held before the actual startup, and I remember feeling my self-confidence grow as she patiently led us through various subjects pertaining to the care of compromised infants. It wasn't only the technical information that was so helpful but also all of us together learning, talking, and building a team. When I think back over the years during which I took care of sick newborns, that remains one of the most valuable lessons.

You see, every time a baby came to our unit, it wasn't just one person providing care; it was many who contributed. I remember one particular baby who arrived unexpectedly back in the early days of the unit. This infant's mother was quite ill, and it was anticipated that the baby would have other problems in addition to her prematurity. Dr. Kaur and I attended the delivery, and many other people were involved: the nurses preparing the equipment in the unit, the unit clerk preparing the chart, the respiratory therapist assisting in the delivery as well as in the NICU, and all the nurses who helped at the bedside after the baby was admitted. Although this infant's mother later died, the baby survived to become a comfort to her family.

Thinking back to the early days of the NICU, the teamwork among nurses, and also between the nurses and doctors, was amazing. The technology we had seems somewhat primitive compared to what exists now, but then, as now, it wasn't the machines that made the NICU so special—it was the passion that we all shared to give every infant in our care the very best chance of life, and his or her parents the blessing of taking their child home.

[Sherry worked in the NICU from 1984 until her retirement in 2015.]

Deborah Hess, RN — "The NICU Family"

I've often wondered if Dr. Kaur knew she was birthing a new family, the "NICU family," when she started the NICU. Being a part of that family has been a wonderful part of my life for the past thirty-one years. Dr. Kaur has been a brilliant mentor and friend to me all that time. She has always encouraged me to do my best, and has placed a high value on continuing education.

The NICU family loves its patients. We care for the smallest and most vulnerable. Their families are frightened, and face so many uncertainties. I have watched the NICU family wrap their arms around these families and love the babies and their families back to health. The people I work with are some of the most compassionate professionals I've ever met.

The NICU family works together. When there's a busy day in the NICU, we help each other out. I've had parents watch the admission of a "micro-preemie" from across the room and comment on the way everyone works together to get that infant admitted and stabilized. One parent described it to me as "a well-oiled machine," another as "the NICU dance." Not many words are needed—we all know what must be done and we pitch in and do the job.

The NICU family loves and supports each other. We have cried together and have had many laughs together. We've celebrated each other's accomplishments, births (children and now grandchildren), and weddings of staff and children together. We've cried together during the trying times of loss and life's difficulties. We have prayed together. Hugs are given freely on a tough day.

We spend many holidays in the NICU, and this staff knows how to throw a good party! Holidays always bring decorations, food, and fun. If you can't be home for Christmas, you might as well celebrate with your other family. Beyond NICU parties, there have been garden tours, lunches, breakfasts, retirement parties, showers, and swim parties.

The members of the NICU enjoy each other's company. You can't work in this NICU without falling in love with the staff, who bring so many talents to the family. I've been asked how I could work in the NICU for so many years. It's the NICU family. They are more than my coworkers and friends—they are my NICU family.

[Deb has worked in the NICU since 1986 to the present time in 2018.]

❧

> "The NICU family loves its patients. We care for the smallest and most vulnerable. Their families are frightened, and face so many uncertainties. I have watched the NICU family wrap their arms around these families and love the babies and their families back to health.

"When I consider what stands out most … it has to be the amazing strength and resilience of the NICU mothers. Parents don't choose this path; babies are born prematurely or ill for many reasons.

Kathleen Warfel, RN — *"Strength of the NICU Mothers"*

When I consider what stands out most as a NICU RN, it has to be the amazing strength and resilience of the NICU mothers. Parents don't choose this path; babies are born prematurely or ill for many reasons. Initially, most mothers are deeply shocked by the fragility of their babies and the immensity of the equipment surrounding the newborn, yet mothers quickly bond, fall in love with, and take on an active role in caring for their tiny children.

I recall one mother who, after her twenty-four-week twins were born, was so concerned about how far away they were from each other in the room. One was born missing a lobe of her right lung, and later was diagnosed with cerebral palsy. Mom came in daily and did skin-to-skin when her daughters were more stable. She remained an advocate for her girls after discharge, so each could have a full life.

Another set of twins I cared for were born at thirty-one weeks. The boy went home and was diagnosed with cerebral palsy. As he grew, he took dance class with his sister and joined the Cub Scouts. Mothers continue to be the strength and hope for their children, pursuing whatever will help them to reach their full potential and achieve some of the dreams children have for themselves.

Another infant was born at twenty-six weeks. She was ventilator dependent for a long time. Her mother came in every day to play an active role in her care. She wanted to do kangaroo care daily, and her goal was to breastfeed. She pumped patiently for ten weeks before she could put her baby to breast. The baby did go home on medications, oxygen, and a monitor. Her wonderful mom changed her own lifestyle so she could devote herself to caring for her fragile little girl. She was devoted to providing the best care a mother could.

One twenty-seven-week infant was on respiratory support throughout her entire NICU stay. Her parents would come on their lunch break to provide her hands-on care. She also went home on many medications, oxygen, and a home monitor. Her father became a stay-at-home dad to fulfill her many complex needs.

I had cared for one little boy from birth until discharge. Seventeen months later, his mother delivered premature twins whom I also cared for until discharge. While discharging those twins, I teased the mother, who was a twin herself, that I'd see her next time with triplets. Well, a year and a half later, she came back with another set of premature twins, giving the family five children under four. The parents were just calm, loving, and amazing.

This is the theme throughout the NICU: Mothers adapting to their new role as caregiver to a medically fragile child because of their love and devotion. Many parents are well educated and many are not, yet families rise to provide outstanding medical care for their sons and daughters so that the children can have rich, full family lives.

When my son, Joel, was a junior in high school, he had to shadow someone in a profession that he was interested in. Joel came to the NICU to shadow Dr. Kaur. She was kind and gracious, and willingly sat with Joel to orient him to her role as a physician, and more specifically as a Neonatologist. Joel came home excited and full of enthusiasm. He was even more determined to become a doctor, and was amazed that such a busy physician would spend time teaching and sharing with him.

In the summer between Joel's junior and senior years of college, he shadowed Dr. Kaur again. He had a wonderful day—going to C-sections, seeing his first delivery in labor and delivery, and just relishing spending the day with someone who truly cared about his future and wanted to share knowledge with him. Dr. Kaur also contacted some of her colleagues in other fields, and Joel was able to shadow them and learn about different types of physician roles.

Dr. Kaur always asks about Joel, and he has such a deep love and admiration for her. As a junior at Drexel Medical School, Joel had a rotation at Lancaster General. Dr. Kaur again took him under her wing, and he learned so much more because Dr. Kaur is such a gifted, loving teacher and there is a special bond between the two of them. These experiences are one of the highlights of Joel's education. He positively glowed with excitement because of Dr. Kaur's kind and caring ways. I am so thankful for the positive influence she's had on Joel's life. She inspired him as a physician, and she inspired him as an educator.

❝ This is the theme throughout the NICU: Mothers adapting to their new role as caregiver to a medically fragile child because of their love and devotion.

Margi Bowers, MSN, MHA, RN, NE-BC — *"Heading a NICU"*

In 1982 I was a young, ambitious nurse starting what I didn't then realize would be a loyalty to Lancaster General Health and a satisfying nursing career. Two years later, excitement spread throughout the pediatric unit, in which I had my first RN position after graduation, about Dr. Kaur, a new physician in town, opening a Neonatal Intensive Care Unit (NICU). Administration was soliciting nurses with an interest in being cross-trained to this new unit of isolettes, ventilators, the tiniest of patients, and parents trying to stay supportive and hopeful through their fear and uncertainty. I jumped at the opportunity.

I recall working alongside these "NICU nurses" in the sunlit nursery. My experience as a cross-trained nurse in the preemie nursery was enhanced as Dr. Kaur shared her knowledge, compassion, and skills with anyone who would listen. The impact of working each day with a mentor who is so positive, kind, and willing to educate has led me to where I am today, the nurse manager for the twenty-nine-bed level-3 NICU at Lancaster General Health/Penn Medicine. My life's journey took me away from maternal child health nursing for thirteen years but never away from the profession of nursing. Not surprising, many of the same nurses that I assisted as a young newcomer to that sunlit preemie nursery during the 1980s are still working in the NICU today. As technology and healthcare rapidly evolved over the years, what remained constant was the super power of the NICU nurse. To be one of these nurses requires a balance of strength and compassion, empathy, skill, confidence, and unwavering dedication to the babies whose lives literally depend on them.

I've witnessed these nurses' ability to detect from across the room when a one-pound infant just doesn't seem right. The nurses stay focused in this unique world of the NICU where it's mostly happy and positive, but can occasionally be devastating. I'm honored to lead this dedicated group of professionals, to witness the joy, support the fear, celebrate the milestones, and counsel the sadness that surrounds the tiniest and most fragile patients at LGH/Penn Medicine. As our patients grow strong and graduate from the NICU to their homes, I'll always feel a positive connection to Dr. Kaur and the NICU. My daughter will soon marry one of Dr. Kaur's first NICU patients. Thank you, Dr. Kaur; thank you, nursing team; and thank you to the countless parents who reinforce for me why I'm a nurse. I am forever grateful.

[At the time of writing, Margi continues to serve as Nurse Manager of the NICU.]

> " The nurses stay focused in this unique world of the NICU where it's mostly happy and positive, but can occasionally be devastating.

Sandra Campbell, RN — *"Thanks"*

Legendary is a word I use to describe Dr. Kaur. She has made our NICU what it is today and has been for the past thirty-plus years. Her compassion, dedication, and never-ending kindness live on and are felt in the NICU every day. I've worked closely with Dr. Kaur for over twenty-three years and all memories of her make my heart smile. Some of my earliest thoughts of her include seeing her sit side by side with families, holding their hands, while giving them updates on their babies. Whether it's positive or difficult news, she's there to offer support and respect.

After meeting Dr. Kaur, the families in our NICU know that they're in good hands. They feel her presence watching over their sick neonate, which is very comforting to them. Dr. Kaur has compassion not only for our NICU families but for staff members as well. She offers herself to those in need, and helps staff achieve personal and professional goals. As I said, she's a legend! Her dedication to the NICU continues every day. She loves to hear updates about families old and new. Dr. Kaur goes above and beyond getting to know the families connected to our ill neonates. The kindness she shows is unsurpassable. She hasn't a negative bone in her body and always has a beautiful smile on her face. These smiles are contagious in the NICU, and all who encounter her feel her love. I've never met a doctor who could remember names and stories as well as Dr. Kaur. She remembers all the micro-preemies who pass through the NICU at Women and Babies Hospital. Her legend continues as time goes on. Thank you, Dr. Kaur, for your service in the NICU!

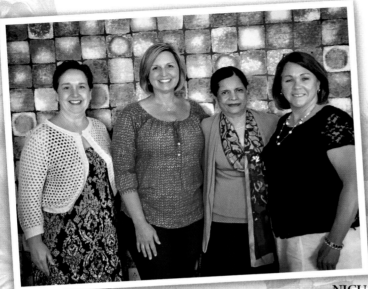

NICU Staff
(l-r): Janice RN, Judy RN, Manjeet MD, Brenda RN

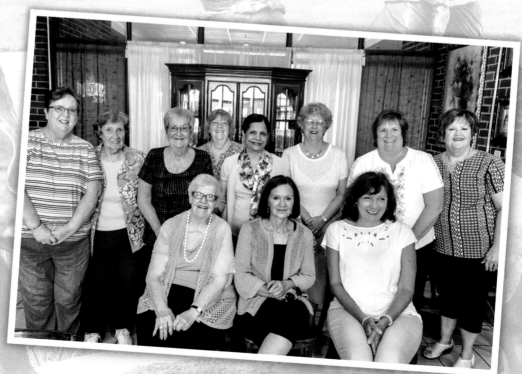

NICU Staff
Front: (l-r): Cleo LPN, Brenda RN, Sherry RN
Back: BJ RN, Pat RN, Vicky RN, Judy RN, Manjeet MD, Debbie RN,
Karen RN, Lynn RN

Ode to a Baby

A sweet poem, a melodious lark,
From a heavenly abode, to a mundane park.
What ethereal beauty, what innocent bliss,
Thine soft arms, thy wet tender kiss.
What ails thee little angel, tell me O, do!
With dew drops on thine brow and dry red lips too.
What hold you in thine fist, a destiny so tight,
With love and prayers we'll try our best to right.
So this sweet little cherub shall sing sonnets anew
Frolic on the mountaintop in colorful hue!
Amongst daisies and lilies and morning glory blue
With the Lord's blessings "Little one"… …
Let us help you !

—Manjeet Kaur

PART III

Neonatal Intensive Care

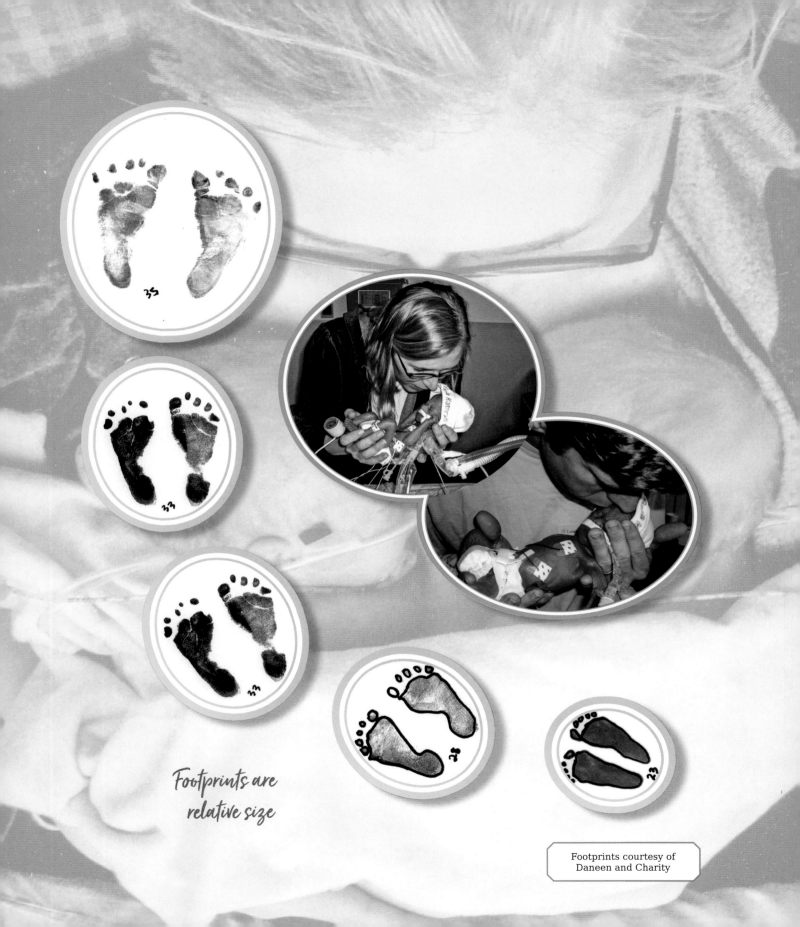

Footprints are
relative size

Footprints courtesy of
Daneen and Charity

Neonatal Intensive Care

*T*he birth of a baby—the blossoming of new life, the fulfillment of parents' hopes and dreams—is a joyous event. However, sometimes things don't go as planned, and some babies have a tough start in life.

The **Neonatal Intensive Care Unit** (NICU) is a facility designed to provide specialized care for babies experiencing problems at the time of birth. The most common admissions to the NICU are **premature** babies, who are born early—we call them "preemies." Sometimes **term** babies also need specialized care due to problems detected at the time of birth.

Being thrown into this unexpected ocean of technology, surrounded by beeps and alarms, can be frightening and unnerving. However, parents can feel empowered, and better equipped to face the challenges of a NICU admission when they are armed with prior knowledge.

A common theme in the stories of the second-time NICU parents is "I knew what to expect; I felt so much better than the first time."

It always seems easier if you are prepared and know what to expect if your baby needs special care at the time of birth. The information throughout this section describes the most common situations for babies needing NICU care and answers questions that parents most commonly ask, such as:

"What happened at the time of delivery?"

"What now?"

"What can I do?"

"What do I need to know?"

"How can I handle things?"

Here's a brief description of the sequence of events, starting in the delivery room, and then describing what happens if your baby needs to be moved into the NICU.

> " Parents can feel empowered, and better equipped to face the challenges of a NICU admission when they are armed with prior knowledge.

In the Delivery Room

Resuscitation—A Tough Start

Every delivery room is equipped to resuscitate (revive) an infant as needed. About 10 percent of babies will require some resuscitation, and 1 percent will require aggressive resuscitation with medications after birth.

After delivery, be it vaginal or via cesarean section (C-section), the infant is placed on a bed called a **resuscitation bed**—also called a warmer bed (**radiant warmer**). This is a bed on wheels with an overhead heating lamp and a special light, so that the infant can be assessed. It is fitted with suction equipment and oxygen-administration terminals, which need to be attached to an oxygen cylinder or wall oxygen in the delivery room (DR) or operating room (OR). The resuscitation bed is also equipped with a timer and a push button, so the birth scores (called **Apgar scores**), which measure the wellbeing of the infant, can be timed and recorded at one minute, five minutes and, if needed, at ten minutes.

Suctioning

The baby is often suctioned (suctioning) via a bulb syringe or a suction **catheter** to remove mucus from the mouth, nose, and throat. The suction catheter is connected to a wall suction outlet that is set to a specified pressure.

Supplemental Oxygen

Normal room air, which is what we all breathe, has 21 percent oxygen. Supplemental oxygen is usually needed for a high-risk or preterm infant. The infant may require up to 100 percent oxygen, which is weaned as appropriate based on a pulse oximeter. Oxygen from the oxygen source flowing to a bag can be delivered to the infant via a mask placed over the infant's nose and mouth.

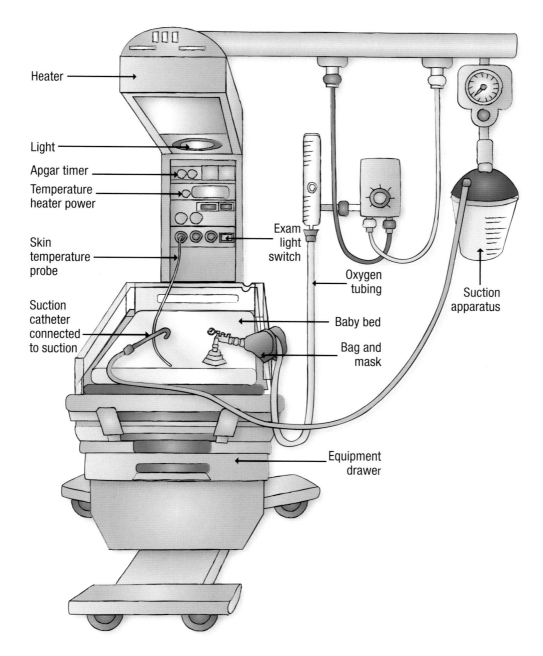

Heater

Light

Apgar timer

Temperature heater power

Skin temperature probe

Suction catheter connected to suction

Exam light switch

Oxygen tubing

Baby bed

Bag and mask

Suction apparatus

Equipment drawer

Figure 1: Resuscitation Bed

Pulse Oximeter

The pulse oximeter is a very useful, noninvasive tool to monitor the infant's blood-oxygen status. A transducer sensor is attached, usually to the right wrist, to measure preductal or unmixed blood. This pulse oximeter sensor is then secured with a wrap, and the lead is connected to a monitor that reads the oxygen carried by the hemoglobin in the blood. The pulse oximeter can read up to 100%. Saturation numbers above 90% are generally acceptable. However, saturation levels may be lower in the first ten minutes after birth, even in term births with no complications.

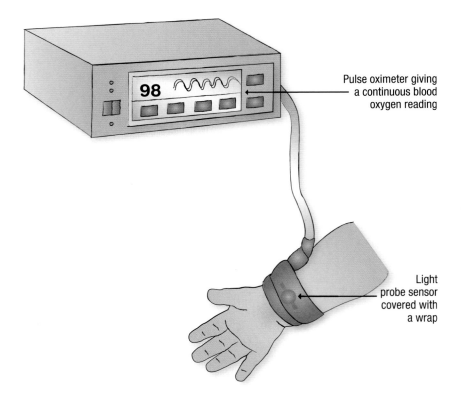

Pulse oximeter giving a continuous blood oxygen reading

Light probe sensor covered with a wrap

Figure 2: Pulse Oximeter

Bag and Mask Ventilation

If a baby does not have spontaneous breathing or respirations despite stimulation, it may be necessary to administer oxygen via a mask over the mouth and nose, connected to a breathing bag and an oxygen source. The bag is compressed or pumped at a certain number of breaths (about forty) per minute. This is called **bag and mask ventilation.** Sometimes this is enough to establish respirations.

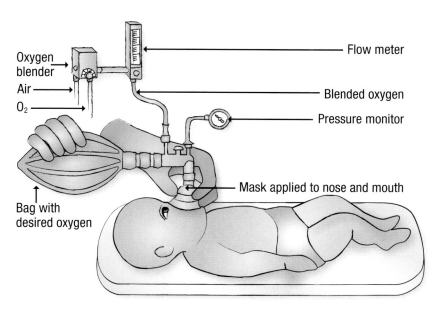

Figure 3: Bag and Mask Ventilation

If this is all that is needed, I often tell parents, the baby just needed a "jump start," though we always try to ascertain the cause. Sometimes just bagging in room air is sufficient, and additional oxygen is not needed. This is called **room air resuscitation.** The resuscitation team is careful regarding monitoring the amount of oxygen administered, especially to a preterm infant, as inadequate oxygen can cause brain injury, and excess oxygen in preterm infants can be associated with retinopathy and chronic lung disease.

Mask CPAP (**continuous positive airway pressure**) may also be given at this time to give additional respiratory airway stenting.

Intubation

If the infant is unable to establish spontaneous respirations despite bag and mask ventilation, an endotracheal intubation will be needed. This is done using a **laryngoscope,** an instrument that has a handle and a thick blade with a bright light at the tip, which helps to visualize the vocal cords and thus the airway.

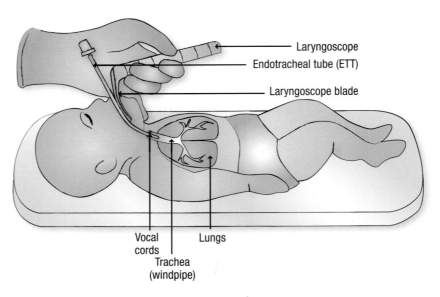

Figure 4: Intubation

The **endotracheal tube** (ETT) is a marked plastic "breathing tube" that is inserted into the windpipe or trachea after visualizing the vocal cords with the laryngoscope. The markings on the ETT help to determine the right depth for insertion depending on the size of the infant. The other end of the ETT is attached to the resuscitation bag so that mechanical breaths can be given with the bag.

If spontaneous breathing is not established, the ETT can then be connected to a **ventilator** (breathing machine) to give ventilator-initiated breaths.

Extremely preterm babies who are unable to breathe may be electively intubated and connected to a ventilator soon after birth.

Apgar Score

The Apgar score (a scoring system named after Virginia Apgar) assesses five parameters: the heart rate, breathing, color, tone, and reflexes.

Key Elements:

- A baby can receive up to two points for each category.
- Scoring is done at one minute, five minutes, and if low, at ten minutes as well.
- Scores of seven to ten are considered normal.
- Scores of four to six indicate a need for some resuscitative efforts.
- Scores below four indicate a definite need for aggressive resuscitation.
- Preterm babies may get somewhat lower scores due to their immaturity.

Cardiac Compression

An infant with little or no heart rate may require cardiac compressions, which involves giving a rhythmic pressure over the chest until an acceptable heart rate is attained.

Normal heart rate in a newborn is 120–140 beats per minute, which is almost double that of an adult. *Normal respiratory rate of a newborn is about forty breaths per minute,* almost twice of an adult's as well.

Umbilical Venous Catheter (UVC)

In case of a need for emergency medication and fluids despite the above resuscitation measures, an umbilical venous catheter is placed. The umbilical cord is cut and a thin tube (umbilical catheter) is threaded in a sterile manner into the umbilical vein, so that drugs and fluids can be administered to the baby, directly into a large vein going to the heart. Blood samples can be drawn from the UVC as well.

Epinephrine

Epinephrine is the drug most commonly used in the delivery room when medications are needed for resuscitation. This can be given via the UVC, or if the line is not yet in place, into the endotracheal tube using a syringe. Epinephrine stimulates the heart to pump more efficiently, and it may be necessary to administer repeat doses.

Additional Fluids

If there was a known loss of blood prenatally or otherwise and the baby appears to be very *pale* and dry, then additional fluids may be needed, which are administered via the UVC.

Failure to Resuscitate

The American Academy of Pediatrics' current guidelines recommend discontinuing resuscitation in those unfortunate circumstances when all the above resuscitation efforts fail, and no heart rate is detected after ten minutes following birth.

Transfer to the NICU

A baby requiring further intensive care after stabilization will then be transferred to the NICU.

The baby is placed with monitoring leads into a **transport isolette (incubator),** and is often connected to a ventilator and pulse oximeter to provide manual or ventilator breathing support and monitoring of the heart rate and oxygen during transport.

Admission to the NICU

The NICU admission team quickly whirls into action upon the baby's arrival. If Dad is accompanying the transport team, we briefly explain what is happening and invite him to sit nearby or in the waiting room; alternatively, he may elect to stay with Mom in her room.

- Depending on the infant's requirements, the baby is transferred to either a **radiant warmer** (open bed where infant can be observed and procedures performed as needed) or an **incubator** (closed bed that provides isolation and warmth).
- Small sticky patches/shields are placed on your little one's chest and connected to a **cardiorespiratory monitor,** which displays both the heart rate and respiratory rate.
- A **temperature probe**—a small wire with a sensor tip—is taped on the skin to record the baby's skin temperature while under the radiant warmer.
- **A small cuff** is placed on the arm to record the **blood pressure.** Blood pressure can also be monitored through the umbilical arterial catheter (UAC). Normal blood pressure range for a baby varies with the gestational age.
- If not already in place, a **pulse oximeter** transducer that gives continuous preductal or unmixed blood oxygen saturation readings is usually placed on the baby's right wrist.
- An **intravenous** (IV) line is placed immediately on admission to the NICU since the sick newborn is initially unable to take oral feeds. Sick babies drop their blood sugar very quickly as the scanty reserves of a sick/extremely preterm baby are consumed rapidly. **Glucose** or sugar, a primary fuel for the brain, needs to be monitored closely.
- **Umbilical catheters** are routinely placed in the VLBW (**very low birth weight or extremely premature**) or very sick neonates. There are two umbilical arteries and one umbilical vein.
- A **peripheral intravenous line** may also be started, although this is usually not required if an umbilical catheter is already in place.

Procedure for placement of umbilical catheters

Sterile drapes are placed over the baby, and while heart rate and respiration are continuously being monitored, an umbilical vein and/or umbilical arterial catheter are inserted in the cord and advanced in the large blood vessels; the umbilical venous catheter (UVC) is inserted into the **inferior vena cava**

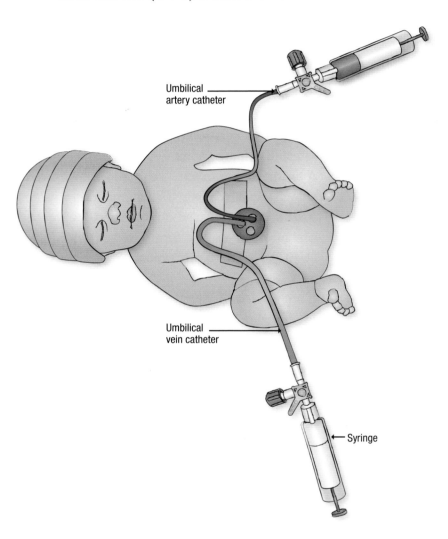

Umbilical
artery catheter

Umbilical
vein catheter

Syringe

Figure 5: Umbilical Catheter

through which fluids are administered; and the umbilical arterial catheter (UAC) is inserted into the large artery of the heart, the aorta, through which blood samples, especially for blood gases, are obtained to give an accurate measure of the oxygenation of the arterial blood. These catheters are then secured, and placement is confirmed by obtaining x-rays to determine the position of the catheter tip. The catheters are then connected to intravenous fluid bags.

The umbilical catheters are necessary for the frequent sampling of blood gases and other blood work needed for monitoring blood sugar, electrolytes, calcium, etc. of these tiny/ sick infants. The umbilical venous catheter is also used to administer fluids, nutrients, and medications to the baby.

Each umbilical catheter is attached to a three-way connector (or stop-cock). The second port of the umbilical catheter is connected to intravenous fluids, and the third port is capped or connected to a syringe. This end is used for drawing blood samples. Blood for testing arterial blood gases (ABGs), etc. is drawn from the umbilical arterial catheter (UAC). A blood thinner medication, **heparin,** is added to the intravenous fluids going into the catheter to prevent blood from clotting and blocking the catheters.

Nasal Cannula (NC)

If the infant needs only supplemental oxygen (O_2), and does not require intubation, this may be administered via soft plastic tubing with prongs that are placed in the nose. This is called a nasal cannula. The NC does not interfere with activity such as feeding and holding.

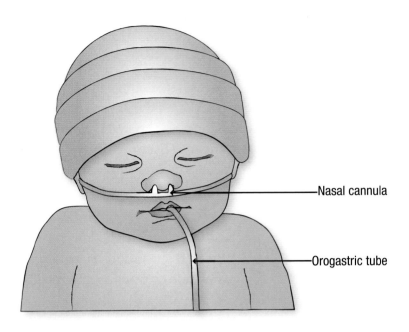

Figure 6: Nasal Cannula

Nasal Continuous Positive Airway Pressure (Nasal CPAP)—see Figure 7

If the infant needs assistance in breathing, he or she may be placed on continuous positive airway pressure or CPAP. This delivers air or oxygen steadily at a specific dialed pressure. Oxygen or air can be delivered via nasal tubes or a nasal mask attached to a coiled tubing, which is in turn connected to the CPAP machine or a respirator.

If CPAP provides adequate oxygenation, then a mechanical ventilator or invasive ventilation s unneccessary.

Nasal Intermittent Positive Pressure Ventilation (NIPPV)

Nasal intermittent positive ventilation, provided via nasal prongs or nasal mask, may be the next step if further assistance is needed for breathing.

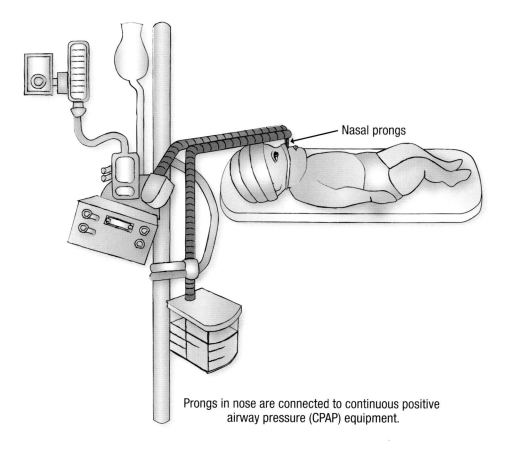

Nasal prongs

Prongs in nose are connected to continuous positive
airway pressure (CPAP) equipment.

Figure 7: Nasal CPAP

Mechanical Ventilation

If the infant is very sick or very premature, nasal cannula, NCPAP, or NIPPV may not be adequate. The baby may need to be *intubated with an ETT* and placed on a mechanical ventilator or a respirator. The ventilators are very sophisticated today and provide measured breaths at a certain rate with humidified oxygen at desired levels very efficiently.

However, very sick babies or those with severe **respiratory distress syndrome** (RDS) have very stiff lungs and may require higher oxygen at increased pressures. They may also require a different mode of ventilator support. In very preterm or sicker infants, a liquid called **surfactant** may be administered via the ETT in the NICU to facilitate lung expansion, if

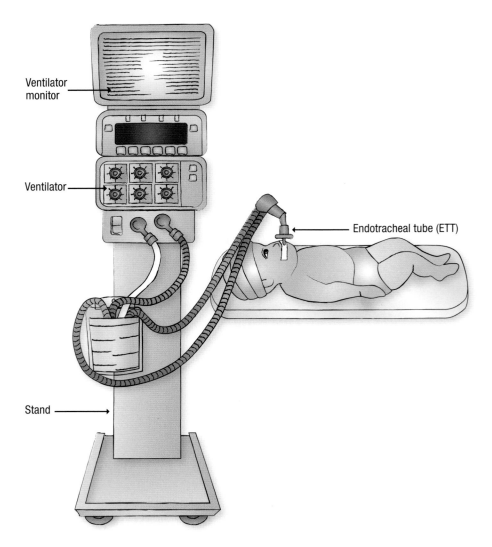

Figure 8: Baby Intubated on Ventilator (Respirator)

this has not already been given in the delivery room. As the infant's breathing improves and oxygenation (PaO_2) and carbon dioxide (PCO_2) in the blood gases become acceptable, the settings are weaned, and **extubation** (removal of the endotracheal tube) may be attempted. However, very sick and especially extremely preterm infants can require ventilator (vent) support for a long time.

Lab Tests

As soon as the infant's airway is stabilized and the umbilical or intravenous lines are placed, a series of blood tests are done. These typically include a **complete blood count** (CBC), **blood culture, blood glucose** (if not already done), **blood gas,** CBG (capillary blood gas), or ABG (arterial blood gas).

- **Complete Blood Count** (CBC) measures the hemoglobin (oxygen-carrying protein in the red blood cells), white blood cell count (germ-fighting cells), red blood cell count (cells containing the hemoglobin), and the platelets (cells that help the blood to clot).
- **Blood culture** tests the blood for any infection.
- **Blood gas** measures the oxygen, carbon dioxide, and acid in the blood, all of which depict the well-being of the lungs and circulation.

X-rays

X-rays are obtained to document the various tube placements (the ETT and umbilical catheters) and to assess the lung status.

Antibiotics

Antibiotics are administered as needed.

Intravenous Fluids

Intravenous fluids are then started through the peripheral intravenous line (or umbilical catheter if one has been placed) to provide nutrition as needed in the form of glucose water and salts such as sodium, potassium chloride, and calcium.

The above procedures mostly take place rather quickly, and by the time you come to the NICU after the delivery, you may find your little cherub cocooned amidst tubes and wires attached to respiratory equipment and beeping monitors. *Rest assured, this cute little alien is your precious bundle who has landed in the NICU cradle of technology and will get loving care by the NICU family.*

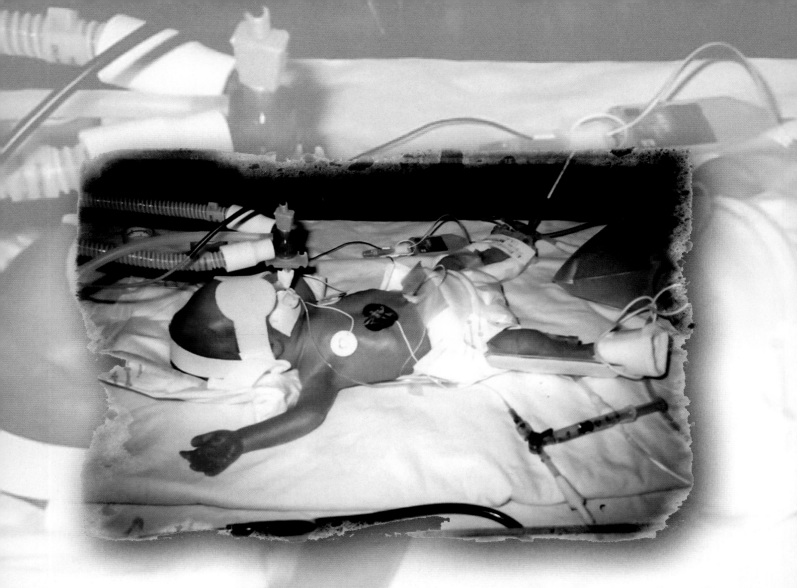

For us, the more knowledge we had,
the more we felt connected, calm, and
prepared to handle whatever came.

—Susan Deatrick (parent)

Common Medical Problems of Neonatal Intensive Care Babies

Prematurity and Related Issues

The major diagnosis of any Neonatal Intensive Care Unit is *prematurity*.

Gestation is another term used for pregnancy time periods.

Term gestation was previously considered to be 37 to 42 weeks. New research shows that each week of gestation can affect the baby's development, and the definition of **Term gestation** has been revised as follows:

Early Term—37 to 38 weeks and 6 days gestation

Full Term—39 to 40 weeks and 6 days gestation

Late Term—41 to 42 weeks and 6 days gestation

Post Term—over 42 weeks gestation

Babies born at or less than thirty-seven-weeks gestation are referred to as preterm or premature infants. *Ten to welve percent* of all babies are born prematurely. The lower the gestation of the babies, the higher the likelihood that there will be problems. So, the onus is always on prenatal care and prolonging the intrauterine environment as much as possible with safety to the mom and baby remaining of primary concern. The best incubator for a baby is certainly the uterus, so every attempt is made to prevent a preterm birth unless there are maternal or fetal issues that warrant a premature delivery. If a preterm delivery is imminent, **prenatal steroids** may be used to decrease the complications of prematurity such as respiratory distress syndrome and intraventricular hemorrhage.

The common issue is that the organs have not yet developed sufficiently to fully cope with the everyday environment of life outside the womb. As I often tell the parents, "All the organs are formed in preterm infants, but the systems are immature."

Problems of prematurity include the following:

- Lung immaturity—leading to **respiratory distress syndrome**
- Immature immune system with fragile skin—leading to increased risk of **sepsis** or **infection**
- Cardiac immaturity—persistence of a **patent ductus arteriosus** (PDA) leading to shunting of oxygenated blood
- Gut immaturity—risk of **necrotizing enterocolitis** and nutritional issues
- Liver immaturity and immature liver enzymes—increased risk of jaundice or **hyperbilirubinemia**
- Neurologic immaturity—With fragile blood vessels that rupture easily, there is increased risk of **intraventricular hemorrhage** or **bleeding** in the cavities of the brain (in babies less than thirty-two-weeks gestation).
- Immature respiratory center—**apnea** and **bradycardia**
- **Anemia**—in stressed preterm infants requiring frequent blood drawing for tests
- **Retinopathy of prematurity**—due to abnormal growth of blood vessels in preterm babies, especially those less than thirty-weeks gestation
- **Bronchopulmonary dysplasia** or chronic lung disease.

Respiratory Distress Syndrome (RDS)

Premature babies have deficient surfactant in their lung sacs or alveoli. **Surfactant** is a lipid or fat secreted by lung cells that lines the **alveoli**, reducing the surface tension, thus keeping them open. Surfactant deficiency leads to collapsed alveoli and stiff lungs. The earlier the gestation, the less is the surfactant, and therefore the higher the incidence of RDS.

Presentation

Babies with RDS present with respiratory distress including **grunting, tachypnea** or fast breathing, and **chest-wall retractions,** thus increasing the work of breathing.

Diagnosis

Diagnosis is confirmed by obtaining a chest **x-ray**. In an x-ray, the air-filled alveoli appear dark and the collapsed alveoli appear white, giving the lungs a ground glass appearance. In severe RDS, with a lot of collapsed alveoli, the lungs appear to be "whited out."

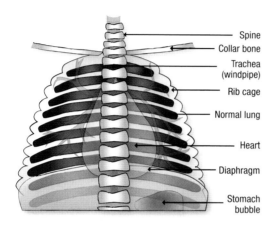

Spine
Collar bone
Trachea (windpipe)
Rib cage
Normal lung
Heart
Diaphragm
Stomach bubble

Figure 9A:
Diagrammatic representation of normal chest x-ray

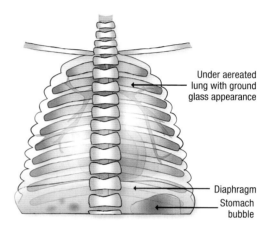

Under aereated lung with ground glass appearance
Diaphragm
Stomach bubble

Figure 9B:
Diagrammatic representation of chest x-ray showing Respiratory Distress Syndrome

Monitoring

It is important to follow the respiratory status, oxygen, and carbon dioxide levels in these tiny infants by meticulously monitoring their blood gases; this requires frequent blood drawing. Maintaining optimal oxygenation is crucial, especially in the extremely premature "fetal infants," in order to protect the eyes and the brain. Too much oxygen can be a risk factor in the causation of retinopathy of prematurity or chronic lung disease, and too little can lead to damage to the developing brain. The pulse oximeter allows us to monitor the infant's blood oxygen continuously. **Oxygen saturation** in these infants is generally maintained between 88 to 95 percent.

Treatment

- **Respiratory support** as needed in order to maintain optimal blood gases depicting the blood oxygen and carbon dioxide.

    The type of support is chosen based upon the baby's individual needs. *Minimally invasive ventilation or breathing support such as nasal cannula oxygen, nasal CPAP, or nasal prong ventilation are preferred to minimize lung injury.*

    Sicker babies may require **mechanical ventilator** support. However, prolonged ventilator assistance can lead to barotrauma (trauma due to the pressure of vent support) and damage to the delicate lung tissues. Therefore, providing the life-sustaining ventilator support and weaning as possible is always a balance for the neonatologist. Multiple modes of ventilation such as oscillators and pressure and volume ventilators are available to provide optimal support and minimize lung injury.

    With advances in technology, the period of vent support required has decreased significantly.

- **Surfactant:** The approval of surfactant administration in the United States in 1990 provided a major breakthrough in the treatment of respiratory distress syndrome. *Surfactant is a liquid phospholipid that can be administered to a baby via the endotracheal tube* in the NICU or even in the delivery room. This is bagged into the lungs via the endotracheal tube. It works by helping to keep the air sacs open (which tend to collapse due to deficient surfactant).

    Various types of surfactant preparations such as Survanta and Curosurf are available today. Often surfactant may be given, and then the baby is extubated and placed on NCPAP if tolerated.

    A frequent question is *"Can we give more of the good stuff—surfactant?"*

    We often see a dramatic response with the oxygen requirement coming down as surfactant is instilled. However, this can gradually go up again due to continued decreased surfactant production in the lungs. Usually one or two, and sometimes three doses are given eight to twelve hours apart. More doses of surfactant have not been found to be effective, and therefore are not recommended.

- **Caffeine:** Extremely preterm infants may be assisted by starting caffeine within the first few days *to decrease the incidence of chronic lung disease, or bronchopulmonary dysplasia (BPD), and neuro developmental delay.*

It is important to understand, however, that each baby is unique and needs to be assessed individually. Even though there are protocols available, neonatology is certainly not a cookie-cutter science. The NICU team will consider various parameters to determine the need for mechanical ventilation support (e.g., weight, gestation, x-rays, and blood gases).

The classical scenario, however, in a preterm (e.g., thirty-two weeks gestation) infant may be worsening of the respiratory distress over the first two to three days and then improvement over the next few days. Surfactant administration helps to stabilize the infant's condition more rapidly. Smaller and sicker babies may require prolonged ventilator support, sometimes for several weeks.

<u>Complications</u>

- **Air leaks or pneumothorax** (pneumo = air, thorax = chest cavity) can occur due to the rupture of air sacs of the lung, leading to air collection around the lung, requiring further respiratory support or a chest tube. This occurs more often in an infant on high vent support with stiff lungs.
- **Pneumonia** is caused by infection in the already immunocompromised baby.
- **Bronchopulmonary dysplasia (BPD),** or chronic lung disease, is due to lung damage due to inflammation and scarring of the air sacs and bronchi. The incidence and severity of BPD has decreased significantly with the use of antenatal steroids before delivery, surfactant, and advancement of non-invasive ventilation.

Sepsis

Immaturity of the preterm immune system may lead to increased incidence of infection in the blood (**sepsis**), other body sites, and sometimes of the protective membranes (meninges) surrounding the brain and spinal cord (**meningitis**).

Another cause of increased infections in preterm infants is an *inadequate transfer of antibodies from the mother.* This transfer generally occurs late in pregnancy, so a baby born early may have missed the transfer of antibodies that would have occurred in the later months.

Group B streptococcus (GBS) and **Escherichia coli** (E. coli) are the most common organisms causing infections in the newborn. Sepsis occurring after one week of age may be due to an acquired infection with organisms such as staphylococcus aureus. Other **bacteria, viruses, or fungi** can also be the causative organisms of infection in the newborn.

If infection is suspected, the infant is placed on treatment right away after obtaining blood cultures and/or spinal fluid as indicated. Babies do not fight infections well and thus the treating physicians do not have the luxury of waiting for culture results before beginning antibiotics. If blood culture remains negative, antibiotics are discontinued after forty-eight hours. If blood culture is positive, antibiotics are continued for ten to fourteen days depending on the organism, and for up to three weeks if the baby has meningitis.

Treatment

The initial antibiotics of choice are usually ampicillin and gentamicin, or ampicillin and cephalosporins, which treat most of the common infections in the newborn. These may be changed, or another added, as the specific organism and sensitivities are identified.

Prevention

Group B streptococci (GBS): *Between 25–40 percent of healthy women may carry GBS in their reproductive tracts.* Fifty percent of babies born to these moms are colonized (carry bacteria on their skin), and only one in a hundred actually develops the infection. However, GBS can cause a serious illness. Therefore, *mothers are screened by obtaining a vaginal swab at thirty-five to thirty-seven-weeks gestation* and treated at delivery if colonized. The awareness of GBS infection and intrapartum (during delivery) prophylaxis has decreased the incidence of GBS in the newborns, and E. coli are now emerging as the infecting organisms more often.

Cardiac (Heart) Problems

Patent ductus arteriosus (PDA) remains the most common cardiac problem encountered in preterm infants (Figure 10).

Prior to birth, the oxygen needs of the fetus are met by the mother. The circulation in the fetus bypasses the stiff, beefy lungs via **foramen ovale** (oval opening) between the two upper chambers of the heart (atria) and **ductus arteriosus** (duct between the two big arteries, the aorta and the pulmonary artery).

- After birth, these two channels, foramen ovale and PDA, normally close within the first day so that blood can get to the lungs, now filled with air (as the baby is breathing). In some infants, the ductus arteriosus remains open (patent).

  Now that the lungs are functioning, PDA leads to increased blood flow to the lungs thus flooding the lungs.
- Thirty to forty percent of babies weighing less than 1,000 grams (2.3 pounds) have a persistent PDA.

<u>Presentation</u>

- A small PDA may cause few problems other than a **heart murmur** and require no treatment.
- A medium-to-large PDA presents with a heart murmur (often referred to as a machinery murmur), a large heart on the chest x-ray, and **increasing respiratory problems**.
- Untreated PDA will lead to an extra volume of blood flooding the lungs, with leakage into the lung fields (pulmonary edema), both of which increase the work of breathing and make the heart work harder.

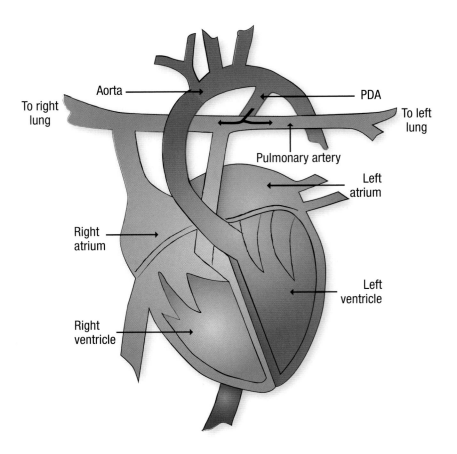

Figure 10: Patent ductus arteriosus (PDA)

Diagnosis

An **echocardiogram,** a study of the heart (like the ultrasound you may have had of your abdomen during pregnancy), is done to confirm the diagnosis.

Treatment

Very often the PDA closes by itself. Further treatment, if required, includes:

- Fluid restriction
- Indomethacin or ibuprofen: If the PDA is symptomatic and causing difficulty in ventilation support or is large, indomethacin or ibuprofen treatment is used. These

drugs are inhibitors of prostaglandin[1] and help close the ductus or PDA.

- If medical treatment is unsuccessful, **surgery** is a treatment option. The surgical procedure is referred to as **"PDA ligation."** A small incision is made in the infant's left chest wall, and a suture or clip is placed around the ductus. Surgery may take up to an hour and requires a chest tube for one to two days afterward, which drains air and fluid to assist the healing. This procedure is done in the operating room, or can be done at bedside in NICUs with adequate surgical support.

Congestive Heart Failure (CHF)

Any condition increasing the work of the heart, such as a significant PDA, other congenital heart disease, sepsis, arrhythmia, severe anemia, and fluid overload can all lead to congestive heart failure (CHF). In this condition the heart muscle weakens, thus decreasing the optimal functioning of the heart.

Treatment is medical, including diuretics (remove excess fluid), digoxin (strengthens the heart), and supplemental oxygen.

Necrotizing Enterocolitis (NEC)

Necrotizing enterocolitis (NEC) is an inflammation of the intestines that can occur in 6 to 10 percent of preterm infants and rarely in term infants. NEC typically occurs within the first two to three weeks, usually as oral feeds are begun, though the cause is not always understood. Lack of oxygen to the gut along with bacterial invasion and early feeds (especially formula) may be some of the risk factors associated with NEC.

---

1   Prostaglandins are vital, hormone-like secretions in the body tissues that can have varied effects, one of which can be to keep the PDA open. Prostaglandin inhibitors thus help to close the PDA.

Presentation

The baby starts to show **abdominal distension** (swelling), intolerance of feeds, vomiting, **blood in stools**, and appears ill. An x-ray is needed to show overt evidence of NEC, which may show distended bowel, or classically air bubbles in the bowel wall, referred to as **pneumatosis**. The swollen bowel may get necrotic as bacteria invade the bowel wall. At surgery,

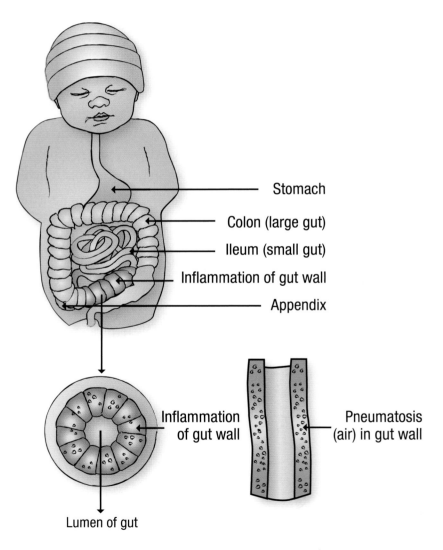

Figure 11: Necrotizing Enterocolitis

this dying segment of the bowel may appear to have a purple to a blackish hue.

Often there is some intolerance of feeds, but there is no x-ray evidence of NEC except for bowel distension. This is referred to as "possible NEC."

Treatment

- **NPO** and observation

   (NPO is a term that translates to "nil per os," which is Latin for nothing per oral, or mouth).

   For "possible NEC," feeds are held for forty-eight to seventy-two hours.

   If the diagnosis is certain, baby may remain NPO for one week or more, allowing time for bowel healing.

- **Bowel decompression**

   An **orogastric** or OG (oro = mouth gastric = stomach) tube from mouth to stomach, or **nasogastric,** or NG (from nose to stomach) tube is inserted to relieve the tension of the distended bowel (bowel decompression). A **replogle** tube may be used instead; this is a larger tube with a vent that is connected to low intermittent suction to further relieve the built-up bowel distension.

- **Intravenous antibiotics are started**, as infection may be a causative factor of NEC.

- Babies with documented x-ray changes of NEC are often very sick and may require **follow-up x-rays** to look for intestinal rupture or perforation.

- **Parenteral (intravenous) nutrition** is continued until recovery, at which time feeds are introduced very gingerly.

Complications

- **Bowel rupture** (intestinal perforation) may occur, requiring emergency surgery where a part of the dead bowel is removed and an opening or stoma is made in the abdominal wall (ostomy), so that bowel secretions and stool can drain out. If the hole is in the large intestine, or colon, this is called a **colostomy**. If it is in the small intestine, or ileum, it is called an **ileostomy**. Another surgery will be needed to close the ostomy and reanastamose (reconnect) the two ends of the bowel at a later date.

- If a large portion of the sick gut needs to be removed at surgery, this can lead to **"short gut syndrome,"** where infants may need total parenteral nutrition (TPN) for a prolonged period. They may need special formulas and special nutrients to be supplemented as the absorption of these nutrients from the short gut is reduced.

Nutritional Issues

Intravenous Nutrition

Optimal nutrition with adequate **nutrients** is an essential part of the care of a NICU infant.

Suck-and-swallow coordination does not occur until thirty-three to thirty-four weeks, so an infant born at twenty-five weeks may require nutritional support for eight weeks before being able to begin oral feeds. At first, intravenous nutrition is initiated with glucose water—glucose with salts such as sodium chloride, potassium chloride, calcium, and then very soon **total parenteral nutrition** (TPN) with a calculated amount of protein, glucose, fats, vitamins, electrolytes, and minerals. Intravenous fluids or TPN are given initially via a peripheral vein or umbilical venous catheter (if in place) and later via a PCVC—peripheral central venous catheter. A PCVC is a long catheter placed in a vein in the arm or leg, as an aseptic procedure and then threaded into a larger vein. The placement is confirmed by obtaining an x-ray. A PCVC can be maintained in place for a longer period. If necessary babies can be provided adequate nutrition with intravenous TPN for weeks.

Enteral Nutrition

Trophic feeds

As the baby's clinical status improves, very tiny feeds called trophic feeds are introduced via a gavage tube (**feeding tube**) as early as tolerated to stimulate the growth of the immature gut. During **gavage feeding** or **tube feeding**, a thin plastic tube (marked for ease of placement) is introduced through the mouth (**orogastric**) or through the nose (**nasogastric**) into the stomach after appropriate measurements. Placement is confirmed clinically. A pacifier may be given to the infant during gavage feeds, referred to as **non nutritive sucking**, which increases digestion and strengthens the sucking process.

Bolus feeds

Bolus feeds[2] are then introduced via a gavage tube in small volumes and increased slowly. In very small babies, the volume of feeds may be started with as little as one to two ml per feed every two to three hours. This may be breast milk or preemie formula such as special care or Enfamil Premature. As the feeds are increased, TPN is decreased.

Continuous feeds

In a very small or very sick baby having difficulty in accepting periodic or bolus feeds, continuous feeds may be given via a gavage tube. This decreases the sudden distension of the stomach and may be better tolerated by some infants.

Nasojejunal feeds

If spitting up or feeding intolerance continues, **nasojejunal (NJ) feeds** may be instituted. A nasojejunal tube is a special weighted tube that is passed from the mouth into the stomach and then advanced to the duodenum and jejunum by appropriate positioning of the infant. The NJ tube position is then verified by an x-ray. The feed thus bypasses the stomach (especially if there is delayed gastric emptying) and **gastroesophageal reflux** is prevented.

---

2   Bolus feeds: This is a feeding method using a syringe to deliver a certain amount of milk periodically through a feeding, or gavage tube.

Breast milk

> **Breast milk** is the optimal food for both term and preterm infants; therefore, every attempt is made to use breast milk as much as possible. *Breast milk has twenty calories per ounce.* However, in very preterm mother's milk, the protein, calcium, and phosphorus are not adequate, and **fortifiers** or supplements (Enfamil or Similac) are added to the breast milk.
>
> With fortifiers, the caloric value is usually advanced to twenty-four calories once regular breast milk is tolerated well. Prolacta, or human milk fortifier is now being used in NICUs. Prolacta is available as Prolacta+4, +6, +8, and +10 to give extra calories per ounce. Prolacta+4 will give four additional calories per ounce and so on.
>
> **Donor breast milk** may also be an option if needed.[3]

Formula

> If breast milk is not available or the mother does not wish to breastfeed, preemie formulas such as Similac Special Care or Enfamil Premature are used. These formulas are available as 20, 24, and 30 calories per-ounce versions as needed.
>
> **Weight gain** is always an exciting event for a parent. Babies are weighed in the NICU daily, traditionally after midnight, and weights are charted. These can be followed on graphs every week to document appropriate weight gain on the optimal curve for that gestation.
>
> Term babies can lose up to 10 percent of their birth weight within the first few days; this weight loss can increase to 15 percent for preterm babies. Sicker babies may lose even more weight. Most of this is retained water weight, or excess body water.
>
> After that, babies gain, on average, fifteen to thirty grams (one-half to one ounce) per day.

---

3   Donor breast milk is obtained from milk banks where excess milk donated by breastfeeding mothers is collected, tested, and stored.

If the preterm baby is still not gaining adequate weight, 24 Cal formula may be initiated as mentioned earlier, or breast milk feeds are fortified to twenty-two or twenty-four calories per ounce and on occasion to thirty calories per ounce.

Kangaroo Care

Kangaroo care, so called due to its similarity to the natural kangaroo pouch, can be initiated as soon as the infant is stable. Parents will note that the nurses are highly encouraging of this practice of skin-to-skin care, which is beneficial to both infant and parent.

The diapered, unclothed baby, with monitors still attached, is held between the mother's breasts or on the father's bare chest, and both are covered with a blanket. Babies maintain their warmth, appear to spend more quiet and alert time, maintain a regular heart rate, and have a better weight gain per reports.

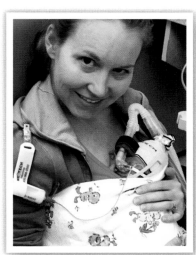

Parents isolated from their preterm babies have found that kangaroo care has brought a special closeness and bonding with their baby, reduction in stress, and improved breast milk production in mothers. Parents can ask when they may start doing kangaroo care with their infant.

Hyperbilirubinemia (Jaundice)

Jaundice (jaune = yellow) is a yellowish coloration of the skin that is caused when red blood cells break down and produce **bilirubin,** which gets deposited in the skin.

Causes

- The most common form of jaundice is **physiologic jaundice,** which occurs in almost 50 percent of term and 80 percent of preterm infants.

  Physiologic (or normal) jaundice occurs due to increased bilirubin production due to larger volume of red blood cells (RBCs) in the newborn, less processing of the bilirubin due to immaturity of liver enzymes, and less clearance from the gut. Thus, the serum bilirubin level increases. If it is more than 5 mg percent it produces visible yellowness of the skin or jaundice. Physiologic jaundice is usually seen on day two or three of life in term, and later in preterm infants. Physiologic jaundice can cause bilirubin to be as high as 12 mg percent in term, and even higher in preterm, infants.

- **Breast milk jaundice** is another question mothers often ask about. This form of jaundice, which presents after three to five days of life in a few breast feeding mothers, can cause prolonged jaundice. Rarely though, does one need discontinuation of breast milk feeds for forty-eight hours. The exact cause of breast milk jaundice is not known.

- **Blood group incompatibility:** A common cause of jaundice in the newborn is blood group incompatibility such as **ABO** or **Rh**.

  If Mom is Rh negative, and fetus Rh positive, fetal red blood cells (RBCs) can cross into maternal circulation—seen as a foreign substance, this can trigger the production of antibodies that travel to the fetus and destroy fetal RBCs (hemolysis), leading to increased bilirubin and jaundice. These antibodies may stay in the system for several days after birth.

  Similar dynamics occur if Mom is blood type O and fetus is A or B. Other minor blood group incompatibilities can occur such as Kell, Duffy, etc.

- Other causes of jaundice include red blood cell breakdown due to a different red blood cell shape, such as **spherocytosis,**[4] enzyme disorders such as **G6PD deficiency,** infection, decreased RBC production, congenital liver enzyme deficiency, and so on.

---

4   Spher-cytosis is a congenital disorder that causes the production of red blood cells that are sphere shaped rather than normal bi-concave disk shaped.

<u>Processing of Bilirubin</u>

Bilirubin gets broken down in the liver in the presence of an enzyme, glucuronyl transferase, to a form that can be excreted in the stool and urine. This enzyme is deficient in newborns, more so in preterm infants, a factor leading to increased (hyper) bilirubin and thus increased jaundice (physiologic jaundice).

Very high bilirubin can stain the central nuclei of the brain and cause **kernicterus** (kern = nuclei, icterus = jaundice), and lead to deafness, abnormal movements, and neurodevelopmental issues later in life. Therefore, bilirubin needs to be monitored and treatment instituted if levels are high.

<u>Presentation</u>

- Icterus, or yellowish skin discoloration, is seen in newborns in a head-to-toe progression (seen on the face first)—usually, the higher the bilirubin level, the more yellow the skin.
- A baby with jaundice may also be less active and feed poorly.
- The bilirubin level can be recorded using a **bilirubinometer** (a simple, large, thermometer-like instrument), which is placed on the forehead and displays the bilirubin reading with a good degree of correlation. However, a blood test will also be sent to the lab for confirmation.

<u>Treatment</u>

- **Phototherapy:** Hospital staff in the late 1950s noted that infants close to the window in the nursery were less jaundiced than those in the center of the room. This led to research of the light spectra and thus arose the concept of phototherapy. However, it was a decade later before controlled trials led to acceptance of phototherapy, which is now the mainstay of treatment for jaundice in the newborn. A certain wavelength of light (blue light) is used to break down the bilirubin to soluble products that can then be excreted in the urine and stool.

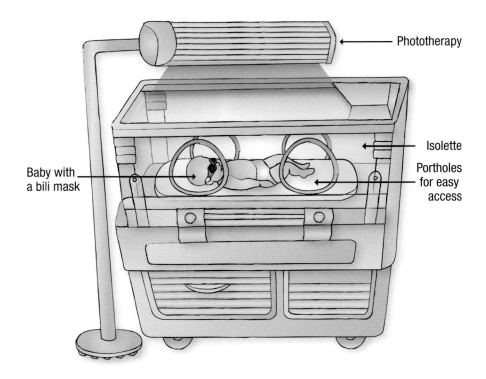

Figure 12: Phototherapy

Phototherapy works well in newborns and, usually, no further treatment is needed.

Sometimes if a premature baby is very small and bruised, preventative phototherapy may be started so that the bilirubin level does not increase rapidly.

<u>Problems</u>

- Problems associated with phototherapy are minimal. However, the infant's eyes are covered with eye patches known as a "bili mask" (which we lovingly refer to as "sunglasses") during the therapy, since phototherapy has been associated with **possible retinal effects in animals.**
- Another problem associated with the use of phototherapy can be **diarrhea,** as bilirubin byproducts are excreted through the gut.
- **Dehydration** may occur due to increased water loss through the skin exposed to light.

- **Exchange transfusion:** The need for exchange transfusions has plummeted, with the advent of phototherapy. However, sometimes the bilirubin level continues to remain high even after phototherapy, and an exchange transfusion is needed.

<u>Procedure</u>

A catheter is placed in the **umbilical vein** with a three-way connector. Fresh blood is obtained, and a double volume exchange (blood volume being about eighty ml/kg) is done. At one time, ten to twenty ml of blood is removed via the catheter and then replaced. The procedure may take one to two hours to complete. The blood glucose, electrolytes, calcium, complete blood count (CBC), and repeat bilirubin levels are all measured before and after the exchange.

Complications that can arise from an exchange transfusion include possible blood clots and emboli (where blood clots can travel to different organs), infection, electrolyte abnormalities, and in some cases even necrotizing enterocolitis, as with the blood drawing and replacement, gut perfusion can be affected. These are very rare complications.

- **Gamma globulin** is another medication more recently being used in certain situations. Gamma globulins block the antibodies, decreasing hemolysis (red cell breakdown) and bilirubin production, therefore decreasing the likelihood that an exchange transfusion might be required.

Intraventricular Hemorrhage (IVH)

Ventricles are chambers in the brain that contain a fluid called cerebrospinal fluid (CSF) that bathes the brain and spinal cord. (Note that the lower two heart chambers are also referred to as ventricles.) There are four ventricles in the brain—two lateral

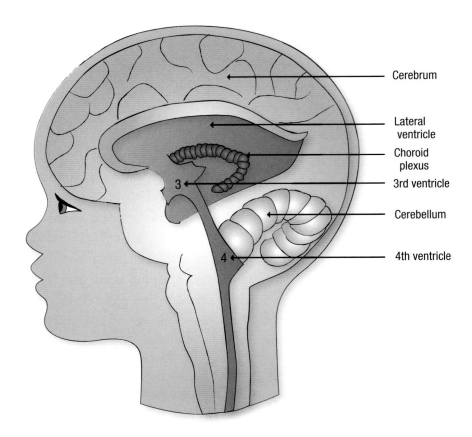

Cerebrum

Lateral ventricle

Choroid plexus

3rd ventricle

Cerebellum

4th ventricle

CSF is produced in choroid plexus → Lateral ventricle → 3rd ventricle → 4th ventricle → spinal canal

Figure 13: Diagrammatic representation of ventricles of the brain and CSF circulation

ventricles (in the forebrain), a third ventricle (in the midbrain), and a fourth ventricle (in the brainstem).

Cerebrospinal fluid is produced in the choroid plexus—a network of blood vessels in the lateral ventricles in the forebrain-and flows to the third ventricle, on to the fourth ventricle, and then bathes the space around the brain and spinal cord (Figure 13).

Blood vessels in the developing brain, especially in an area called **germinal matrix,** are immature and very fragile. In the sick preterm infant exposed to either low or high cerebral blood flow, these fragile blood vessels can rupture, leading to blood collecting in the ventricles. This may lead to enlargement of the ventricles, and in more severe cases blood flows into the brain tissue outside the ventricles destroying it, leading to cysts, damage, and **periventricular leukomalacia** (PVL) or softening of the white matter.

About 20% of babies less than 1,500 grams may have an intraventricular hemorrhage.

More than 50% of the ventricular bleeds occur in the first twenty-four hours and about 95% by the first week.

<u>Risk Factors</u>

- **Prematurity:** Risk is inversely related to gestational age. The more preterm the baby, the higher the risk of IVH. Autoregulation of brain blood flow is also poor in preterm infants, which can lead to fluctuating flow, especially with any adverse events.
- Some of the **other risk factors** include stressors such as prolonged labor, requirement of prolonged resuscitation, intrauterine infection or sepsis, and pneumothorax.

<u>IVH is Categorized into Four Grades (Figure 14)</u>

- Grade I   Blood limited to the germinal matrix
- Grade II   Blood in the ventricle
- Grade III   Blood in the ventricle with ventricular enlargement
- Grade IV   Bleeding in and injury to brain tissues around the ventricle
  - ◆ Grades I and II generally have a good outcome.
  - ◆ Grades III and IV are at risk for neurologic disabilities.
  - ◆ PVL is associated with injury, and a high risk of disabilities.

<u>Presentation</u>

Presentation of an IVH may be silent, or there may be a sudden deterioration of status with a drop in blood pressure and increasing respiratory support or a sudden drop in hemoglobin.

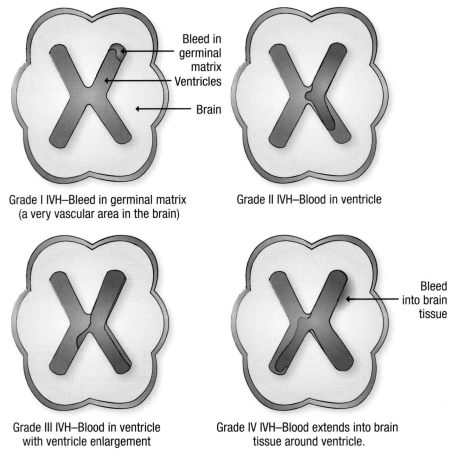

Grade I IVH–Bleed in germinal matrix
(a very vascular area in the brain)

Grade II IVH–Blood in ventricle

Grade III IVH–Blood in ventricle
with ventricle enlargement

Grade IV IVH–Blood extends into brain
tissue around ventricle.

Figure 14: Grades of Intraventricular Hemorrhage

Diagnosis

A head ultrasound (HUS) from the anterior **fontanelle** (soft spot of the skull) gives a good bedside diagnosis of an IVH. Initial HUS screen is done by one week of age in preterm babies less than thirty-two-weeks gestation (or earlier in very sick or extremely preterm infants). If normal, HUS is repeated at thirty-six to forty weeks.

If HUS is abnormal, a close follow-up is recommended.

Outcome

It is very hard to predict the neurologic outcome in an infant with IVH. Usually it's a "let's wait and watch" approach. In general, however, a mild case will have no or few problems, and a more severe IVH (III or IV) may lead to long-term neurodevelopmental complications.

Having said that, newborns can be very resilient, and I've seen many different outcomes, as some of the stories depict.

Periventricular Leukomalacia (PVL)

Peri = around; leuco = white; malacia = softening: This translates to softening of the white matter around the ventricles.

This is a brain injury in mostly premature infants where an area around the ventricles is injured. This injury most commonly occurs due to leakage or decreased blood flow leading to cell death in this area.

Causes of periventricular leukomalacia (PVL) are often unknown, but may be related to IVH (as above), temporary lack of oxygen, brain infection (e.g., meningitis), seizures, or at times it may be an intrauterine event. The more severe the PVL, the higher the likelihood of significant motor or cognitive developmental delay.

Complications

- **Hydrocephalus** (hydro = water; cephalus = head) occurs due to too much cerebrospinal fluid (CSF) in the ventricles. This can be congenital due to a deformity, causing an obstruction of the CSF drainage, or acquired, for example, following IVH.

  Normally the cerebrospinal fluid flows from its site of production in the choroid plexus in the lateral ventricles (brain chambers) to the third and fourth ventricle. This then bathes the brain and spinal cord and is constantly absorbed (Figure 13).

  An obstruction or blockage in this pathway can occur due to a congenital narrowing of the flow pathway such as third ventricle stenosis (narrowing), obstruction in fourth ventricle, or due to blood clots following IVH, and in some cases meningitis, causing adhesions and blockage.

In either case the obstruction can result in collection of the fluid leading to large ventricles and a large head size or hydrocephalus, often referred to in lay terms as "water head."

Treatment

- **Serial spinal taps** may be done in an attempt to remove excessive spinal fluid to relieve pressure on the brain. Sometimes a reservoir is placed in the head to periodically drain fluid from the lateral ventricles of the brain.
- **Medications** may be used temporarily to decrease the spinal fluid production.
- If other treatments fail, a **shunt** (thin tube) may be inserted to drain CSF from the brain ventricle. This is done by threading a tube underneath the skin from the brain ventricles into the heart or peritoneal cavity of the abdomen, so that the fluid drains there. These shunts or channels may need to be lengthened or revised with the child's growth.

Cerebral Palsy (CP)

An injury to the brain before, during, or shortly after birth can cause cerebral palsy. The cause of CP in preterm babies is usually due to lack of oxygen to the brain, brain hemorrhage, or PVL. Preterm infants are at an increased risk for development of cerebral palsy, with an increased incidence in VLBW (very tiny) babies. Cerebral palsy can especially affect body movements, muscle control, coordination, muscle tone, and balance.

After discharge, a close monitoring of milestone achievements, muscle exams, and coordination may detect CP earlier. Early diagnosis and **early interventional programs** providing **occupational, physical, and speech therapy** can assist in a better outcome. Thus, early interventional follow-up programs are always recommended when a preemie is discharged.

Drugs such as muscle relaxants and surgery may help problems of spasticity. Orthopedic devices (i.e., splints and walkers) may be needed in some cases.

Apnea of Prematurity

The respiratory system of a premature infant is immature, as is the firing center for respirations or breathing in the brain. As we often tell parents, "The respiratory center in the brain is immature and babies thus often forget to breathe." This leads to pauses during breathing. If the pause is twenty seconds or more, it is called "**apnea**." Apnea may be associated with a drop in the heart rate, which if less than eighty beats per minute is called **bradycardia**. Apnea may be accompanied by "cyanosis" or a blue spell as oxygenation drops. This can certainly be a very scary sight for a parent.

Causes

Apnea remains one of the most common problems of prematurity. The more preterm the infant, the higher is the incidence of apnea, being seen in *over 90 percent of infants less than twenty-eight weeks, and in about 50 percent of babies between thirty-three to thirty-five-weeks gestation.* Apnea can be **central** due to immaturity of the respiratory center or **obstructive** due to obstruction or blockage of the airway due to immaturity and decreased tone of upper airway musculature. **Mixed apnea** is a combination of both, which is often the case.

Apnea, however, can be a symptom of some other illness such as an infection, IVH, or electrolyte or glucose abnormalities, all of which need to be investigated and ruled out.

Treatment

- "**Stimulation**" by flicking the toes or rubbing the back, in other words "reminding the baby to breathe," is all that is generally needed to reinstate regular breathing.
- Sometimes the baby may need **supplemental oxygen** given with an oxygen tubing or "bag and mask" ventilation, often referred to as **"bagging,"** where a mask is applied to the nose and mouth and gentle mechanical breaths are given to the infant, usually for a few seconds, before the baby starts breathing normally.

- **Continuous positive airway pressure (CPAP)** or **ventilator support** may be needed in some cases. CPAP stents the fragile collapsible airway, whereas the ventilator provides mechanical breaths.
- **Medications:** Central apnea may be treated by using **medications such as caffeine** (as in coffee) or **theophylline**, which stimulates the respiratory center. These medications are discontinued by thirty-three to thirty-four weeks as respirations improve, and the baby is then monitored in the hospital prior to discharge.
- Babies are usually observed for *five to seven (apnea or bradycardia) alarm-free days* before being cleared for discharge. On occasion infants may have to be discharged on caffeine.
- If the infant is having brief apnea episodes, but is otherwise ready for discharge, the baby may be sent home on a **home monitor.** The respiratory center usually matures by the time infant achieves forty-weeks gestation or term status. Parents are given monitor training and infant **cardiopulmonary resuscitation training (CPR).** You will then be set up with a close follow-up, usually by monitor-company nurses. I usually tell parents, "It would be great to have all parents trained in infant CPR. You probably will not need it, but it is an invaluable tool to have in an emergency."
- If there is a family history of **sudden infant death syndrome (SIDS),** a home monitor may be requested. Apnea, however, does not predispose to SIDS.

Anemia of Prematurity

Anemia is a common problem in the NICU and is caused by a lack of adequate red blood cells (RBCs) or hemoglobin (Hgb) in the RBCs that carry oxygen throughout the body.

Causes

Most babies experience what is called physiologic anemia as their growth exceeds the red blood cell production. This is more marked in the preterm infant with excessive catch-up growth and less iron reserves, often referred to as *physiologic anemia of prematurity.*

Frequent blood drawing is necessary in these tiny neonates whose *blood volume is only about eighty ml (two and a half ounces) per kilogram of weight.* Loss of blood is a significant cause of anemia.

Monitoring

Hemoglobin and **hematocrit** are thus monitored regularly in the NICU. If these fall too low, a blood transfusion is required so that optimal oxygen carrying can continue to the tissues for healthy functioning of all the organs.

Hemoglobin or hematocrit will be monitored frequently in the first week and at least once weekly while infant is in the hospital.

Treatment

- **Oral iron** supplementation is started early in preterm infants, they are once on full feeds.
- **Blood transfusion** may be needed if hemoglobin remains low despite iron supplementation.

Preterm infants often require multiple blood transfusions during a NICU stay, in spite of iron-supplemented formula and supplemental iron, especially during the acute care period.

The hemoglobin or hematocrit should be monitored for some time after the infant is discharged as well. An iron-enriched formula is usually used during the hospital stay as well as after discharge if the infant is being formula fed, and iron supplementation if being breast fed.

Retinopathy of Prematurity (ROP)

Retinopathy of prematurity (ROP), as the name implies, is a disease of the retina in preterm infants caused by an excessive and abnormal growth of blood vessels in the retina (the membrane lining the inner side of the back of the eye, which is the light-sensitive screen).

ROP can lead to vision problems such as nearsightedness requiring glasses; strabismus, or even blindness.

See Figures 15, 16, and 17.

Risk Factors

- ROP is felt to be associated not only with prematurity-associated risk factors, but also with a high concentration of supplemental oxygen.
- The smaller and earlier the preterm infant, the more is the risk of developing ROP.

Normally, blood vessels in the retina begin to develop at sixteen weeks of gestation and continue to grow from the optic disc at the center of the eye to the periphery of the retina. However, their growth is interrupted with preterm birth. Abnormal growth of these blood vessels can continue after birth. This abnormal growth can be accompanied by blood and fluid leaking into the eye, which is even more serious, and can lead to scarring and eventually even retinal detachment and blindness.

Screening

- All preterm babies born at less than thirty-weeks gestation and less than 1,500 grams (three and a half pounds) birth weight are scheduled to have an ophthalmology (eye) check-up at four to six weeks of age, and then every two weeks until the blood vessel growth is complete.
- If any issue is recognized, the follow-up may then be done weekly.
- Other very sick preterm infants may also be eligible for an ophthalmology exam.

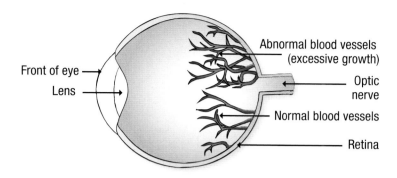

Figure 15: Eye showing normal and abnormal blood vessels in
Retinopathy of Prematurity (ROP)

Stages of Retinopathy of Prematurity (ROP) figure 16

The stages of ROP are categorized from stage 1 (abnormal blood vessel growth) to stage 5 (retinal detachment):

- Stage 1: Mildly abnormal blood vessel growth in retina
- Stage 2: Moderately abnormal blood vessel growth with a ridge in retina
- Stage 3: Severely abnormal blood vessel growth with extra retinal fibrous growth
- Stage 4: Fibrous tissue attaches to lens, pulling the retina away from the wall of the eye
- Stage 5: Completely detached retina

Zones

In addition to "staging," Ophthalmologists also refer to "position or zones" of ROP by concentric circles around the optic nerve. (Figure 17).

Plus Disease

Plus disease is another term used in addition to staging. In Plus disease, blood vessels are more dilated and convoluted, indicating a more severe retinopathy.

Outcome

ROP resolves in almost 75% of cases. There may be mild vision issues such as nearsightedness and strabismus or squint; however, sometimes blindness can result due to complete retinal detachment.

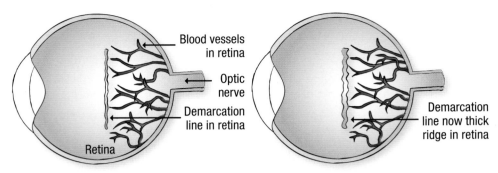

Stage 1: Vascular retina   Stage 2: Vascular retina forms a ridge

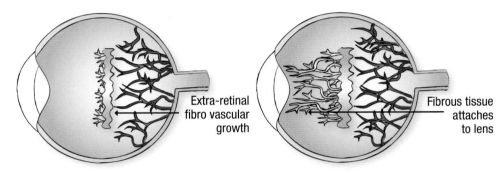

Stage 3: Extra retinal fibro-vascular growth   Stage 4: Fibrous tissue attaches to lens

Figure 16: Stages of Retinopathy of Prematurity (ROP)

Treatment of Advanced ROP

Cryopexy or laser treatment is recommended in babies where ROP monitoring indicates worsening ROP with a risk of retinal detachment.

- **Cryopexy** is when a probe is used to freeze the abnormal vessels with liquid nitrogen.
- **Laser therapy** in which a laser beam destroys the abnormal blood vessel growth—this requires sedation, though usually no anesthetic is needed. Baby's eyes may remain swollen for a few days after treatment.
- **Avastin** (bevacizumab—a blood vessel growth factor inhibitor) injection may be used. More research trials are underway for use of this treatment.

Close oxygen monitoring in the NICU has decreased the incidence and severity of ROP over recent years.

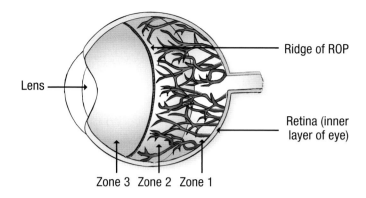

Figure 17: Zones of ROP
Zone 1: around the optic nerve
Zone 2: circle surrounding Zone 1
Zone 3: remainder of the retina

Bronchopulmonary Dysplasia (BPD)

Bronchopulmonary dysplasia (BPD) or chronic lung disease (CLD) refers to damaged and scarred breathing tubes and lungs occurring mostly in preterm infants following prolonged respiratory support and oxygen. Any preterm infant still requiring oxygen, or on any form of respiratory support, at or beyond thirty-six-weeks gestation meets the criteria for BPD.

<u>**Risk Factors**</u>

- **Prematurity:** Preterm infants on prolonged ventilator support are at the greatest risk for BPD.
- **Barotrauma** (pressure trauma) or **volutrauma** (trauma due to volume) from ventilators, especially for those on prolonged high ventilator support as well as **high oxygen concentration,** are the main risk factors causing damage to the immature lungs.
- **Bacterial infections** may worsen the scarred, narrowed bronchi or windpipes.
- Other respiratory problems such as **meconium aspiration** can also result in chronic lung disease or BPD.

<u>Prevention</u>

- Use of **non-invasive ventilation** such as nasal CPAP and nasal prong ventilation may preclude or shorten the duration of invasive ventilator support.
- Wean ventilator support as soon as possible.
- Use of **caffeine** soon after birth also seems to decrease the incidence of BPD.

<u>Treatment</u>

- **Optimal nutrition:** Additional calories may be needed to provide adequate nutrition to infants with BPD with higher energy requirements due to increased work of breathing.
- **Diuretics** to rid the body of fluid, especially from the lungs.
- **Bronchodilators** such as albuterol puffs may be needed to assist adequate ventilation.
- Babies with severe BPD may receive **low-dose steroids** for a short duration after a discussion with the parents.
- Some babies with chronic lung disease are sent home on monitors and home oxygen, as they require **prolonged respiratory support.** These patients will need to have a close follow-up and home care with ancillary support, such as respiratory care and home nursing assistance.

<u>Complications</u>

- Infants with BPD are more prone to upper respiratory infections as well as pneumonia.
- Re-hospitalization may be required and parents are usually pre-warned about this possibility.
- An increase in mucus resulting from the prolonged support, with the diaphragm being pushed down by the lungs with air trapping and scarring, may lead to **reflux and aspiration,** which can contribute to increased infections.
- BPD leads to a strain on the heart as well as the lungs, often leading to congestive heart failure and **right ventricular hypertrophy** or thickening. An echocardiogram may be

done to rule out right ventricular thickening and pulmonary hypertension.

- **Hypoxia episodes** may occur in BPD patients, leading to cyanosis or **"blue spells,"** during which the infant requires increased oxygen or bagging with a bag and mask.
- **Feeding problems** can result due to **oral aversion** (association with tubes, suctioning).

Prognosis

The outcome of BPD is mostly positive, though time intensive. "There is certainly light at the end of the tunnel as the alveoli continue to grow until eight years of age," as I often tell parents, adding, "Not that it's going to take that long."

With patience and support, improvement is seen in most babies in weeks to several months. Some may, however, continue to have reactive airways, or asthma.

Other Common Issues

Transient Tachypnea of the Newborn (TTN)

The most common cause of respiratory distress is Transient Tachypnea of the Newborn (TTN) in term and sometimes preterm infants that occurs due to retained lung fluid. As the name implies, it is transient and the baby is tachypneic (has rapid breathing).

TTN usually lasts for twelve to twenty-four hours, and sometimes up to seventy-two hours. Only a few babies need admission to the NICU due to TTN.

Recent data shows some association of TTN with reactive airway disease such as asthma.

Risk Factors

Cesarean section, rapid birth, or infant of diabetic mother may be some of the factors associated with retained lung fluid.

Presentation

- Rapid breathing with minimal chest retractions that develop soon after birth.
- A chest x-ray may show increased lung fluid.

Treatment

- Babies needing NICU admission may require supplemental oxygen via nasal cannula or occasionally nasal CPAP.
- Intravenous fluids are often needed due to the risk of aspiration with the fast breathing.
- Infection will need to be ruled out.

Hypoglycemia

Glucose is a major source of energy for newborns, especially for the brain. With delivery, the maternal supply of glucose is cut off and the newborn compensates by drawing on body reserves. Though the definition of hypoglycemia remains a contentious issue in the newborn, glucose less than forty mg/dL in the first twenty-four hours and less than fifty mg/dL after twenty-four hours is considered as hypoglycemia.

Prolonged hypoglycemia can have neuro developmental effects. Thus, we need to monitor glucose in infants at risk for hypoglycemia.

<u>Causes and Risk Factors for Hypoglycemia</u>

- **Transient Neonatal Hypoglycemia**

  Preterm, **small for gestational age (SGA)** infants have low body reserves and higher needs.

  Large for gestational age (LGA) infants with a larger brain have a greater glucose requirement.

  Stress, i.e., infection, generates a higher energy requirement.
- **Hyperinsulinism,** for example, **infant of a diabetic mother (IDM)**: High glucose levels in the mother lead to increased insulin production by the fetus. At delivery the glucose supply is cut off, but high insulin may persist leading to hypoglycemia for hours or days.
- Other causes include **metabolic errors, endocrine causes, polycythemia** (high hematocrit) with a higher glucose use by the increased red blood cell mass, and so on.

<u>Presentation</u>

- Most are asymptomatic and are picked up by frequent glucose monitoring of the "at-risk" infants.
- Symptoms include jitteriness, sweating, tachypnea (rapid breathing), apnea, abnormal cry, low tone, or even seizures.

<u>Diagnosis</u>

- Documentation of low blood glucose
- Glucose screening needs to be done in preterm, term SGA, IDM, LGA, and other at-risk infants soon after birth usually through the first twenty-four hours of age. Further screening may be needed as indicated by the glucose levels.

For persistent hypoglycemia, further testing, such as serum insulin, serum cortisol, and other tests, are done to rule out rarer causes.

Treatment

- Provide glucose as frequent feeds if tolerated.
- If hypoglycemia is not corrected by feeds, intravenous fluids may be administered and a bolus of glucose given.
- Some infants need frequent intravenous glucose boluses and up to 20% continuous intravenous glucose for correction of persistent hypoglycemia, and require monitoring for several days in the NICU. If more than 12.5% glucose is needed, an umbilical venous line is placed to administer the higher concentration of glucose that can be abrasive to the peripheral veins.
- Rarely, other medications may also be needed.

Meconium Aspiration Syndrome (MAS)

Meconium is the dark green, tarry substance that represents the first few stools of a newborn infant. If meconium is passed by the fetus inside the uterus, the amniotic fluid becomes green-tinged and is referred to as **meconium-stained amniotic fluid (MSAF).**

Ten percent of deliveries have MSAF, which may be (though not always) a sign of fetal distress, as babies often pass meconium in response to stress such as cord entanglement, cord compression, placental dysfunction, maternal infection, etc.

Meconium is sterile, yet if aspirated, it can cause blockage of breathing tubes (bronchi), breathing problems, and later chemical pneumonia with a continued decrease in surfactant production. Thus respiratory distress ensues.

The incidence of meconium aspiration has decreased due to improved prenatal care and support processes through delivery.

Presentation

Babies present with **respiratory distress** with rapid breathing or tachypnea, chest retractions, usually requirie supplemental oxygen and other respiratory support, such as CPAP, intubation, and ventilator assistance.

<u>Complications</u>

- **Pneumothorax** (air leak) is a complication of MAS. As air sacs get over-distended due to blockage by meconium and continued high ventilator support, they may rupture, leading to air collection in pleural cavity (space between the lungs and the chest wall) or pneumothorax.
- Air may collect in the sac around the heart and major blood vessels causing what is called a **pneumomediastinum.**
- **Pneumonia**—Though meconium is sterile, its aspiration provides a good medium for bacterial infection. Meconium aspiration can also induce a chemical pneumonitis.
- **Persistent pulmonary hypertension (PPHN)**, due to clamped or constricted lung capillaries, can be a serious complication.

<u>Treatment</u>

- **Respiratory support**, as needed
- **Antibiotics** are started, since infection cannot be ruled out.
- Severe cases with **pulmonary hypertension (PPHN)** may require **nitric oxide therapy,** which dilates the lungs' tiny blood vessels or capillaries; or, in extreme cases, **extra corporeal membrane oxygenation (ECMO)**, a procedure in which blood is taken out of a blood vessel, oxygenated outside, and then returned.

Pneumothorax

Pneumothorax (pneumo = air; thorax = chest cavity) is an air collection in the thorax due to an air leak from the lungs in the pleural space surrounding the lung. The infant is often on ventilator support.

<u>Causes</u>

- Spontaneous pneumothorax can occur in one percent of all live births for no known reason.
- Complication of respiratory distress syndrome (RDS) in preterm infant
- Complication of pneumonia or meconium aspiration syndrome (MAS)

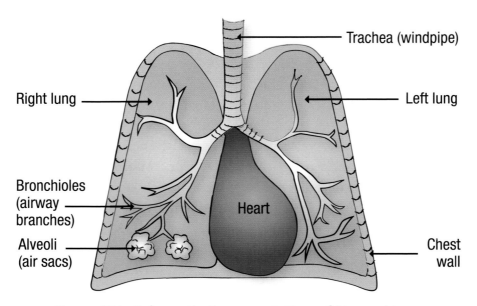

Figure 18A: Schematic Representation of Normal Lungs

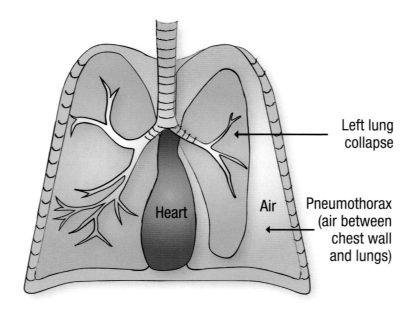

Figure 18B: Schematic Representation of Lung
with Pneumothorax

Symptoms and Signs

- Babies developing a pneumothorax may remain asymptomatic or present with respiratory distress with rapid breathing (tachypnea) and chest wall retractions.
- If large and producing tension, a sudden deterioration of respiratory status with a drop in heart rate and oxygen occurs.

Diagnosis

- **Transillumination** can be used in the NICU in an emergent situation—a bright light over the chest that lights up the side with the air collection (pneumothorax).
- Diagnosis is confirmed by **chest x-ray.**

Treatment

- Pneumothorax may resolve spontaneously.
- **Trial of nitrogen washout:** if stable, the infant is placed in a high oxygen concentration for twelve to twenty-four hours. The trapped air may be reabsorbed, and can be checked on a repeat chest x-ray.
- If pneumothorax is causing a tension on the heart and mediastinum (heart and big blood vessels in the center of chest), air may be removed by inserting a needle in the space between the lungs and chest wall (**needle aspiration**). If there is further concern regarding re-accumulation of air, a **chest tube** will need to be inserted. Babies requiring chest tube placement are managed with pain medication. The chest tube is connected to a pleur-evac drain, which pulls air out by a measured gentle pressure, documented by bubbling in the pleur-evac drain fluid. The chest tube is often required for two to three days or more. The lung heals after the chest tube is removed, and there are usually no long-term issues due to the history of pneumothorax.

Persistent Pulmonary Hypertension (PPHN)

While in the uterus, the blood circulation is called **"fetal circulation,"** where the stiff beefy lungs (with no air) are bypassed by two channels called **foramen ovale** (an opening between atria or upper two chambers of the heart) and **ductus arteriosus** (a channel between the aorta—a large artery coming from the heart—and the pulmonary artery).

After birth, in the presence of lungs now filled with air and oxygen, the blood must flow to the lungs; the lung capillaries open up; and the two channels (the foramen ovale and the ductus arteriosus) begin to close.

In **persistent pulmonary hypertension of the newborn (PPHN)**, this normal process does not occur and lung capillaries remain constricted (as in the uterus) causing pulmonary hypertension (PPHN) and reverse flow of the oxygenated blood results. So the baby may turn blue due to the mixing of the oxygenated (red) blood with the deoxygenated (blue) blood.

Causes

- Idiopathic—no known cause
- Asphyxia or lack of oxygen
- Meconium aspiration or pneumonia
- Respiratory Distress Syndrome
- Congenital malformations, e.g., congenital diaphragmatic hernia/lung hypoplasia

Presentation and Diagnosis

- Baby presents with respiratory distress with tachypnea or rapid breathing, chest retractions, and cyanosis.
- Baby may remain hypoxic (low oxygen) despite good ventilation and needs high ventilator support.
- A chest x-ray may, or may not, reveal the underlying cause.
- An echocardiogram is used to confirm the diagnosis.

<u>Treatment</u>

- **High ventilation**, maintaining high oxygenation and lower carbon dioxide levels, helps to open the tight lung capillaries (or small blood vessels).
- On occasion, **a high frequency ventilation** with an **oscillator**—a different mode of ventilation—may help.
- **Medications** such as **dopamine** and **dobutamine** administered as intravenous drips may be used for maintaining optimal blood pressure. Babies may need to be sedated during this time.
- **Inhaled nitric oxide** (iNO) administered via the ETT has been used in recent years; this is a gas that dilates the constricted (narrowed) lung capillaries.
- **Extracorporeal Membrane Oxygenation** (ECMO) (when none of the above work): This procedure uses a modified heart and lung machine, where blood from a large vein is taken, oxygenated outside the body in the ECMO circuit, and then transferred back to a large artery or back to a vein. The blood thus bypasses the lungs. As the infant's condition improves, the ECMO flow is decreased and more blood goes to the lungs. Infants may remain on ECMO for five to seven days, up to a maximum of two weeks.

PPHN infants can be very difficult to ventilate due to the clamped lung capillaries that continue to shunt back the oxygenated blood. Some of the family stories in Part II are examples of the seriousness of PPHN. When I am teaching, I often tell resident doctors that PPHN babies were some of the sickest infants that I have taken care of over the years.

Pneumonia

The airway and the lungs are common sites of infection in a newborn. Pneumonia (infection of the lungs) can be **congenital**, where the infection occurs from the mother in utero, or it may be **acquired** from respiratory or other equipment, family, or nursery personnel.

<u>Causes</u>

- Pneumonia may be bacterial (most commonly Group B streptococci, Escherichia coli, staphylococcus aureus, or other bacteria), viral, and, rarely, due to fungal infection.
- Chorioamnionitis—infection of the amniotic fluid and membranes enclosing the fetus in the mother—may be an associated factor.

<u>Presentation</u>

- Babies with pneumonia present with respiratory distress with fast breathing, chest retractions, and temperature instability.
- Infants born with congenital pneumonia are usually very sick at birth, requiring not only respiratory and nutritional support, but also medications to support the blood pressure.

<u>Diagnosis</u>

- Chest x-ray to document the pneumonia
- Blood gases for respiratory management
- Blood culture and viral tests such as TORCH (toxoplasma, rubella, cytomegalovirus, and herpes) to identify the infection.

<u>Treatment</u>

- **Antibiotics** are started. The antibiotics for bacterial pneumonia are usually continued for ten days.
- **Respiratory and nutritional support**
- Treatment of cause
- May need **intravenous vasopressors** to support blood pressure.

Neonatal Seizures

The brain is a complex computer composed of billions of neurons (nerve cells). The upper part of the brain (cerebrum) is the major nerve center, whereas the lower part (cerebellum and brainstem) controls balance and vital body functions, such as breathing and heart rate. Neonatal seizures are a symptom of possible brain irritation or injury.

Neonatal seizures are stereotypical, uncontrolled, rhythmic movements of muscles resulting from abnormal electrical discharges of the brain.

<u>Causes</u>

- Seizures may be due to lack of oxygen (asphyxia), or cerebral blood supply (ischemia).
- Intracranial hemorrhage
- Chemical imbalance, i.e., low glucose (hypoglycemia), low calcium (hypocalcemia), or electrolyte abnormality
- Secondary to an infection (i.e., meningitis)
- Secondary to a congenital malformation
- Idiopathic or no known cause

<u>Presentation</u>

Seizures may present as jerking movements of one or more limbs, arching, stiffening, unusual eye movements (staring, blinking, eye movements in one direction), excessive sucking or apnea and bradycardia, or the seizure may be subtle.

<u>Diagnosis</u>

- Blood chemistries to rule out low sugar, calcium, or electrolyte abnormalities
- Blood culture is obtained to rule out blood infection.
- Lumbar Puncture (spinal tap) to rule out meningitis

<u>Procedure</u>

- Infant is placed in lateral, fetal, or sitting position and bent forward or flexed. A spinal needle is then inserted into the lower back in the lumbar part of the vertebral column (backbone). Spinal fluid is collected from the spinal needle in sterile tubes and sent to the lab for tests.
- An electroencephalogram (EEG) is obtained where electrodes are placed on the skin of the scalp and the electrical activity of the brain is recorded. Seizures present as abnormal activity in specific areas of the brain. If seizures are due to severe asphyxia, they may persist for a long time. Continuous EEG monitoring may be needed in some cases.

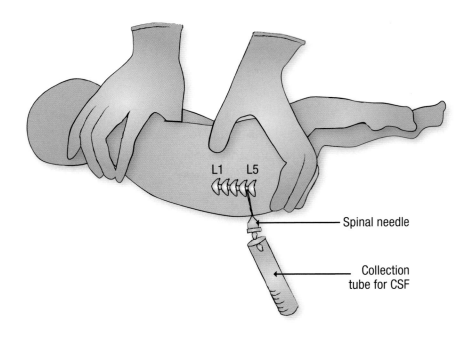

Figure 19: Lumbar Puncture (Spinal tap)
Baby is held in flexed position to widen the gap between the
bones (vertebrae) of the spine. (L1—L5 represent lumbar vertebrae.)

<u>**Treatment**</u>

- Seizures can cause the brain to use up nutrients quickly, especially glucose and oxygen, and can be harmful to the neurons. Thus seizures do need to be treated.
- **Medications** used for seizures are phenobarbital and Dilantin, and on occasion Ativan (a brand of lorazepam).
- It is important to **restrict fluids** to decrease brain swelling and watch for other signs of hypoxia.
- **Respiratory support** as needed
- Investigation and further treatment of possible underlying cause.

<u>**Outcome**</u>

- Will depend on underlying cause.

Perinatal Asphyxia

Perinatal (peri = around, natal = delivery) asphyxia is derived from a Greek word *sphyzein* that means "stopping of the pulse."

Perinatal asphyxia indicates impaired blood supply and impaired gas exchange around delivery. If this persists it can lead to **hypoxia** (lack of oxygen) or **ischemia** (decreased blood supply), which can lead to **hypoxic-ischemic encephalopathy (HIE)**—pathy (disorder) of the encephal (brain). This may occur *before, during, or after birth.*

<u>Causes</u>

- Maternal: toxemia, infections, abdominal trauma, substance abuse, and other illnesses
- Fetal congenital brain malformations, chromosomal abnormalities, infection
- Cord accidents such as entanglements, compression, true knots or prolapse of the cord, placental abruption (tears)
- Delivery: Prolonged, difficult delivery

<u>Presentation</u>

- Fetal hypoxia may present as fetal distress with a drop in the heart rate and acidosis (detected by fetal scalp blood sampling).
- These babies often require prolonged resuscitation, including intubation, chest compression, and emergency medications.
- Poor respiratory effort, poor tone
- Pallor and hypotension (low blood pressure)
- Seizures

Asphyxia is akin to the diving reflex; blood supply is shunted to the brain and heart—the vital organs, the kidneys, gut, liver, skin, etc., receive less blood.

- Decreased renal (kidney) blood leads to **acute tubular necrosis**, resulting in decreased urine and abnormal kidney function, which usually improves.

- Decreased gut supply makes the intestine prone to hypoxia, poor motility, and inflammation with **risk of necrotizing enterocolitis.** So, feeds are held and abdominal status is observed closely. This is a transient effect only.
- Decreased blood supply to the skin presents as extreme pallor with poor perfusion.
- Decreased blood supply to the heart leads to heart rate irregularities or **dysrhythmias** and heart ischemia. Blood pressure is monitored closely.
- Finally, prolonged hypoxia results in low brain blood supply, leading to **seizures** and possibly **hypoxia-ischemic encephalopathy.**

Management

The goals of the mother-baby team are to monitor high-risk situations (picked up from prenatal care or at arrival for delivery) closely and intervene for emergent delivery by cesarean section if necessary. However, often asphyxia may not present with recognizable symptoms in the mother and may remain undetected until she comes in for an exam.

Monitoring Babies with Possible HIE

The infant is monitored in the NICU for complications from the hypoxia/ischemia.

- Blood tests, including kidney and liver function—blood urea nitrogen (BUN), creatinine, liver function tests (LFTs) to detect compromised function of kidneys and liver
- Electroencephalogram (EEG) for any evidence of seizures and to record brain activity
- C.T. scan or MRI as feasible to investigate the cause and effects of HIE; MRI—usually after a few days—to demarcate areas of brain that show evidence of lack of blood supply or bleeding.

NICU Management

- **Maintaining optimal ventilation** and oxygenation, usually with ventilator support

- **Maintaining good perfusion**—with medications like dopamine (to treat low blood pressure) as needed
- **Correcting chemistries** such as low blood sugar and acidosis
- **Control of seizures**—phenobarbital is first drug of choice.
- **Prevention of brain swelling**—moderate fluid restriction or medication
- **Head or whole body cooling** is another modality used. Hypothermia (low temperature) is thought to protect the brain from further injury by preventing the decline of high-energy phosphates. Whole body or head cooling is instituted within six hours of age and infants need to be over thirty-six-weeks gestation. Head cooling is generally done to 33.5 to 34.5 degrees centigrade for about seventy-two hours and then a gradual rewarming is done over four hours to 36.5 to 37.0 degrees centigrade. If eligible for hypothermia protocol, infant will need to be transferred to a facility where this service is available.

Outcome

The outcome is varied depending on the causation, duration, and the extent of damage. Most survivors of perinatal asphyxia have less sequelae or neurodevelopmental issues after head or whole body cooling as depicted by studies.

In recent years, the incidence of HIE has declined due to better prenatal care and perinatal monitoring.

Anemia

Anemia in the newborn means a low hemoglobin (red blood pigment in RBC or red blood cells) or low hematocrit (RBC percentage).

Causes

- **Loss of RBCs or hemorrhage** (bleeding)
  - Within the uterus: placental abruption, tears, cord abnormalities, twin-to-twin transfusion syndrome

- ◆ Around delivery: **feto-maternal bleed** (fetus loses blood into the mother's circulation), cesarean section, cord rupture
  - ◆ Neonatal period: **intracranial hemorrhage** (bleeding in brain), clotting defect
- **Decreased production of RBC,** congenital defects or nutritional issues
- **Increased destruction of RBC**—various causes leading to RBC breakdown, e.g., blood group incompatibilities such as Rh or ABO incompatibility, RBC shape and RBC enzyme defects, and hemoglobin disorders such as sickle cell disease (does not usually present in newborn period due to presence of fetal hemoglobin), and clotting defects
- **Iatrogenic**—caused by needed blood drawing with decreased production in the sick and preterm infant

Diagnosis

- CBC and diff (differential), blood smears
- Other select blood lab studies
- Maternal blood test KB (Kleihauer-Betke test)—testing for fetal cells in case of feto-maternal bleed

Management

- Blood transfusions, if severe
- Respiratory support, as needed
- Nutritional supplements, such as iron
- Appropriate treatment, depending on the cause

Outcome

The outcome will vary, depending on the cause, and most babies improve after treatment. Although those with fetomaternal bleeds appear extremely pale and sick at birth, most will be like Mandy's story in Part II; their condition will improve rapidly, and they will go home with no long-term effects.

Thrombocytopenia

Blood contains a variety of cells. The **red blood cells** are primarily responsible for carrying oxygen to the body tissues; the **white blood cells** for fighting infections; and the **platelets** control bleeding or help in blood clotting.

Thrombocytopenia (thrombo = clotting, cytes = cells, penia = less) indicates a low count of the clotting cells or platelets.

The lifespan of platelets is normally seven to ten days and a normal platelet count is greater than 200,000/ml. *A platelet count of less than 150,000/ml is called thrombocytopenia.*

Presentation

Babies with thrombocytopenia look healthy (unless low platelets are due to illness such as infections, etc.), but show bruising and a purplish spotted rash called petechiae, resulting from tiny hemorrhages under the skin due to low platelets.

Causes

- **Maternal disorders** such as infections, drugs, severe hypertension, associated HELLP syndrome, a condition in the mother associated with preeclampsia (hypertension, often with swelling of legs, feet, and arms), liver dysfunction, and low platelets
- **Platelet antibodies** are often a cause of low platelets in babies. The antigens or immune response substances on the surface of platelets called PLA (platelet antigens) are determined by genetics. Just as the well-known Rh antigen in red blood cells, the fetal platelets can cross into maternal circulation and if seen as a foreign substance can produce antibodies that travel to the fetus and destroy fetal platelets. Infants can thus be born with very low platelets **(isoimmune thrombocytopenia)**.
- **Idiopathic thrombocytopenia purpura** (ITP) is a condition caused by antibodies produced by the mother affecting all platelets, and causing low platelets in her as well as in the fetus.

Most antibody problems continue as long as the antibodies last in the baby's circulation—usually for a few days.

Diagnosis

- Blood tests—CBC, platelet counts, tests for infection
- Tests for maternal platelet count, PLA (platelet antigen), and for antibodies that may have caused the platelet destruction. The father's blood may be tested as well.

Treatment

- The goal is to keep platelets high enough to prevent bleeding especially intracranial hemorrhage.
- Platelet transfusion given in isoimmune thrombocytopenia are platelets lacking the incompatible antigen. Platelets have a short lifespan, so repeated transfusions may be needed.
- Intravenous gamma globulin may be useful in isoimmune thrombocytopenia.
- Short-term steroids may be helpful.

Outcome

Once treated, without complications, term babies with low platelets due to conditions such as isoimmune thrombocytopenia do well with no long-term effects. Miles' story in Part II is one such testimonial.

Neonatal Abstinence Syndrome (NAS)—Drug Withdrawal

Maternal drug use remains a significant issue in the United States. In 2011–2012, 5.9 percent of pregnant women reported the use of illicit drugs, and almost one in ten reported drinking alcohol during pregnancy.

Almost four million babies are admitted every year with history of withdrawal, or neonatal abstinence.

Drug use during pregnancy can lead to birth defects and long-term neuro developmental issues.

Infants born to mothers dependent on opioids, such as heroin and methadone, however, are especially at risk for withdrawal known as Neonatal Abstinence Syndrome (NAS).

Over 50 percent of these babies require treatment and, therefore, will be admitted to the NICU.

Presentation

Most babies with maternal history of drug use are admitted to the newborn nursery where they are observed for signs and symptoms of withdrawal with the **NAS scoring record** for *at least five days.*

Babies may present with:

- Neurologic symptoms—a high-pitched cry, irritability, sleeplessness, marked tremors, and increased muscle tone and, sometimes, seizures
- Gastro-intestinal symptoms such as poor feeding, vomiting, and loose stools
- Respiratory and other symptoms—rapid breathing, nasal stuffiness, sneezing, yawning, sweating, and fever.

Preterm babies less than thirty-five-weeks gestation are at a lower risk for developing symptoms of withdrawal due to their immature neurological system, lower fat deposition, difficulty in identifying the signs, and, of course, they have less exposure to the drugs due to their preterm birth.

Diagnosis

Confirmed by urine (detects recent use) and meconium for drug screen.

Treatment

- If NAS scores are high, the baby is transferred to the NICU and placed on medications such as morphine alone or phenobarbital and morphine to ride out the period of withdrawal.

- Morphine is gradually weaned and then discontinued. Some of the babies with withdrawal may need to be in the NICU for weeks.
- Social services are involved for rehabilitation and family support.
- The mother is allowed to breastfeed in case of opioid abuse, if the mother plans to continue substance-abuse treatment and is able to maintain sobriety.

    Breastfeeding is contraindicated in situations such as history of cocaine abuse or HIV.
- Caretakers must be made aware that some symptoms can persist for four to six weeks.

❡ Readers should be aware that there are many other NICU issues such as congenital malformations, chromosomal problems, and other respiratory, cardiac, gastric, and neurology issues, which have not been touched on here, as they are beyond the scope of this succinct review.

§ Just a word of caution—the Internet is a wonderful resource, and there's an enormous amount of data available online today; but sometimes that can be overwhelming and confusing, may be out of date, use technical jargon, and may not apply to your own situation. Always be sure to consult with your own health care professionals to validate what you find online.

Disclaimer

The content in this part is not intended to be a substitute for medical advice, diagnosis, or treatment.

The goal here is only to provide a concise understanding of some of the problems of an infant admitted to the NICU, and to give families some insight into the workings of the NICU.

Supporting You!

"First NICU was an acronym—then it was a place—and then it was home.—Amy Hynes

Coping Tips

It can be very intimidating and stressful when the anticipated time of joy has culminated in a whirlwind of activity and the babe that has landed in that cradle of love has come with wires, beeps, and whistles. It is only natural to wish to distance yourself from any calamity, even if in this case it was to be the love of your life. It's very normal to feel overwhelmed, guilty, fearful, sad, and even alienated.

Often a preterm baby may remain in the hospital for two to four months.

Remember, there are many in the same scenario. You are not alone! Over the years, all of us at the NICU have worked with other families in your situation, and in this section, I'm sharing a few tips that have worked well for them and helped them to cope in just the same circumstances as you are experiencing.

1. **Get involved—ask questions!**

   Even though the NICU staff tries to explain things so you can understand, there may be terms and "NICU language" that you feel hesitant to ask about. I often tell NICU parents, "There are no questions that are too basic or trivial." Get involved—ask what you can and absorb what you can.

"There are no questions that are too basic or trivial.

2. Learn all you can.

Knowledge is empowering.

You probably feel overwhelmed, but try to focus on the issues at hand and learn all you can. Empowerment leads to strength and acceptance. Acceptance leads to peace. Peace brings an amazing courage—a courage that brings the ability to act and support—and a reconciliation that gives you the strength to go on. Everyone deals with difficulties and adversity differently. One set of parents will want to know all the details about the quantity of medications and fluids; whereas others just listen quietly and happily acquiesce with all that is told to them. Most, however, are right in between. *There is no right or wrong way. Whichever way makes you more comfortable is fine.*

> "There is no right or wrong way. Whichever way makes you more comfortable is fine.

Learn from your physicians, nurse practitioners, nurses, brochures, or brief review booklets. You do not need any extensive reading. *Just know some basic information to understand your child's problems and what to expect!*

3. Accept and participate in daily care.

As one parent put it, "First NICU was an acronym—then it was a place—and then it was home."—Amy Hynes

I recall one patient telling me, "My car automatically turns towards the hospital." Parents often call and come back after discharge to visit and send nostalgic notes.

When an infant is stable, touch and hold. *Do whatever you are allowed to do for your infant's care,* whether it is recording a temperature, or holding a pacifier. Make recordings of your voice: you can read some nursery rhymes and stories, sing a lullaby, or pray. The nurses can play these recordings when you are not there.

Pray if you wish. When visiting your baby, ask when you can give skin to skin or "Kangaroo Care." If the baby is stable, this may be an option for you and your baby (see page 329).

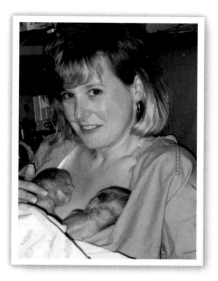

Your nurse will place the baby on your chest, next to your skin, and will cover the baby with your gown or blanket and leave the monitor on. This has been reported by most mothers and fathers as a very satisfying mode of bonding and is beneficial for the baby as well.

4. Provide baby's groceries.

Breast milk still remains the best nutrition for your preterm infant. You are still in charge of your baby's groceries. One of the first things I tell a mom if she is planning to breastfeed is to pump and bring us that "good stuff" (nourishment) for the little one. It brings a quick smile and strength for a mom lost in the ocean of technology that she is still in charge of her baby's care. Talk to your nurse about pumping and storage of breast milk. It can be extremely helpful to talk with your lactation consultant if you are having problems or have questions. Discuss the other options if you are unable to breastfeed for any reason.

" Breast milk still remains the best nutrition for your preterm infant;
—you are still in charge of your baby's groceries.

5.   Don't be afraid of your feelings.

All parents go through worry, fear, and negativity as their organized plans for the birth of their baby go awry. It is normal to feel sad, angry, and resentful. Accept the situation and your feelings. It is fine to cry, express your anger, and vent your frustrations. Talk to the staff and other parents, and realize that you are not alone. There are others in similar or worse situations. Only then can you move forward and go on.

> "It is normal to feel sad, angry and resentful.

6.   Remain positive.

I often call it cautious optimism, remaining realistic, but positive. *Celebrate every milestone, no matter how small,* on that roller-coaster ride that we so often talk about. Celebrate weight gain, fewer alarms, weaning vent support, or the removal of a tube, whether it is a breathing tube, a feeding tube, or an intravenous line.

> "Celebrate every milestone, no matter how small.

7.   Accept help.

Most of us today are very independent. In our current nuclear family environment, it is hard to ask for or accept support from family, let alone friends. I have found the Amish in the Lancaster community with their fantastic family support to be most accepting and stoic during challenging times. Their families are by their side on most occasions. It is fine to accept support as offered, be it from relatives, friends, your church—and maybe from total strangers. As one parent wrote:

“ *My advice to parents going through this experience is, when people offer to help, take them up on their offer.*

“Of particular help to me at the time were all the people who sent meals to us. Almost every evening for months on end, our church, our friends, and our relatives cooked a meal for us. *My advice to parents going through this experience is, when people offer to help, take them up on their offer.*

“I truly appreciated having one less thing to think about each day, yet you need the sustenance to keep up the busy schedule. To this day, I jump at the chance to take a meal to a family in their hour of need. It is all about the 'paying it forward' movement!”—Pam Sherts.

8.   **Establish routines.**

We are all creatures of habit. If we form certain routines, we manage better.

“Whenever possible, I tried to keep some sense of normalcy in our lives.”—Pam Sherts

“We created a schedule.”—Rita Getzloff

Balance your home, hospital visitation, and work. Use a planner to schedule your visitation to coincide with feeding times if your baby has reached that milestone. There are only certain times during the day that are kept for reports and change of shift. Otherwise the NICU visitation is usually allowed all day. Write down those times scheduled for reports, and when you can visit.

Routines are an excellent way of coping when your life seems to be wrought with challenges.

9. Create NICU diaries and journals.

Even in today's media world, journaling whether via paper or electronic is helpful. Write down the diagnosis, daily weights, and gestation. One parent wrote about her journaling experience.

> "Journaling was a support on a daily basis. We continue to this day, once a year, for Jacqueline. We started it the day she was born and looked forward to putting down thoughts and emotions each day in it and closing it to the world. It was a place to get it all out and then stay focused on her."—Amy Hynes.

Record your thoughts and feelings.

Writing down your thoughts and feelings can be very therapeutic for you, and writing down celebratory milestones as they occur, similarly, will bring positivity to your baby's NICU journey.

You can write down milestones in your journal like "umbilical catheter removed," "breathing by self," "held for first time," "starting feeds," "graduated to a crib," etc.

Journal entries are a quick reminder of how far your baby has come.

10. Take care of yourself.

Before takeoff in an aircraft the flight attendant always announces, *"In case of a need for oxygen, please place the oxygen mask on yourself and then help place it on your child."* If you are not doing well yourself, how will you help others? This is an

"
Take care of yourself … In case of a need for oxygen, please place the oxygen mask on yourself and then help place it on your child.

> **Recognize and accept that your partner and you will react differently.**

analogy I often give to families. Make sure you take care of your meals (eat, drink), exercise, and obtain adequate sleep as much as possible—if not for your sake, then do it for your little one's sake.

If things appear overwhelming—take a day off!

If you are feeling depressed, speak to your doctor, the baby's doctor, or your primary care nurse. They can help you to connect to the proper resources.

11. **Get involved with support groups.**

Ask regarding parent support groups at the hospital and, of course, online. These are a great way for you to share feelings of helplessness, anger, frustrations, and concerns. Remember that your best support on a day-to-day basis is always your NICU staff. Voicing concerns or questions and finding solutions and the NICU has great resources, and our NICU social workers and case managers can often connect you with the appropriate groups and provide answers. This time in the NICU is stressful to you as well as your spouse. Talk to your spouse about your concerns and issues. Recognize and accept that your partner and you will react differently.

12. **Trust in faith, hope, and prayer.**

Faith is always a major support especially during adversity. Explore and lean on your spirituality. Speak to a pastor, priest, rabbi, or imam appropriate to your faith. "More things are wrought by prayer than this world dreams of," wrote Alfred Tennyson.

Prayer can certainly bring you not only peace and comfort, but also a renewed strength to face the challenges ahead of you. As some parents have written:

"Without our faith in the Lord, I do not know where we would be!

"When we felt helpless, we would pray, when things went well we'd pray.

"When things took a turn for the worse we would pray. Our family spent countless hours on our knees."—Kimberly Eltman

"Our personal relationship with God, our prayers and those of others were our biggest support."—Susan Deatrick

"My faith and prayers are what got us through this difficult time."—Janice Oree

"Our faith is the beginning and end of the story."—Terra Hussar

Though parents talk about the support of families, NICU staff, and friends, the reverberating theme—the common thread that carried them through—always comes back to acceptance, trust, faith, and prayers.

Accept, learn, have faith, and stay involved on this tumultuous roller-coaster ride! You are certainly not alone!

Breast Feeding and Lactation Support

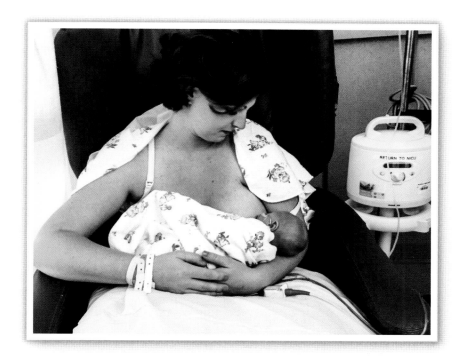

Let the Elixir Flow

As natural as the rising sun,
Diana's moonlight, when the day is done.
Commences, as the peonies bloom,
A robin's song, a nightingale's tune.
A mother's love, rhapsody galore.
Provides milk, for her babe evermore.
I'm little, I am tiny, I'm unable to eat,
So mother dear, stockpile it neat.
As soon as I'm able, I promise I do,
I'll guzzle down the last drop and some more too!
—Manjeet Kaur

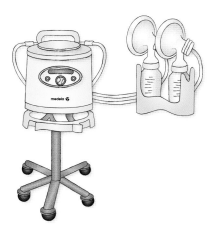

Figure 20: Medala Symphony
Breast Pump

Breastfeeding

Planning how to feed your baby may have been a thought that you've had for quite some time, or perhaps it is something you are only now considering. Since your baby has been born prematurely, he or she needs the best nutrition available to support his/her immune system and to promote growth.

Breast milk is the best nutrition for babies, and each mother's milk is especially suited for her own baby's needs. A mother of a premature baby makes milk designed for a premature baby, and this milk changes as the baby grows so that the baby receives what he or she needs at that time.

If you are planning to breastfeed, it is important to start expressing your milk right away, at least within a few hours after birth, so that your body learns to make lots of milk for your growing baby. Even if you were not planning to breastfeed, you might consider pumping to provide milk for your baby while the baby is in the NICU so that your baby can benefit from the extra advantages that breast milk provides.

Breast milk is powerful stuff! It has hundreds of benefits for your baby and to you. Here are just a few of them:

<u>Benefits to Your Baby</u>

- As a mother, you can help your baby fight infection by feeding him/her your breast milk. Breast milk has special proteins called antibodies that help to fight infection.

  These antibodies are your way of passing your own immunity on to your baby and, as a mother, you can help your baby fight infection by feeding him/her your breast milk. The first milk that you make in the first few days is especially full of these antibodies, but the benefit doesn't stop there. As long as you breastfeed, you are providing some immunity to your baby.

- Your milk is made especially for your baby. The milk that you make in the first few days is called colostrum. Colostrum has more protein and less fat and carbohydrates than mature milk. Mothers that deliver premature babies make milk that is higher in protein, fat, and certain minerals than milk from others who have delivered full-term babies.

- Breast milk is the perfect nutrition that your baby needs for his/her brain growth. In fact, some studies show that breastfed children on average have higher IQ scores than those that are formula fed.
- Your milk is very easily digested and absorbed without much waste, so your baby's bowel movements will be softer and looser as a result.
- Breast milk helps to protect against the development of diabetes and some cancers such as leukemia as per some literature.
- Breast milk reduces the occurrence of ear infections, diarrhea, and respiratory infections. Babies that are breastfed are less likely to become sick!

Benefits to You, The Mother

- Breastfeeding helps you to lose any baby weight and will help your uterus to return to its original size more quickly.
- Studies show that breastfeeding helps to protect you against breast cancer and reduces the risk of developing diabetes if you have had gestational diabetes and obesity.
- Breastfeeding helps you to bond with your baby.

Calories in Breast Milk

The amount of fat and calories in breast milk varies from woman to woman, from day to day, and even differs throughout the day. Breast milk on average has about twenty calories in each ounce, but some mothers have much higher calorie milk.

Fortifiers

Premature babies often need extra protein and minerals to support their bones and growth. Your baby's healthcare provider may request that your milk be fortified for a period of time while the baby is in the hospital. Fortification means that extra protein and minerals are added to your milk.

"*Premature babies often need extra protein and minerals to support their bones and growth. Your baby's healthcare provider may request that your milk be fortified for a period of time.*

The NICU currently uses a human milk–based fortifier called Prolacta to add to your milk when necessary. This substance is made up of human milk that has been pasteurized and tailored to a specific amount of calories. When added to your milk, it will increase the calories in each ounce and will help your baby to grow faster. Older babies can tolerate a fortifier that is made from cow's milk.

Supplements

The best way to make a lot of milk is to empty your breast early and often! Emptying your breasts by breastfeeding, pumping, and hand, expressing frequently (as much as eight to ten times per day) will help you to make enough milk for your baby. Most mothers can make all the milk that their babies need if they follow these guidelines.

Still, some mothers have difficulty making the amount of milk that the baby needs at each feeding. When a mother's milk supply is low, the baby may need to be supplemented. Supplementing means that a food other than breast milk is offered for feedings. Formula is available to supplement the extra amount that is needed for a feeding. Donor human milk may also be available in some areas. **Donor milk** used in a NICU is milk that other mothers have donated to a milk bank where it is pasteurized and packaged to be distributed to those who need it.

Your Diet

<u>Calories</u>

Producing breast milk requires about 500–600 extra calories per day. Any extra weight that you gained during your pregnancy will be used for this purpose when you are breast-feeding. It's still a good idea to increase your calories so that you are nourishing your body to be able to make milk. It's great news to know that, even if you don't have the best diet, your breast milk will still have all the nutrients that are needed for your baby.

<u>Protein</u>

It is a good idea to have two to three servings of protein per day. Good sources of protein include meat, poultry (chicken), fish, eggs, milk, nuts, and legumes. Meats are a good source of vitamin B12 as well as iron and zinc. If you follow a vegetarian diet, it is best to take a vitamin B12 supplement while breastfeeding.

<u>Fruits and Vegetables</u>

Eating five to six servings of a variety of fruits and vegetables of different colors helps to replenish your body of vitamins and minerals. Dark green leafy vegetables provide a source of iron, while yellow and orange fruits and vegetables are rich in vitamin C and A, and help to boost your immune system. The more colorful your plate, the better!

<u>Grains</u>

Include whole grains in your daily diet. Sources of whole grains include whole wheat pasta, cereal, oatmeal, and whole wheat bread.

<u>Dairy</u>

Remember, you don't have to drink milk to make milk. You may continue to enjoy dairy foods as you did before your pregnancy, but there is no need to increase the amount of dairy in your diet. Some babies are sensitive to the amount of dairy in your diet, and if this is identified, you may need to eliminate or reduce dairy for a period of time.

Calcium

Milk is rich in calcium; your own milk is rich in calcium, too, and that comes from your body. It is a good idea to eat calcium-rich foods when you are breastfeeding to replace the calcium that is needed for healthy bones. Calcium-rich foods include milk, yogurt, cheese, shellfish, leafy greens, broccoli, bok choy, figs, oranges, sardines, salmon, white beans, tofu, and almonds.

Making Milk

Your breasts have been preparing to produce milk throughout your pregnancy. You will have colostrum, the first milk, available immediately after birth. Colostrum comes in small quantities but has everything that your baby needs for those first few days. Your breasts will start to feel fuller a few days after your baby is born, but this milk supply will decrease unless you empty your breasts frequently and consistently.

Pumping and hand expressing are the best ways to empty your breasts if your baby can't feed at the breast. *Premature babies can feed at the breast as early as thirty-three weeks if their medical condition allows.* Even then, it is recommended to continue to pump to be sure that your breasts are completely emptied while the baby practices this skill.

Your goal is to pump eight to ten times every twenty-four hours. By one to two weeks, you should be making at least 500–750 ml of breast milk per day. The baby's feeding amounts will increase and will catch up with you, so making more than enough milk is a good thing. If you have twins, the milk amounts will be higher.

Your baby's nurses and lactation consultants will help you along the way regarding your milk supply and pumping.

Storage and Handling of Breast Milk

- All milk brought to the NICU must be labeled. Each time you pump, put that milk in a container, and then label it with the date, and time. The nurses will provide you with labels with your baby's information. In addition, you will be given orange numbered stickers that should be placed on each container of colostrum. Colostrum is identified with orange stickers so that the nurses feed this milk first whenever possible in the order in which it was pumped.

- Fresh milk is best and preferred over frozen milk when it is available. Bring all of your milk into the hospital so that it is ready for the baby when the baby can feed. The nurses will tell you if you are making enough milk so you can start to leave some milk at home.
- The following table gives guidelines for handling and storage of human milk.¶

Human Milk	Room Temperature	Time in Refrigerator	Time in Freezer
Fresh (never frozen)	≤ 4 hours	≤ 2-4 days	**Ideal:** 1 month **Optimal:** ≤ 3 months **Acceptable:** ≤ 12 months in a deep freezer (-20°C)
Previously frozen, thawed but not warmed	≤ 4 Hours	≤ 24 hours	Do not refreeze
Previously frozen and brought to room temperature	For completion of current feeding	≤ 4 hours	Do not refreeze
Infant has started feeding	Completion of current feeding and then discard	Discard	Discard

¶Source: Human Milk Banking Association of North America, 3rd ed. 2011 Rev. 2012

Which Pump Is Best?

There are many types of breast pumps on the market. Which type is best for you depends on your pumping situation. Pumping works best when hand expression is added to pumping. Your nurse or lactation consultant will show you how to hand express your milk.

- Rental Pumps: For mothers who are separated from their babies and/or managing their milk supply by pumping alone, a hospital-grade electric pump is best. These pumps are powerful, durable, and efficient in milk removal. Due to the high cost, they are usually rented monthly. Some insurances will pay for pump rentals when babies are in the NICU.

  Medala Symphony breast pumps are available for you to use while you are in the hospital and when you are visiting your baby in the NICU (See Figure 20).

- Returning to Work Pumps: These pumps are designed for mothers who are pumping at least half the time and feeding directly at the breast as well. These pumps may be sufficient for mothers with babies in the NICU after their milk supply is well established. They are double electric pumps, and many insurance companies will cover this type of pump if you are breastfeeding.

- Handheld Pumps: These can be single or double pumps that are battery or manually operated. They are for occasional use. Mothers who are breastfeeding healthy term babies who need to pump here and there for appointments, etc., may do well with this pump. This would not be ideal for mothers of babies in the NICU.

Breast Pump Rental Locations

Note: The following product, price and location details were current at time of publication, and may have changed since.

- Wellspan Medical Equipment: $65/month + tax (also $49.50 + tax for a kit − one-time purchase). Two locations: Ephrata, PA and New Holland, PA (717) 733-0405; (888) 290-4363.

- Superior Oxygen: $75/month + tax (can purchase a pump kit at Babies RUs) from Lancaster, PA (717) 509-0202.

Other Frequently Asked Questions

Q: Can I have caffeine while breastfeeding?

A: Yes, you may have caffeine. Caffeine does enter the breast milk but, in most cases, moderate amounts of up to two to three servings per day (in an average-size cup) are tolerated by babies.

Q: Can I breastfeed if I smoke?

A: Yes, you can. While smoking is not recommended for your health, the benefits of breast milk outweigh the risks of smoking to your baby. Nicotine does pass through the breast milk, so it is best not to breastfeed for at least twenty minutes after smoking a cigarette. Never smoke around the baby and consider wearing a covering over your clothes when you smoke.

Q: Can I have an alcoholic drink while breastfeeding?

A: You can safely manage occasional small amounts of alcohol while you are breastfeeding. Drinking excessive amounts of alcohol while breastfeeding is not recommended. The American Academy of Pediatrics recommends that you wait two hours before pumping or breastfeeding for each serving of alcohol that you drink.

Q: How long should I feed my baby?

A: The benefits of breastfeeding continue as long as you breastfeed. **The American Academy of Pediatrics recommends exclusive breastfeeding for about the first six months of life.** This means that your baby needs no other foods or fluids unless medically indicated. Babies should continue to breastfeed for a year and for as long as is mutually desired by the mother and the baby.

Encouragement

Having a baby in the NICU can be a stressful time for you and your family. It is important to take care of yourself, get enough sleep, eat well, and take breaks when you need them.

Pumping may seem like a chore sometimes, but only you can make this special milk for your little one. Many mothers find that providing their breast milk is a way to feel close and to connect with their baby, even when they are not with him or her.

Taking the time to sit down and pump for twenty minutes every few hours gives you an opportunity to relax and think about your baby. If this is your first baby, breastfeeding will be a new experience for you. Trust your body! Your body has been a perfect home for your baby inside and now knows what to do to make milk for him or her. You just need to help it along by emptying your breasts as often as the baby feeds.

Premature babies aren't mature enough at first to suck, swallow, and breathe, so they are fed through a tube. Babies are very comfortable in their mother's arms, and when you practice skin to skin, your baby will learn your scent and know how to find your breast when that time comes. When he or she is old enough, you will be able to directly breastfeed your baby. Whatever your goals are for feeding your baby, the NICU staff wants to help you to succeed.

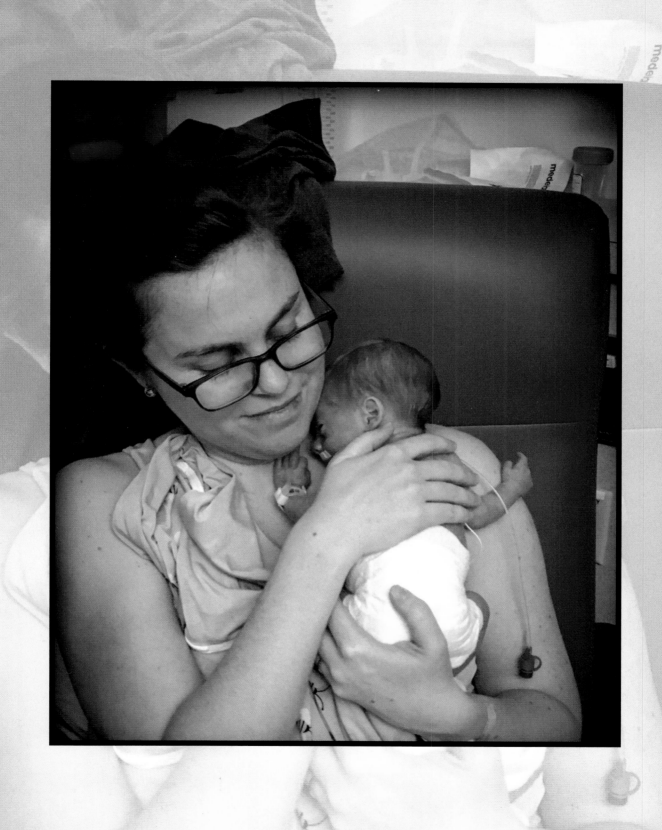

Only Love

A joyful heart,
A spring of love
A ray of sunshine
A gentle dove
A fragrant flower
A twinkling star
A bubbling brook
A purple mountain top
A simple smile …
Brings
"ONLY LOVE"
A love that heals
A love that feels
A love that conquers
A love that cures
A love that rejoices
A love that flows
A love that forgives
A love that embraces
A love that connects
A love that reflects
On "Serenity amidst chaos"
On "Perfection in imperfection"
"ONLY LOVE"
—Manjeet Kaur

PART IV

Discharge: Homeward Bound

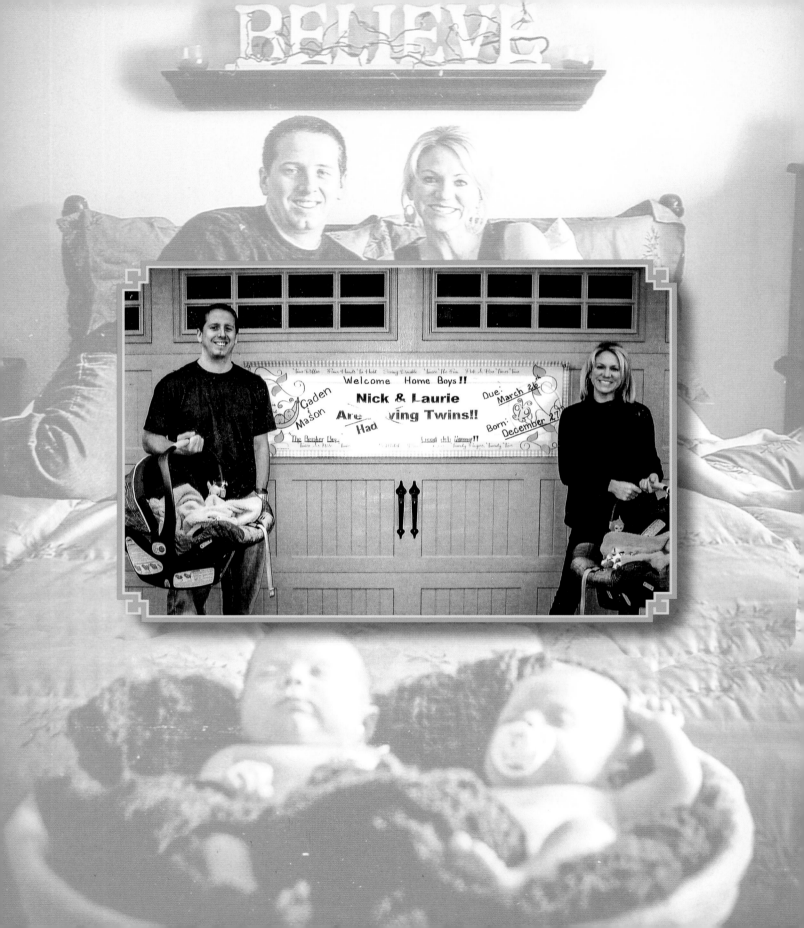

*W*ith great celebration and anxious anticipation, a NICU baby comes home. "Now what?" is often a parent's unvoiced question quickly followed by, "How am I going to manage? Am I up to caring for this fragile little precious bundle who has been looked after by so many professionals?" and, "What do I need to know?"

First—know that it is normal to feel anxious and stressed, but following an orderly format may facilitate the discharge with more ease and make the transition smoother.

Here are some suggestions!

Discharge Planning

NICU Night Experience

Try to spend a night or two in the NICU prior to discharge. This will give you a lot more confidence in feeding, giving medications, caring for your baby, and using equipment such as a home monitor, if indicated.

There are special rooms available for this purpose, and you can sign up to use them. In fact, Ross, one of our very own NICU graduates, helped with the construction of those rooms. You can read his story in Part II.

Family Conferences

Family conferences are specially arranged for you. Discharge from the NICU needs a team approach with parents or caregivers, physicians, nurse practitioners, nurses, care manager, and social workers. The team during these meetings will discuss the approaching discharge and medical issues; suggest and coordinate follow-up, depending on your residence and insurance; and answer any of your questions. They will also discuss with you the need for Synagis for RSV[1] prevention during RSV season (usually between October and April); the arrangement for a home monitor, if needed; and CPR training for caregivers, etc. You should make every attempt to come on time for these meetings and to participate actively!

Discharge Planning Checklists

Follow your discharge planning checklists. These are a great help to get organized while your baby is still being looked after in the hospital. Having this done ahead of time will make the transition to home life much easier.

Here is a ten-point checklist:

1. Review Baby Care

Your nurses may already have gone over baby care such as recording temperature, giving a bath, feeding, giving vitamins and medications, storing and thawing breast milk, etc. Anxiety aside—are you comfortable with caring for your little one? Now is the time to ask questions!

Most of the appointments and arrangements may have already been made by your care manager or nurse, but going through the following checklists will give you confidence and control.

2. Review Appointments

1. Have you selected and arranged for an appointment with *your follow-up doctor?*

2. Have appointments been made with *specialists* as required for neurology, gastroenterology, pulmonology, urology, cardiology, and pediatric surgery?

3. Have you arranged a follow-up appointment with *Early Intervention?*

4. Does your baby need to have a follow-up *ophthalmology* appointment?

---

1   RSV (respiratory syncytial virus). This virus is an important cause of lower-respiratory infections in neonates and children—especially preterms.

5. Ask if you qualify for home *visiting nurses*. Do you have an appointment scheduled?

6. Has your baby passed a *hearing screen*, and if not, what follow-up is needed?

7. Has your baby had a *newborn genetic (neogen)* screen? Is any repeat testing needed?

8. Are any other follow-up tests—such as *head ultrasound, repeat echocardiogram, hip ultrasound* (if your baby was a breech presentation), *blood tests* etc.—needed?

3. Review Discharge Records, Medication, and Equipment Needs

1. Learn how and when to administer medications.

2. Learn about any equipment that the baby may need at home, such as a home monitor and home oxygen. Make sure you are comfortable with usage as much as possible.

4. Check Immunizations

1. Has your infant received the hepatitis B vaccine?

2. If it is the RSV season (fall through spring), does your infant qualify for **Synagis** for the prevention of respiratory syncytial virus infection?

3. Is a repeat dose needed, and when is it due?

4. Has your little one received any other immunizations?

5. Ensure Your Infant's Groceries

1. For nursing mothers, take any stored breast milk home. Speak with the lactation consultant or your nurse regarding the breast pump, storage, thawing, etc. Preterm babies will require some additional supplements as well.

2. Make sure you have the same formula that the infant is getting in the NICU at home.

3. Ensure that you have multivitamins, medications, and other supplies available in a clean container close at hand.

6. Plan Safe Travel

Make sure you have an appropriate car seat, as premature infants may have special needs due to their size, strength, and other issues, such as apnea and oxygen needs. Bring in your baby's car seat, and a car seat testing will be done in the NICU as per the American Academy of Pediatrics' recommendation. On occasion the infant may need to go home in a car bed.

7. Review Social Issues

1. Determine your eligibility for any programs. Ask your care manager if you qualify for a local or state public health support program, such as **WIC** (Women, Infants and Children), so you can take care of any paperwork needed.

2. Speak with your social worker if you have any issues with **electricity, phone, transportation,** or any other needs related to baby care.

3. Ascertain and complete the necessary paperwork if baby needs to be added to your **health insurance.**

4. Ask if **home visiting nurses** are needed and available for you.

8. Check on Home Monitor and CPR Training

1. If a home monitor is needed, make a note of the company's name and their contact phone number and e-mail. Ensure that all who will be watching the baby are comfortable with the monitor and have received the necessary training.

2. Make sure that you and other caretakers have received infant CPR training as well.

9. Plan Your Journal

Make a paper or electronic journal if you have not already done so. Include the following:

1. Enter baby's *measurements* (weight, length, and head circumference) at birth and discharge.

2. Enter *diagnosis* as you understand it.

3. Note *medications and vitamins* to be given and when.

4. Record *immunizations* given.

5. Record *follow-up appointments.*

10. Keep Information at Your Fingertips

1. Note *feeding times* in the NICU.

2. Record all the important *medical phone numbers*—pediatrician, NICU, visiting nurses, early intervention, specialty follow-up as needed, e.g., neurologist, cardiologist, etc.

3. Make a note of *general phone numbers* of friends that you have made in the NICU, be they parents or others. You may wish to keep in touch with both as resources and support.

4. Make a note of any *future resources* (speak with the care manager and the social worker if you have any special needs). Add any other needed phone numbers, internet resources, or notes. These are great references as needed.

Review!

1. Ask any questions while the support is staff available.

2. Ask how to recognize illness and symptoms.

3. Make notes—it's easy to forget many of the instructions.

"Soon there would be no one but my husband and me to care for him.

Were we up to the challenge?—Pam Sherts (parent)

A Benediction

A sweet cherub,
A melodious melody.
An entrancing fragrance,
A darling parody!
A smile so angelic, a laughter that rings bliss.
That drunken gaze, where nothing is amiss.
Ushers in a joy, so unique, so rare,
Where only little goblins and angels dare.
Life stops,
Life giggles!
Life dances,
Life wiggles!
As this ethereal chub ogles with love galore,
In precious adoration, so dear, so pure.
An oasis in a desert,
A rainbow amidst a tempest.
A dazzling heavenly light,
An endearing sight.
A boon! A blessing!
A benediction!!
—Manjeet Kaur

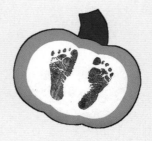

Your Pumpkin is Coming Home

Home Preparation for Baby's Arrival

1. Obtain supplies such as clothing, diapers, blankets, formula, bottles, lactation supplies, and a digital thermometer.

2. Prepare the crib or another sleep option.

3. Clean your home of any dust, pet hair, or smoke.

4. Have hand sanitizers and/or hand cleansers available, and ensure good hand washing.

5. Have a separate area where the baby's milk supplies are cleaned, assembled, and poured.

6. Have all nutritional needs, supplements, vitamins, medications, and supplies close at hand in a clean container.

7. Post phone numbers near your phones and the crib. For emergencies, you may call 911 or go to the hospital emergency room.

Additional Instructions after Discharge

1. Avoid crowds (e.g., shopping malls, grocery stores, social gatherings, and churches) for the first three months, especially in the winter.

2. Restrict visitors, especially children, and anyone with colds.

3. Everyone should practice good hand washing, including your family and visitors.

4. Keep hand sanitizer nearby.

5. Do not allow smoking around the baby.

6. Notify the physician if the baby is not feeding is sleepy, difficult to awaken, extremely fussy, has vomiting or has

diarrhea, or a fever of more than 100.4°F (rectal). If the temperature is more than 99.5°F (axillary), obtain a rectal temperature if you have learned how to do that.

After-Discharge Care

Growth and Nutrition

- Growth is generally measured by the baby's weight, length, and head circumference. Growth charts will be used in your doctor's office.
- Growth tracking will need to be adjusted to take account of the fact that your little infant came into the world early. Therefore, calculation of age for a premature infant is adjusted as per gestation (also called corrected age, post-conceptional age, or adjusted age), in order to track growth appropriately.
- Term pregnancy is 40 weeks; therefore, a baby born at 24 weeks is 16 (40–24) weeks, or four months, premature. So, if the baby is now nine months old, the corrected age or adjusted age is five months.

   Corrected Age = Actual Age – Months Premature

   For example, if baby is four months premature, then:

   Corrected Age = 9 months – 4 months = **5 months**
- Corrected age is used for growth tracking up to two years of age.

Growth Evaluation

- The infant should *gain weight at one-half ounce to one ounce per day* (or four to six ounces per week) for the first six months.
- Length usually increases one half to one cm per week (0.2 to 0.4 inches per week) initially with a total increase of about twelve inches (thirty centimeters) in the first year.
- Usually catch-up growth occurs by two years for weight and length, and by the first year for head circumference. Your doctor will follow growth on a growth chart.

Refer to the growth charts in the Appendix. These will enable you to track your infant's growth if you wish to do so. The Fenton Growth Charts (pp 420–423) are specifically designed for use with pre-term infants up to fifty weeks. After that, the CDC/WHO charts can be used.

Growth charts are not intended to be used as a sole diagnostic instrument. Rather, they are tools that contribute to forming an overall clinical impression for the child being measured.

Copies of the CDC growth charts can be freely downloaded at the following website, which also includes an online training course in their use:

cdc.gov/growthcharts/who_charts.htm

Nutrition and Feeds

Nutrition

Nutrition needed for growth is about 110–120 calories per kilogram per day. Breast milk or regular formulas have twenty calories per ounce.

Breastfed Babies

Breastfeeding remains the best nutrition for the growing preterm infant. Note the following:

- Breastfed infants should be fed on-demand every one and a half to three hours (at least eight to twelve times per day).
- They should not have more than one prolonged period of sleep (four to five hours).
- Feed for approximately ten to fifteen minutes initially, and gradually increase feed time with maturity.
- Pump after feeds for the first several weeks to stimulate milk supply.
- At discharge, a four to five-pound infant should be taking one and a half to two ounces per feed every two and one half to three hours (about twelve to fifteen ounces per day).

- Supplement with formula such as NeoSure or Enfacare or preterm formula equivalent for two to three feeds per day, or as recommended by your physician.
- Provide multivitamins with iron, one ml per day. Continue as advised. (This will provide the required vitamin D and iron for breastfed babies.)
- A way to see if your baby is getting enough milk is to ensure that your baby is having six to eight wet diapers per day.
- If the baby is experiencing inadequate weight gain despite good feeds, your doctor may recommend a concentrated formula of twenty-four calories per ounce or more.
- Regurgitation of feeds may be caused by:
  - Overfeeding: Decrease volume, and increase frequency.
  - Swallowed air: Burp the baby frequently; the nipple of the bottle should be filled with milk.
  - Reflux: Keep the infant semi-upright thirty to sixty minutes after feeds. Try smaller, more frequent feeds.

The above are guidelines only. Recommendations will be as from your follow-up physician.

Formula-Fed Babies

Preterm discharge formulas, e.g., NeoSure or Enfacare or equivalent, provide increased protein, calcium, phosphorus, and vitamins, and they have more easily digestible fat and sugar as compared to regular infant formula, and with a higher caloric amount per ounce (twenty-two calories per ounce). Your pediatrician will probably recommend the preterm discharge formula for *nine to twelve months* instead of standard formula to provide the needed additional calories and mineral supplements.

Development and Intervention

- Increased survival of the extremely preterm infants emphasizes the need for better developmental assessment screens, so as to hone in on the optimal potential of these tiny babies, and any others with a tough beginning.
- Intellectual difficulties and mental retardation may only be diagnosed with some certainty in later preschool years.
- Hearing impairment, blindness, and cerebral palsy can usually be diagnosed during the first two years.
- Standardized screening for developmental assessment will be done by the pediatrician at every visit, starting from the first visit.
- Follow-up with early intervention programs is extremely important. These programs aim at exercises and management as needed in order to obtain optimal potential.
- A lot can be achieved with therapy, OT/PT/speech therapy, especially involving motor and behavioral skills.
- Family members can also be taught how to best help their child.

Developmental red flags include the baby not achieving milestones for adjusted age or if the baby is stiff or floppy, or not responding to sounds or following objects.

Gastrointestinal Problems

Gastroesophageal Reflux

Reflux and spitting up are very common problems in newborns, especially preterm infants. This is a real risk for some infants leading to poor weight gain or even aspiration.

Symptoms

- Gagging, retching, and vomiting
- Irritability after feeds
- Failure to gain weight
- Repeated respiratory infections or apnea

Diagnosis may be made clinically or with tests.

Management Tips

- Positioning during and after feeds can be helpful. Keep head elevated (semi-upright) for one-half hour to one hour after feeds.
- At the discretion of the follow-up physician, thickening feeds with rice cereal may be recommended.
- Provide smaller volume, but more frequent feeds. Allow adequate time to burp frequently and minimal stimulation after feeding.
- Make sure the nipple of the bottle is filled with milk at feeds to avoid excess air.
- Although these are suggested feeding recommendations, the infant's condition may require further evaluation or treatment with medications.
- Very rarely, surgery (fundoplication) may be indicated.

Constipation

Constipation is a common problem in preterm infants. This is often due to decreased abdominal muscle strength, decreased motility, and less intake. But occasionally it may be due to anatomical problems or an obstruction.

Symptoms

- Hard, small stools that are difficult to pass
- Any blood in the stool (It is important to check your baby's stool and know what is normal!)
- Significant decrease in number of bowel movements (The baby should typically have a bowel movement at least once a day.)

Management Tips

- It is important to review concerns of constipation with a physician, particularly in case any urgent workup needs to be done to rule out obstruction or anatomical issues.
- Occasional rectal stimulation may be needed.
- If necessary in severe cases, the pediatrician or specialist may recommend medications to relieve the constipation.

Jaundice

Jaundice or "yellow" coloration of the skin or eyes can be a common problem that develops due to cholestasis (slowing of the bile flow) or liver disease. Often a problem in infants with long-term TPN (total parenteral nutrition), cholestasis and gallstones may be a challenge in the NICU and post-discharge. Neonates can also suffer from other liver or anatomical biliary tract conditions.

Take-Home Points

- Diagnostic tests may include blood tests to measure bilirubin levels and abdominal ultrasound.
- It is always good to check that your baby's stool is a healthy normal color; white or pale, clay-colored stools are something that require a doctor's evaluation!
- Medications such as Actigall may be prescribed for some babies.

Respiratory Issues

Bronchopulmonary Dysplasia (BPD)

- A small percentage of preterm babies develop BPD, especially those who have required prolonged ventilator support and oxygen.
- Some of these babies may go home on oxygen, cardio respiratory monitor, medications such as diuretics, and bronchodilators.

Take-Home Points

- Ensure good nutrition for optimal weight gain.
- Ensure adequate respiratory support.
- Administer medications as recommended.
- Avoid infections.
- Avoid crowds during RSV season (fall through spring).
- RSV prophylaxis will need to be given, especially through RSV season (fall through spring).
- The flu vaccine will be given at follow-up visits after six months, at your physician's discretion.

- Home nursing will probably be needed and arranged prior to discharge.
- Maintain good hand washing and keep hand sanitizer nearby for quick use. Babies born early are at risk not only for RSV but also other bacterial or viral infections such as a cold, or the flu.

Apnea and Bradycardia

- About 25 percent of preterm infants have apnea and/or bradycardia.
- If monitoring is needed, an event or memory monitor is chosen, so that events can be recorded and reviewed.
- Usually the baby will remain on the home monitor for a couple of months after discharge, and then reevaluated for further need for monitoring by the follow-up physician.
- If an infant is sent home on medication (e.g., caffeine), any change will be based on the clinical course.

Central Nervous System (CNS)

Intraventricular Hemorrhage

Intraventricular hemorrhage (IVH) is a bleed from the germinal matrix in lateral ventricles of the brain. About 20 percent of babies less than 1,500 grams may have IVH. The smaller the gestation period, the higher the incidence of IVH.

Generally, IVH is categorized as Grade I to Grade IV.

- Screening is done by obtaining head ultrasound (HUS) at the bedside. No radiation is involved.
- Magnetic resonance imaging (MRI) gives more details, but is more expensive and usually requires sedation.

Follow-up

- If IVH is noted, close follow-up with a HUS screen will be needed.
- Head circumference should be followed at each visit and at least monthly. Rapid head growth may indicate increased intracranial pressure, and repeat cranial imaging may be required.

- Increasing head circumference may be due to "catch-up growth," which is normal. In this case, development is normal with no evidence of increased intracranial pressure. If head circumference increases *more than one and a quarter centimeters per week*, imaging of the head may be recommended.
- If hydrocephalus with shunt is in place, it must be observed for obstruction or infection.

Hernias

Umbilical hernias occur in 10 to 20% of newborns. An umbilical hernia is a protrusion covered by skin in the region of the navel or umbilicus; it can be small, the size of a golf ball, or even larger. *Most hernias resolve spontaneously by two years of age.* Surgery is only considered if large and persist beyond five years.

Inguinal Hernias

Three to 30% of preterm infants may develop inguinal hernias (a protrusion covered by skin in the groin). *A referral to pediatric surgery* needs to be followed due to the risk of obstruction and strangulation of the bowel in the inguinal hernia.

Screening and Follow-up Blood Tests

Note: Guidelines may differ from hospital to hospital.

1. **Genetic screen**, also referred to as newborn screen, is a blood test for various genetic disorders that is *done on all babies*. This screen includes PKU (Phenylketonuria), hypothyroidism, hemoglobin disorders, combined immune deficiency, cystic fibrosis, galactosemia, maple syrup urine disease (MSUD), G6PD deficiency, and other metabolic errors. If abnormal, you will be asked to bring the infant back for a repeat testing.

2. **Hearing screen** is done on all babies prior to discharge from the NICU and repeated in the NICU if abnormal. If the infant failed the hearing screen in the NICU, an

audiology referral for BAER (brain audiology evolved response) is mostly made by six weeks.

3. **Ophthalmology screen** is recommended in NICU for babies less than thirty weeks gestation or under 1500 grams birth weight or other sick preterms at four to six weeks of age as per protocol and then every two weeks until the blood vessel growth in the retina is complete. If your child has been diagnosed with retinopathy (ROP), close follow-up will be needed. Make sure to keep these appointments! Ophthalmology follow-up of all preterm babies is also generally recommended at nine to twelve months, and a repeat at two to three years of age because of the increased risk of additional ophthalmology problems such as squint, myopia, and other refraction errors.

4. **Head ultrasound (HUS)/ CT scan / MRI HUS** is done on premature infants less than thirty-two weeks gestation at one week of age, or earlier for very sick or extremely premature infants. If normal, HUS is repeated at thirty six to forty weeks. If HUS is abnormal, close follow-up is recommended.

5. **Hemoglobin/hematocrit** is done at discharge and then again a few weeks after discharge with follow-up as recommended. Physiologic anemia of prematurity occurs at one to two months. Infant may need to continue iron supplementation per pediatrician.

6. **Electrolytes** may be assessed every two weeks if infant is on diuretics. Once stable with no dose change, an electrolyte check will be done as recommended by your physician.

7. **Nephrocalcinosis** screen may be recommended if baby has been on long-term diuretics. Tests of urine for blood and protein may be obtained and, if needed, renal ultrasound.

8. **Critical Congenital Heart Disease screen (CCHD)** is a recently added testing to screen for critical cyanotic congenital heart disease and is recommended for all babies over 1,500 grams or thirty-week gestation by twenty-four to forty-eight hours of life. A pulse oximeter is placed on baby's right wrist or foot, and blood oxygen saturations are recorded.

   Note: This screen does not rule out all congenital heart disease.

General Guidelines

Dental Care

Preterm infants are prone to dental and, especially, enamel problems and cavities.

- Wipe gums daily and teeth as they emerge with a wet washcloth, especially at night.
- First visit to the dentist is recommended as per AAP (American Academy of Pediatrics) guidelines at twelve months of age.
- Toothbrush should be introduced no later than the molar eruption.

Sleep

Sleep recommendations include the following:

- Establish a routine: place the infant in bed/crib at a particular time on the back.
- Adjust medication to sleep schedule.
- Minimal stimulation at sleep time is recommended. However, babies are used to the sounds of the beeps and hustle-and-bustle of the NICU!

Travel/Socialization

- Baby may be taken outside if weather is appropriate.
- Good hand washing must be continued at home.
- Avoid crowds for the first three months, and during flu season.
- Do not expose the infant to visitors with infections in the first few months, even if they are relatives or friends.

- Dressing should be comfortable, i.e.; what is comfortable for you is comfortable for the baby—with a light blanket added.
- Avoid smoke and strong perfumes.
- Call if you have any other concerns regarding the infant.

⁋ The above are guidelines only! Recommendations will be as per your follow-up pediatrician.

Immunization in Preemies

Immunizations

Vaccines can protect your child from dangerous diseases.

Immunizations are based on the child's actual birthday. Premature babies get their immunizations at the same age as full-term babies, with no age correction done for prematurity.

- **Hepatitis B** is a serious infection of the liver, which can be prevented by the Hepatitis B vaccine. Three doses are generally given to all babies. For term and preterm babies over two kilograms birth weight the first dose is given at birth, the second at one to two months of age, and the third at six to eighteen months.

  All other preterm babies will receive their first dose of Hepatitis B vaccine at discharge or by thirty days of age. The second and third doses are given as above.
- **Routine immunizations**—such as DTaP (diphtheria, tetanus, and pertussis), Hib, pneumococcal vaccine, polio, Rotavaccine—are done in the office as per routine. Mumps, measles, rubella (MMR) are given later.
- **Influenza vaccine** is given each year to all children between six months and eighteen years of age.
- Preterms are at increased risk for **respiratory syncytial virus (RSV)** infection as well as development of sequelae.

  Babies *less than* thirty-two-weeks gestation and younger than one year should receive RSV prophylaxis monthly at the start of the RSV season (fall through spring).

Babies thirty-two to thirty-four weeks gestation with additional risk factors may also qualify for the immunization.

Other indications for RSV prophylaxis are *severe congenital heart disease, BPD, fibrosis, and neuromuscular disorders.*

Your physician will assess the risks and advise accordingly.

Readmission Risk

- Preterm babies have a higher risk of readmission with infections as well as respiratory or feeding problems. Your threshold for calling your doctor will be and should be lower.
- Call if the baby is not feeding well, has diarrhea or is vomiting, as the risk of dehydration is greater.
- Call if the baby is extremely fussy, sleepy, or difficult to awaken; has coughing, apnea, breathing difficulty, or a fever of more than 100.5 degrees Fahrenheit (38°C) rectally. Axillary temperature (measured under the armpit) is usually less by 1°F and 0.5°C.

Especially in the winter, the baby has a higher risk of bronchiolitis due to RSV or other viruses.

Time

There are a myriad sagas, numerous joys, yet much sorrow,
On the slate of today, only to be washed out on the morrow.
Time is timeless, it waits for none, quotidian or sublime,
Yet invariably we place fetters … of a timeline on time!
—Manjeet Kaur

Resources for NICU Families

*I*nfants, parents, and families in the NICU need additional support and services during and after their NICU stay. These are some of the local support services for Lancaster County (Pennsylvania) and the surrounding area. If you're not from Lancaster County, your local area should have many of these supportive services. Ask your NICU team for guidance with these services as you transition home with your infant(s).

Early Intervention

- Early Intervention offers *support-coordination services based on developmental evaluations* for:
  - Special Instruction
  - Occupational Therapy
  - Speech/Language Therapy
  - Physical Therapy
  - Vision Support
  - Hearing Support
  - Other services as specified by law

These services focus on the needs and strengths of your child, and they are coordinated around you and your baby's normal routine to provide developmental support.

- Early Intervention also provides a follow-up program called "Tracking" if your child is not initially eligible for supportive services. Ages and Stages questionnaires are sent out every two months until your child is two years old and then every three months when your child turns three. A developmental score is given to help determine if developmental support is needed from any of the above services.

Your child should be eligible for the Early Intervention Tracking program if he/she:

- Weighed under three and a half pounds at birth

- Was cared for in a Neonatal Intensive Care Unit
- Has high lead levels
- Qualifies for support for other possible reasons.

Local Support Organizations

- **Lancaster County Early Intervention**
  <u>Contact information:</u>

  Address: 150 North Queen Street, Suite 517, Lancaster, PA 17603
  Phone: 717-399-7323
  E-mail: MHIDEarlyInt@co.lancaster.pa.

- **Excentia S. June Smith Center**—provides therapeutic and educational services for children with developmental needs from birth and up.
  <u>Contact information:</u>

  Address: Excentia Main Office, 1810 Rohrerstown Road, Lancaster, PA 17601
  Phone: 717-519-6740
  E-mail: info@ourexcentia.org

- **Schreiber Pediatric Rehab Center** offers premier outpatient physical, occupational, and speech-language therapy to children with disabilities, developmental delays, and acquired injuries.
  <u>Contact information:</u>

  Address: 625 Community Way, Lancaster, PA 17603
  Phone: 717-393-0425
  E-mail: info@schreiberpediatric.org

- **Cleft Palate Clinic** is a not-for-profit organization dedicated to improving the quality of life of infants, children, and adults with craniofacial conditions resulting from birth defects, trauma, and disease.
  Contact information:

  Address: 223 North Lime Street, Lancaster, PA 17602
  Phone: 717-394-3793
  Website: www.cleftclinic.org

- **Mothers of Multiples** offers general meetings the first Tuesday of every month (except July) at Westgate Baptist Church (2235 Harrisburg Pike, Lancaster, PA). The purpose of the club is to address the challenges of parenting and encourage the development of friendships among mothers of multiples in the community; to nurture a positive atmosphere by offering information and speakers who deal with the raising of children and the issues of women; and to promote interest and knowledge with the raising of multiples.
  Contact information:

  E-mail: lancastermoms@aol.com

- **March of Dimes** offers Share Your Story, a place to share your experience with prematurity, birth defects, or loss. Funds raised by the March of Dimes support prenatal wellness programs, research grants, neonatal intensive care unit (NICU) family support programs, consumer and clinician education, and advocacy efforts for stronger, healthier babies. Find a local March of Dimes chapter and walk annually in the March for Babies to give every baby a fighting chance.
  Contact information:

  Local Address: 3544 North Progress Avenue, Suite 204, Harrisburg, PA, 17110
  Local Phone: 717-545-4534

National Address: March of Dimes National Office, 1275 Mamaroneck Avenue, White Plains, NY 10605
National Phone: 914-997-4488

National Support Organizations

There are also many national organizations that provide support and education for NICU families during and after their NICU stay. Here are three popular organizations who offer various means of support services and educational options for NICU families. We have listed only the few that we have received information on.

- **Graham's Foundation** offers support, advocacy, and research for every path of prematurity. Graham's Foundation also offers NICU care packages, preemie parent mentors, and the MyPreemie app.
  <u>**Contact information:**</u>

  Address: Graham's Foundation,
  P.O. Box 755, 1205 Louisiana Avenue,
  Perrysburg, OH 43552
  Phone: 888-466-2948

  Website: www.grahamsfoundation.org

- <u>**Hand to Hold**</u> is a nonprofit 501(c)(3) organization, which carefully matches seasoned parents of preemies (Helping Hands) with parents in need of support. Hand to Hold offers support, information, and education through helpful articles, educational videos, parent-to-parent blogs, sibling support programs, and more.
  <u>**Contact information:**</u>

  Phone: 855-424-6428, Parent Support ext. 712
  Website: www.handtohold.org

- **Peekaboo ICU** offers support and education for families in the NICU. Their goal is to empower the preemie parent.
  <u>Contact information:</u>

  Address: Peekaboo ICU,
  7900-D Stevens Mill Road, Suite #237,
  Matthews, NC 28104

  Website: www.peekabooicu.net

Note: There are many other good national organizations providing support for NICU families that can be found online which we have not discussed here, as we do not have sufficient information and have not used them.

On and On

The lush green grass on the mountaintop,
Speckled with daisies, amongst the thistle ferns.
The mighty eucalyptus trees with the glistening dew drop,
As little lambs frolic and the mountain wren yearns,
For that first rainwater, ready to grope,
Though tranquil waters enrich the slope.
Amidst the hum of the bubbling brook a rhapsody resounds,
A voice in the wilderness, a glorious sound.
A beacon of hope, a beacon of light,
beckoning me on and on and On and On!

—Manjeet Kaur

Appendices

Charts

Weight Conversion Chart

Pounds and Ounces to Grams Conversion Chart

POUNDS

OUNCES	0	1	2	3	4	5	6	7	8	9	10	11	12	13	14
0	0	454	907	1361	1814	2268	2722	3175	3629	4082	4536	4990	5443	5897	6350
1	28	482	936	1389	1843	2296	2750	3203	3657	4111	4564	5018	5471	5925	6379
2	57	510	964	1417	1871	2325	2778	3232	3685	4139	4593	5046	5500	5953	6407
3	85	539	992	1446	1899	2353	2807	3260	3714	4167	4621	5075	5528	5982	6435
4	113	567	1021	1474	1928	2381	2835	3289	3742	4196	4649	5103	5557	6010	6464
5	142	595	1049	1503	1956	2410	2863	3317	3770	4224	4678	5131	5585	6038	6492
6	170	624	1077	1531	1984	2438	2892	3345	3799	4252	4706	5160	5613	6067	6520
7	198	652	1106	1559	2013	2466	2920	3374	3827	4281	4734	5188	5642	6095	6549
8	227	680	1134	1588	2041	2495	2948	3402	3856	4309	4763	5216	5670	6123	6577
9	255	709	1162	1616	2070	2523	2977	3430	3884	4337	4791	5245	5698	6152	6605
10	283	737	1191	1644	2098	2551	3005	3459	3912	4366	4819	5273	5727	6180	6634
11	312	765	1219	1673	2126	2580	3033	3487	3941	4394	4848	5301	5755	6209	6662
12	340	794	1247	1701	2155	2608	3062	3515	3969	4423	4876	5330	5783	6237	6690
13	369	822	1276	1729	2183	2637	3090	3544	3997	4451	4904	5358	5812	6265	6719
14	397	850	1304	1758	2211	2665	3118	3572	4026	4479	4933	5386	5840	6294	6747
15	425	879	1332	1786	2240	2693	3147	3600	4054	4508	4961	5415	5868	6322	6776

Chart 1: Convert pounds and ounces to grams/grams to pounds and ounces

To convert baby's weight from pounds and ounces to grams:

- Select weight in pounds in the blue row.
- Select the weight in ounces in the pink column.
- Read the weight in grams from the cell where the two selections meet.
- E.g., If weight is 4 pounds and 7 ounces, then the weight in grams is 2,013 grams.

Length Conversion Chart

Centimeters to Inches Conversion Chart					
Centimeters	Inches	Centimeters	Inches	Centimeters	Inches
25.4	10	43.2	17	61.0	24
26.7	10½	44.4	17½	62.2	24½
27.9	11	45.7	18	63.5	25
29.2	11½	47.0	18½	64.8	25½
30.5	12	48.3	19	66.1	26
31.8	12½	49.5	19½	67.4	26½
33.0	13	50.8	20	68.7	27
34.3	13½	52.1	20½	69.9	27½
35.6	14	53.3	21	71.2	28
36.8	14½	54.6	21½	72.5	28½
38.1	15	55.9	22	73.8	29
39.4	15½	57.2	22½	75.1	29½
40.6	16	58.4	23	76.4	30
41.9	16½	59.7	23½	77.6	30½

Chart 2: Convert centimeters to inches/inches to centimeters

To convert baby's length from centimeters to inches:

- Select the length in centimeters in the blue column.
- The length in inches is in the next adjacent cell [to the right] in the pink column.
- E.g., If the length is 57.2 centimeters, then the length in inches is 22 ½ inches.

Temperature Conversion Chart

Degrees Fahrenheit to Degrees Centigrade Conversion Chart	
Fahrenheit	**Centigrade**
96.1	35.6
96.4	35.8
96.8	36.0
97.7	36.5
98.6	37.0
99.5	37.5
100.4	38.0
101.3	38.5
102.2	39.0
103.1	39.5
104.0	40.0
104.9	40.5
105.8	41.0
106.7	41.5
107.6	42.0

Chart 3: Convert degrees Fahrenheit to degrees centigrade/
degrees centigrade to degrees Fahrenheit.

To convert baby's temperature from Fahrenheit to centigrade:
- Select baby's temperature reading in the blue column.
- Read the temperature in centigrade from the adjacent cell in the pink column.

E.g., if the temperature is 101.3° Fahrenheit, then the temperature is 38.5° centigrade.

Growth Charts

Growth charts are used to:

- monitor a baby's growth over time
- compare your baby's growth against the expected growth of infants of the same age and sex.

The **Fenton Growth Charts**[1] were developed by Dr. Tanis Fenton of the Cumming School of Medicine, University of Calgary. The Fenton Charts are specifically designed for use with pre-term infants up to 50 weeks, and are used for monitoring babies' growth. After that, the CDC/WHO charts can be used.

Although growth charts are an important tool, they are not intended to be used as the only diagnostic device for monitoring your baby's progress. Rather, they are one of the tools that contribute to an overall clinical impression for the child's growth.

About the growth charts

Separate charts are used for boys and girls because of gender differences.

The Fenton Growth Charts measure three growth factors:

- weight
- length (height)
- head circumference.

Using the Fenton Growth Charts

The following pages show scaled-down versions of the growth charts for both boys and girls.

For ease of use, you can download the full-sized charts free of charge from the University of Calgary website at http://www.ucalgary.ca/fenton/

These full-sized charts can be used to plot the readings week by week as your baby grows.

The website also has details of handy apps that you can use for the Fenton Charts.

---

1   The Fenton growth charts are included with kind permission of Dr. Tanis Fenton.

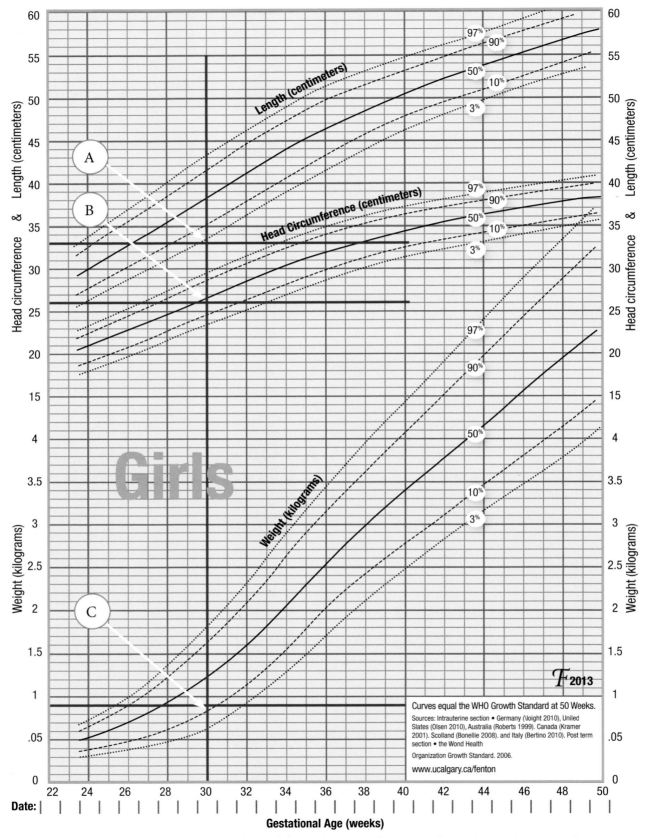

Chart 4: Fenton Preterm Growth Chart for Girls: Weight, Length and Head Circumference.

Fenton Growth Chart for Girls

Using the chart

- Locate your baby's gestational age on the horizontal axis and draw a vertical line on the chart.
- The example on the chart is for a baby with a gestational age of 30 weeks.

To calculate weight percentile[2]

- Locate your baby's current weight in kilograms on the vertical axis, and draw a horizontal line on the chart.
- The intersection of this line with the vertical for gestation will give baby's weight percentile.
- The example opposite shows a baby with a weight of 900 gm.
- Intersection point "C" shows this baby's weight is about the 10th percentile.

To calculate length percentile[2]

- Locate your baby's length in centimeters on the vertical axis, and draw a horizontal line on the chart.
- The intersection of this line with the vertical line for gestation will give baby's length percentile.
- The example opposite shows a baby with a length of 33 cm.
- Intersection point "A" shows this baby's length is in about the 3rd percentile.

To calculate head circumference percentile

- Locate your baby's current head circumference in centimeters on the vertical axis, and draw a horizontal line on the chart.
- The intersection of this line with the vertical line for gestation will give baby's head circumference percentile.
- The example opposite shows a baby with a head circumference of 26 cm.
- Intersection point "B" shows this baby's head circumference is about the 40th percentile.

Percentiles measure where your baby ranks compared with fetuses of the same gestational age. After birth, almost all babies lose some water weight. After they lose this weight, they place lower on the growth chart, which is normal. E.g. if your baby's measurement is in the 10th percentile for length, this means that 10% of fetuses that gestational age weigh the same or less than your baby, and 90% of fetuses weigh more than your baby. Because of this early weight loss, and their challenges adapting to being born early, most babies born prematurely place low on growth charts. Each baby finds their own growth pattern, and their length is usually at lower percentiles than their weight. What you want to see is that most weeks babies show continued growth.

---

2   Length measurements are not easy to obtain in neonatal units, so you may see very jagged patterns, since the measures are not very accurate.

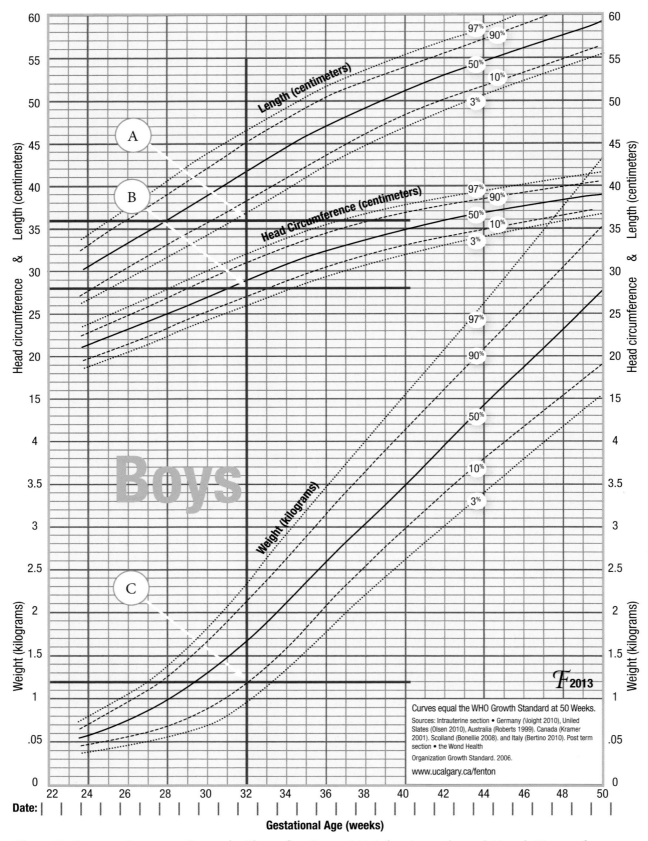

Chart 5: Fenton Preterm Growth Chart for Boys: Weight, Length and Head Circumference.

Fenton Growth Chart for Boys
Using the chart

- Locate your baby's gestational age on the horizontal axis and draw a vertical line on the chart
- The example opposite is for a baby with a gestational age of 32 weeks.

To calculate weight percentile[3]

- Locate your baby's current weight in kilograms on the vertical axis, and draw a horizontal line on the chart.
- The intersection of this line with the vertical line for gestation will give baby's weight percentile.
- The example opposite shows a baby with a weight of 1.2 kg.
- Intersection point "C" shows this baby's weight is about the 10th percentile.

To calculate length percentile[4]

- Locate your baby's length in centimeters on the vertical axis, and draw a horizontal line on the chart.
- The intersection of this line with the vertical line for gestation will give baby's length percentile.
- The example opposite shows a baby with a length of 36 cm.
- Intersection point "A" shows this baby's length is in approximately the 3rd percentile.

To calculate head circumference percentile

- Locate your baby's current head circumference in centimeters on the vertical axis, and draw a horizontal line on the chart.
- The intersection of this line with the vertical line for gestation will give baby's head circumference percentile.
- The example opposite shows a baby with a head circumference of 28 cm.
- Intersection point "B" shows this baby's head circumference is about the 25th percentile.

Percentiles measure where your baby ranks compared with fetuses of the same gestational age. After birth almost all babies lose some water weight. After they lose this weight, they place lower on the growth chart, which is normal. E.g., if your baby's measurement is in the 10th percentile for length, this means that 10% of fetuses that gestational age weigh the same or less than your baby, and 90% of fetuses weigh more than your baby. Because of this early weight loss, and their challenges adapting to being born early, most babies born prematurely place low on growth charts. Each baby finds theirown growth pattern, and their length is usually at lower percentiles than their weight. What you want to see is that most weeks babies show continued growth.

3   Length measurements are not easy to obtain in neonatal units, so you may see very jagged patterns, since the measures are not very accurate.

Nutritionals—formulas and fortifiers

Human milk remains the best nutrition for an infant—both term and preterm, though some fortifiers may be required in preterm infants early on. Human milk has 20 calories (cal) per ounce (oz).

The formulas most commonly used are:

Formulas for term infants

- Enfamil with iron or low iron—20 cal per oz.
- Similac with iron or low iron, both with 20 cal per oz.

Preterm infant formulas

- Similac Special Care 20, 24, 30 cal (per ounce) with iron.
- Enfamil Premature 20, 24, 30 cal (per ounce) with iron.

    Similac Special Care 20 or Enfamil Premature 20 will be used initially and advanced to 24 cal or more as tolerated.

Fortifiers

Fortifiers may be used to add additional calories to the preterm breast milk:

- Similac and Enfamil fortifier may be used.
- Nowadays **human milk fortifiers** such as **Prolacta** are available as Prolacta + 4, Prolacta + 6, Prolacta +8, and + 10, which provide four, six, eight, or ten calories per ounce of breast milk.

Other formulas

Other formulas may be used in specific situations:

- Similac Sensitive (previously called Lactofree) 20 cal per oz for lactose-intolerant infants.
- Similac Spit-up (with added rice starch) for babies with regurgitation and reflux.
- Enfamil-Prosobee and Similac-Isomil—soy formulas for babies with milk intolerance.

Special formulas used for milk protein sensitivity

The proteins in these formulas have *basic protein units(amino acids)* or *broken down proteins* that are more easily digestible.

These are also used in preterm infants in specific situations and have 20 cal per ounce.

- EleCare—has basic amino acids.
- Similac Alimentum—has casein hydrolysate and certain amino acids.
- Neocate—has basic amino acids.

As such these special formulas are tried in babies with allergies and intolerance of regular formulas.

If your baby has been placed on a special formula, a careful consideration would have been given.

There are also *many other formulas* available, such as Nutramigen and Pregestamil.

Preterm discharge formulas:

Preterm infants may need special formula at discharge which give additional calories and mineral supplements:

- Similac Neosure—22 cal per oz.
- Enfamil Enfacare—22 cal per oz.

These are generally recommended for babies till nine to twelve months of age.

Recommended immunization schedule for infants and children⁋

Birth	**Hepatitis B**
2 months	**Hepatitis B, DTaP** (diphtheria, tetanus and pertussis), **IPV** (inactivated polio), **Hib** (haemophilus influenza-B), **PCV** (pnemococcal), **RV** (rota-virus)
4 months	**DTaP, IPV, Hib, PCV, RV**
6 months	**DTaP, Hib, PCV, RV**
6 to 18 months	**Hepatitis B, IPV**
12 to 15 months	**Hepatitis A, Hib, MMR** (mumps, measles, rubella)—first dose, **PCV, Varicella** (chickenpox)—first dose
15 to 18 months	**DTaP**
18 to 23 months	**Hepatitis A**
4 to 6 years	**DTaP, IPV, MMR**—second dose, **Varicella**—second dose
** Annual	**Influenza** vaccine for all children from 6 months through 18 years of age
** Monthly	**RSV** (respiratory syncytial virus) prophylaxis during the RSV season (fall through spring) for high risk babies—born at less than 32 weeks gestation (and younger than one year) or other situations as deemed by your physician)

⁋ Vaccine recommendations will vary in certain high-risk and catch-up situations when immunization have been missed.

Common medications and supplements used in the NICU

Refer to the Glossary for descriptions.

Antibiotics

Amoxicillin

Amphotericin

Ampicillin

Cefotaxime (claforan)

Ceftazidime (Fortaz)

Clindamycin

Cloxacillin

Erythromycin

Gentamicin

Methicillin

Metronidazole

Nafcillin

Nystatin (Mycostatin)

Penicillin

Vancomycin

Cardiovascular medications

Digoxin

Dopamine/ Dobutamine

Epinephrine

Furosemide (Lasix)

Heparin

Hydrochlorothiazide

Ibuprofen

Indomethacin

Prostaglandin E1

Spironolactone (aldactone)

Gastrointestinal drugs

Actigall

Metoclopramide (Reglan)

Ranitidine (Zantac)

Miscellaneous

Erythropoietin

Hepatitis immune globulin

Insulin

Intravenous immune globulin

Tylenol (acetoaminophen)

Naloxone (Narcan)

Nervous system drugs

Anticonvulsants

Dilantin (phenytoin)

Lorazepam (Ativan)

Phenobarbital

Sedatives

Chloral Hydrate

Fentanyl

Midazolam (versed)

Morphine

Respiratory

Caffeine

Dexamethasone (Decadron)

Inhaled nitric oxide(iNO)

Surfactant

Theophylline

Ventolin (albuterol)

Vitamins and minerals

Calcium gluconate

Fer-in-sol (Iron)

Polyvisol

Potassium chloride

Sodium chloride

Vitamin D

Vitamin K

Commonly used abbreviations in the NICU:
"The NICU Lingo"

ABG: Arterial blood

ABO: Blood groups A, B, O, and AB

BP: Blood pressure

BPD: Bronchopulmonary dysplasia (chronic lung disease)

C+S: Culture and sensitivity

CBC: Complete blood count

CBG: Capillary blood gas

cc: Cubic centimeter or ml

CDC: Centers for Disease Control

CMV: Cytomegalovirus

CO2: Carbon dioxide

CP: Cerebral palsy

CPAP: Continuous positive airway pressure

CSF: Cerebrospinal fluid

CT scan: Computed Tomography

ECMO: Extracorporeal membrane oxygenation

EDC: Expected date of confinement

EDD: Expected date of delivery

EEG: Electroencephalogram

EKG: Electrocardiogram

ETT: Endotracheal tube

FiO2: Oxygen percentage

GBS: Group B Streptococci

GIT: Gastrointestinal tract

gm: Gram

h+h: Hemoglobin and hematocrit

HC: Head circumference

hct: Hematocrit

Hgb: Hemoglobin

HMD: Hyaline membrane disease

I&O: Intake and output

IDM: Infant of diabetic mother

iNO: Inhaled Nitric Oxide

IUGR: Intrauterine growth restriction

IV: Intravenous

IVH: Intraventricular hemorrhage (bleed)

LBW: Low birth weight

LGA: Large for gestational age

LP: Lumbar puncture (spinal tap)

Lytes: Electrolytes (sodium, potassium, chloride)

MAS: Meconium aspiration syndrome

MRI: Magnetic resonance imaging

NAS: Neonatal Abstinence Syndrome

NG: Nasogastric

NGT: Nasogastric tube

NICU: Neonatal Intensive Care Unit

NNP: Neonatal nurse practitioner

NPO: Nil per oral or nothing by mouth

O2: Oxygen

OGT: Orogastric tube

OT: Occupational Therapy

PCVC: Peripheral central venous catheter

PDA: Patent Ductus Arteriosus

PIH: Pregnancy Induced Hypertension

PPHN: Persistent Pulmonary Hypertension

PPROM: Premature, prolonged rupture of membranes

PPV: Positive Pressure Ventilation

Preemie: Preterm infant
PT: Physical Therapy
RBCs: Red blood cells
RDS: Respiratory Distress Syndrome
RN: Registered nurse
ROP: Retinopathy of Prematurity
RSV: Respiratory syncytial virus
Sats: Oxygen saturations
SGA: Small for Gestational Age
stat: Immediately
Sz: Seizures

Temp: Temperature
TPN: Total Parenteral Nutrition
TTN: Transient Tachypnea of the Newborn
UAC: Umbilical Arterial Catheter
UVC: Umbilical Venous Catheter
VLBW: Very low birth weight
WBC: White blood cells
Weeker: Weeks gestation
WIC: Women, Infants, and Children Nutrition Program
wt: Weight

Glossary

A

ABG: Arterial blood gas

ABO incompatibility: When mother's blood group is O and baby's is A or B, it may result in antibodies and destruction of fetal red blood cells, leading to jaundice and anemia.

Abruption: Separation of placenta from the uterus causing bleeding.

Actigall: (urosodiol) Used to improve sludging of bile (or cholestasis) associated with TPN (total parenteral nutrition); also, used to dissolve gallstones.

Acute: Illness with a sudden onset and of a brief duration.

Adjusted age (or Corrected age): Number of weeks (or months) since baby's birth (actual age), minus the number of weeks (or months) that baby was born before the due date, is the adjusted or corrected age. This is important for assessing gestation adjusted development. See example on page 396.

Air leak: Caused by tearing of one or more lung air sacs (alveoli) causing air collection in chest cavity.

Alveoli: Air sacs in the lung where oxygen and carbon dioxide are exchanged.

Amniotic fluid: Fluid in the uterus surrounding the baby.

Amoxicillin: Oral broad-spectrum penicillin.

Amphotericin: Antibiotic used to treat fungal infections.

Ampicillin: Broad spectrum penicillin used intravenously in neonates frequently to treat bacterial infections such as Group B streptococci (GBS).

Anemia: Low red blood cells or low hemoglobin.

Antibiotic: Drug that kills bacteria.

Anticonvulsants: Drugs used to treat seizures.

Aorta: A major blood vessel carrying blood from left side of the heart to the body.

Apgar score: Scoring system for evaluation of baby's condition at birth. Scoring is done for heart rate, breathing, color, tone, and reflexes. Lowest score is zero and highest is ten.

Apnea: A pause in breathing for twenty seconds or longer—a common problem in premature babies due to immaturity.

Artery: Blood vessel carrying blood and oxygen to all parts of the body.

Asphyxia: Lack of oxygen to body cells with resultant accumulation of acid waste and carbon dioxide. It can lead to neurologic damage if left untreated for a prolonged period.

Aspiration: Inhaling a foreign material into the lungs, e.g., formula, stomach contents, medication, milk, meconium, blood, etc.

Audiologist: A professional with specialized training to evaluate hearing loss and related disorders, and to rehabilitate these individuals.

B

Bacteria: Microorganisms that can cause infection.

Bag and mask ventilation: Pumping oxygen or air into the lungs using an oxygen bag connected to a face mask (bagging).

Barotrauma: Trauma to lung tissue due to pressure of ventilator support.

Bilirubin: Breakdown product of hemoglobin (substance in red blood cells that carries oxygen in the blood). When bilirubin is in excess, it causes jaundice.

Bleed: Term used in newborns generally for intracranial (head) hemorrhage. However, bleeding can occur in various other parts of the body as well.

Blood culture: Blood test used to look for growth of microorganisms on a culture medium.

Blood gas: Measures oxygen, carbon dioxide, and acid status in the blood. Blood gas can be a *capillary blood gas* obtained from a finger or heel by a needle stick or *arterial* obtained from a large artery such as radial in the arm or from the umbilical artery catheter. The oxygen status is much more accurate from an artery since it carries oxygenated blood.

Blood glucose: Sugar levels in blood.

Bolus feeds: Feedings given by a nasogastric or orogastric tube—usually flows by gravity or pump over a short period—usually 15–30 minutes.

Bowel decompression: Relieving tension on the gut in cases of obstruction or pseudo obstruction, by placing a tube in the stomach (orogastric tube) and connecting it to intermittent suction.

Bradycardia: Slowing of heart rate to less than 100 beats per minute in the newborn.

Brain ventricles: Spaces in the brain where cerebrospinal fluid or CSF circulates.

Breast pump: A machine used to collect breast milk. Hospital-grade breast pump is usually more powerful and can be rented.

Bronchi: Lung airways or divisions from the trachea into smaller branches called bronchi.

Bronchopulmonary dysplasia (BPD): Chronic lung disease (CLD) caused in mostly preterm infants due to a prolonged ventilation and high levels of oxygen. This involves damage of air sacs, scarring of lung tissue, as well as areas of collapse.

C

Caffeine: A medication that stimulates the respiratory center; used in treatment of apnea of prematurity.

Calories: Used to measure energy value of foods; one ounce of breast milk has twenty calories.

Cannula: Soft, thin tube with prongs that deliver oxygen into baby's nose.

Cardiac compression: Rhythmic pressure or compression over the chest given to resuscitate a baby with low or no heart rate.

Cardiopulmonary resuscitation (CPR): Method of reviving someone not breathing or if heart rate has slowed or stopped. This involves artificial respiration and cardiac compression.

Cardiorespiratory monitor: Equipment used to measure heart rate and breathing.

Care manager: Professional nurse overseeing the needs of the family and the baby while baby is in the NICU; also, coordinates discharge follow-up and other needs.

Catheter: A thin, hollow, flexible tube for insertion into a body cavity or vessel; used to drain fluid or administer fluids, i.e., umbilical venous or arterial catheter.

CBG: Capillary blood gas.

Cefotaxime (Claforan): A cephalosporin antibiotic used against bacterial infections.

Ceftazidime (Fortaz): A strong cephalosporin antibiotic.

Central venous line: An intravenous line fed from a small vein into a central location close to the heart as access for intravenous nutrition and medication.

Cerebral palsy (CP): A chronic, non-progressive condition in which posture or movement is affected due to abnormal muscle tone. This may be due to a brain malformation or damage before, during, or after birth. CP can occur due to a lack of oxygen. Cause is often unclear.

Chest tube: Tube inserted in the chest to drain air (pneumothorax) collected between chest wall and lung (caused by rupture of lung sacs).

Chloral hydrate: Oral sedative used to relieve agitation and pain.

Clindamycin: Antibiotic used to treat deep tissue infections.

Cloxacillin: A type of penicillin antibiotic to treat certain infections.

Colostomy: Surgical opening in the intestine to allow drainage of fecal material outside the body.

Complete blood count (CBC): Blood test measuring the cells in the blood: white cells or WBCs (that fight infection); red cells or RBCs (oxygen-carrying cells); platelets (blood-clotting cells); and concentration of hemoglobin.

Computed tomography (CT): Diagnostic imaging using a beam of radiation rotating around the body, constructing with a computer a two-dimensional picture of internal organs; used to diagnose blood and fluid or deformity in the brain or other parts of the body.

Congenital diaphragmatic hernia: Birth defect involving an opening in diaphragm so abdominal organs, i.e., stomach, intestines, etc., are pushed into the chest. This hinders lung development.

Congestive heart failure: Failure of the heart to pump blood adequately, leading to fluid overload.

Continuous feeds: Feeds given continuously via nasogastric tube using a pump with a certain volume being delivered per hour.

Continuous positive airway pressure (CPAP): Air or oxygen is mechanically pumped into baby's lungs to keep air sacs open. This is usually delivered via short prongs in nose (nasal CPAP) or via endotracheal tube (ETT CPAP).

Cord accidents: Any issues with the umbilical cord leading to disruption of blood flow to the baby such as cord tear, cord entrapment, compression, abnormal cord insertion, or prolapse.

Corrected age (CA): Number of weeks since baby's birth, minus the number of weeks the baby was born before the due date, is the corrected age. CA is important for assessing gestation-adjusted development.

CPR: Cardio pulmonary resuscitation.

Cryotherapy (Cryopexy): Freezing abnormal tissue in blood vessels as in the retina in retinopathy to halt their growth.

Cytomegalovirus (CMV): A viral infection that in a pregnant woman can lead to severe newborn illness or chronic disabilities, including vision and hearing problems

D

Dehydration: Significant loss of body fluids.

Desaturation: When oxygen falls below the desired level.

Developmental delay: Failure to meet average motor milestones of development such as sitting, walking, behavioral milestones, and learning skills.

Dexamethasone (Decadron): A steroid with anti-inflammatory properties is given as a short course in chronic lung disease or BPD; also, used to treat tracheal edema.

Diarrhea: Loose or watery, frequent stools or bowel movements.

Digoxin: A medicine obtained from the foxglove plant, used to treat arrhythmias and congestive heart failure (CHF); need to be very meticulous with doses.

Dilantin (Phenytoin): Medication for treatment of neonatal seizures.

Discharge formulas for preemies: These formulas have extra calories, protein, vitamins, and minerals as compared to the routine infant formulas. They are recommended for premature or low birth weight infants for nine to twelve months, such as Neosure (twenty-two calories per ounce), EnfaCare (twenty-two calories per ounce), or other preterm equivalents.

Discharge summary: Brief report transcribed by physician or nurse practitioner summarizing baby's problems in the NICU.

Donor milk: Excess breast milk donated by breastfeeding mothers is collected by milk banks, screened, processed, and stored. This donor milk can then be used as needed.

Dopamine/Dobutamine: Vasopressors used to improve blood pressure and low perfusion.

DPT (diphtheria, pertussis (whooping cough), and tetanus); usually given along with H. influenza, polio, and pneumococcal vaccines: First dose of vaccine may be given to infants who remain in NICU for a longer period.

E

Early intervention program: Interventional services provided for children under three years of age with a potential for developmental delay.

Echocardiogram: Ultrasound of the heart, viewing the structure and function of the heart.

Electroencephalogram (EEG): A test recording electrical activity of the brain, depicting brain function. This is conducted by placing several electrodes on the scalp.

Electrolytes: Chemicals in blood that include sodium, potassium chloride, and bicarbonate.

Endotracheal tube (ETT): A tube placed into a newborn's trachea or windpipe from mouth or nose to deliver warm humidified oxygen to the lungs and assist breathing.

Enteral nutrition: Nutrition or feeding using the gut.

Epinephrine: A medication used to resuscitate a newborn, which stimulates the heart. It can be given intravenously or via the endotracheal tube (ETT).

Erythromycin: Antibiotic used as eye ointment in all babies to prevent possible eye infection; also, used to treat other infections, sometimes as a substitute for penicillin in cases of intolerance.

Erythropoietin: Medication to stimulate red blood cell production in high risk preterm infants.

Escherichia coli (E. coli): Gram negative bacteria, second most common cause of bacterial infection in the newborn.

Exchange transfusion: A procedure where equal amounts of blood are removed from baby and replaced. Used when jaundice remains at high levels that can be detrimental to the brain.

Extra uterine: Outside the uterus.

Extracorporeal membrane oxygenation (ECMO): Oxygenation outside the body in equipment like a heart lung machine; used in babies where lungs are unable to oxygenate.

Extremely low birth weight: Refers to babies with birth weight less than 1,000 grams or two pounds three ounces.

Extremely preterm: Babies born between twenty-three to twenty-eight weeks.

Extubation: Removal of endotracheal tube.

F

Failure to thrive: Failure to gain weight and grow as expected.

Feeding tube: A narrow, flexible tube inserted through the nose or mouth into the stomach so breast milk or formula can be fed using a syringe. This is also called a gavage tube.

Fentanyl: An intravenous opioid used to sedate and relieve pain.

Fer-in-sol (Iron): Helps to treat anemia.

Fetal circulation: The circulation of blood in the fetus. Most of the blood bypasses the fetal lungs due to two open shunts—foramen ovale and ductus arteriosus.

Fever: In an infant (until three months of age) if axillary body temperature is higher than 99.5 degrees Fahrenheit (37.5 degrees Celsius), or if rectal temperature is higher than 100.4 degrees Fahrenheit (38 degrees Celsius).

Fontanelle: Soft spot on top of baby's head, which is a normal opening between the bones of the developing skull.

Fortifier: A commercially prepared substance added to breast milk to provide additional calcium and nutrients.

Full term or Term gestation: Previously considered to be a gestation between 37 to 42 weeks. This definition has recently been revised as research shows that each week's gestation can affect the baby's development.
*Early term is 37 to 39 weeks.
*Full term is now considered to be 39 to 41 weeks.

*Late term is 41 to 42 weeks.

*Post term is over 42 weeks.

Furosemide (Lasix): Diuretic to get rid of additional body water; used in CHF, PDA, BPD

G

Gamma globulins (or immune globulin made from plasma): Contain antibodies that protect the body against disease.

Gastroesophageal reflux (GERD or Reflux): Backward flow of stomach contents into esophagus (food pipe); may lead to discomfort and excessive spitting-up or vomiting.

Gastrointestinal tract: The esophagus, stomach, and intestines.

Gastrostomy tube: Feeding tube inserted into a surgically created hole in the abdominal wall into the stomach; used in babies with long-term feeding problems.

Gavage feeding: Tube feeding via nasogastric or orogastric tube.

Genetic: A feature one is born with.

Gentamicin: Antibiotic frequently used intravenously against Gram negative bacteria; blood levels are monitored.

Gestation: Time between last menstrual period and birth. In humans, forty weeks is the average gestation for a term baby.

Gestational age: The number of weeks between the first day of the last menstrual period and date of birth.

Group B streptococci (GBS): Bacterial infection that a baby can contract usually from mother's birth canal resulting in illness. Screening is done in pregnancy at thirty-five to thirty-seven weeks.

H

Head or whole body cooling: In severe cases of asphyxia, head or whole body is cooled for about seventy-two hours, which protects the brain from further injury.

Heart murmur: A specific swishing sound of blood flow through the heart, which may be benign; indicates flow through an abnormal opening (conduit), or through a narrow valve.

Hematocrit: The percentage of red blood cells in blood; used as a measure of anemia.

Hemoglobin: The component of blood that carries oxygen; also used as a measure of anemia.

Heparin: Medication that prevents blood from clotting; used in umbilical and other catheters to prevent blockage from clots.

Hepatitis: Disease that causes inflammation of the liver caused by different viruses A, B, C transmitted by food (A) and blood or sexually (B, C).

Hepatitis B vaccine: The first of three doses is given to all newborns over two kg at birth and other preterms prior to discharge.

Hepatitis immune globulin: Antibody given to babies born to hepatitis antigen positive mothers.

Hernia: A protrusion of an internal organ through tissues that normally enclose it

Herpes: An inflammatory disease of the skin and mucus membranes caused by a virus that is transmitted sexually. A baby may get infected while passing through the birth canal, resulting in a severe illness in the newborn.

High frequency ventilation: Special form of ventilation that provides rapid respiratory rates.

Hind milk: Breast milk produced at end of feeding. This is higher in fat and calories than foremilk.

Home monitor: Monitor used after baby's discharge to monitor apnea (cessation of breathing) or bradycardia (drop in heart rate).

Human milk: Has twenty calories per ounce; composition varies with lactation—see chapter on Lactation Support.

Hyaline membrane disease: Akin to respiratory distress syndrome. This term is not commonly used nowadays.

Hydrocephalus: Excessive fluid in brain ventricles (chambers) that exerts pressure on the brain and causes baby's head to expand. Literally means hydro = water, cephal = head. Excessive pressure can cause brain damage.

Hydrochlorothiazide: Diuretic—removes excess body water.

Hyperbilirubinemia: A higher than normal level of bilirubin in the blood.

Hyperglycemia: High blood glucose levels.

Hyperinsulinism: High levels of insulin in the blood; can be seen temporarily in an infant of a diabetic mother.

Hypoglycemia: Low blood glucose levels. Blood glucose less than forty before twenty-four hours of age, and less than fifty after twenty-four hours of age is referred to as hypoglycemic in a newborn.

Hypothermia: Lower than normal body temperature. This can result in issues such as breathing problems, low glucose, etc.

Hypoxia: Lack of oxygen in the body.

I

Ileostomy: Surgical opening in small intestine to drain fecal matter outside the body.

Immunization: Vaccination given to reduce a person's likelihood of acquiring an infection.

Incubator (Isolette): A transparent box-like crib where a sick or premature baby is placed; provides isolation and maintains the baby's body temperature in normal range.

Indomethacin: An anti-inflammatory agent; a prostaglandin inhibitor. Prostaglandins are vital, hormone like, secretions in the body tissues that can have varied effects, one of which can be to keep the PDA open. Prostaglandin inhibitors such as indomethacin help to close the PDA.

Infant of a diabetic mother (IDM): Often preterm, large baby born to a diabetic mother; baby may be prone to injuries, metabolic problems, and congenital anomalies.

Infection: Invasion of the tissues by harmful microorganisms (bacteria, viruses, fungi, or protozoa).

Inferior vena cava: Large vein that carries blood from lower body into right atrium of heart.

Inflammation: A biological response of body tissues, usually to trauma or infections, causing swelling, redness, warmth, and pain in the area.

Inhaled nitric oxide (iNO): Inhaled gas used to dilate tiny lung blood vessels in pulmonary hypertension (PPHN).

Insulin: Medication used to treat high blood sugar. High blood glucose may be a transient problem in preterm infants due to immaturity.

Intrauterine growth retardation: Decreased growth of the fetus while in the uterus or womb, causing baby to be smaller than normal.

Intravenous (IV): Needle inserted into a vein that allows administration of fluids, nutrition, and medication.

Intravenous immune globulin: An antibody given in addition to antibiotics in severe sepsis, and in some cases of thrombocytopenia.

Intraventricular hemorrhage: Bleeding into the brain ventricles and possibly the surrounding tissues.

Intubation: A procedure where an endotracheal tube (ETT) is inserted through the mouth or nose into the trachea or windpipe to assist with breathing.

Isoimmune thrombocytopenia: Low platelets in baby due to antibodies in mother's blood against fetal platelets.

Isolette: See Incubator.

J

Jaundice (jaune = yellow): Yellow coloration of skin and eyes due to increased production or decreased clearance of bilirubin. If too high, this can cause neurologic damage. Jaundice can be treated with phototherapy using special lights.

K

Kangaroo care: Practice of holding a NICU infant skin-to-skin (often between mother's breasts or on father's chest) to provide close human contact between parent and baby for bonding. Additional benefits can be increased quiet time, weight gain, and improved feeding.

Kernicterus (kern = nuclei, icterus = jaundice): Rare condition of increased bilirubin that can stain the brain nuclei and cause permanent brain damage.

L

Lactation: Milk production in a woman's breast.

Lactation consultant: A nurse or a health-care consultant who provides information and support regarding breastfeeding and pumping. This is an important resource for NICU mothers.

Lanugo: Fine downy hair that covers the fetus before or shortly after birth.

Large for gestational age (LGA): A newborn whose weight is above the ninetieth percentile of the standard growth chart.

Laryngomalacia: Larynx is abnormally soft or floppy and collapses during breathing, resulting in a stridorous sound.

Laryngoscope: An instrument with a blade and handle, and a light at the tip that helps to visualize the larynx and vocal cords and assist in intubation.

Lead wires: Wires that go from the electrodes (sticky patches) on chest or abdomen of baby to a cardiorespiratory monitor.

Lesion: A patch of abnormal skin that may be present at birth or is due to an infection or injury.

Let-down reflex: Oxytocin (hormone) release that causes a mother's breast milk to go into reservoirs behind the nipples. Milk may start to drip, especially when infant breast feeds.

Lorazepam (Ativan): Drug used for treatment of neonatal seizures.

Low birth weight (LBW): An infant who weighs less than 2,500 grams (five pounds eight ounces) at birth.

Lumbar puncture - LP (Spinal tap): A diagnostic or therapeutic procedure for obtaining cerebrospinal fluid (CSF) from the spinal space. A needle is inserted into the lower back between the lumbar vertebrae into the space between the spine and its membranous coverings. CSF is collected and sent for tests.

M

Magnetic resonance imaging (MRI): Imaging technique that uses powerful magnets and computers to produce very detailed pictures of internal tissues and organs (no radiation is used).

Malformation: An anatomic abnormality present at birth.

Mechanical ventilation: Using a ventilator to help a sick baby breathe. The machine is connected to an endotracheal tube in the baby's windpipe or trachea and delivers a certain number of breaths per minute under a certain pressure or a certain volume.

Meconium: Dark green to blackish bowel movement passed by the newborn baby for the first two to three days.

Meconium aspiration: Meconium can be passed by the fetus in the uterus that may be inhaled into the airway. This may lead to breathing difficulties.

Meconium aspiration syndrome (MAS): Problems caused by meconium (baby's first bowel movement) going into the lungs while baby is still in the womb, or during transit from the womb.

Meningitis: An inflammation of the lining of the brain usually by viral or bacterial infection.

Methicillin: Antibiotic used to treat bacterial infections such as staphylococci.

Metoclopramide (Reglan): Facilitates gastric emptying and motility; improves feeding intolerance and possibly prevents reflux.

Metronidazole: Antibiotic used for specific infections.

Midazolam (Versed): Short acting sedative; also used before procedures.

Milestone achievements (Milestones): Skills most children can perform at a certain age; e.g., smiling, rolling, sitting, crawling, walking, and speaking.

Monitor: A machine that records information such as heartbeat, respiration, and blood pressure.

Moro reflex: A normal reflex to a stimulus or noise, causing a newborn to stretch out and then flex arms and legs; also called "hugging reflex."

Morphine: Narcotic used for sedation and pain relief; also used in drug withdrawal in cases of maternal drug addiction to opioids.

Myopia: Difficulty in seeing distant objects as clearly as near objects.

N

Nafcillin: Antibiotic used to treat certain bacterial infections.

Naloxone (Narcan): Reverses opioid effect in case of maternal use during labor; cannot be used in opioid addiction as it can cause acute withdrawal.

Nasal cannula: Tubes that connect to prongs in nose for giving additional oxygen by blowing humidified air mixed with oxygen into the nose.

Nasal intermittent positive ventilation (NIPPV): A form of non-invasive ventilatory assistance, in which ventilation is provided via nasal prongs or nasal mask.

Nasogastric tube: A tube passed through the nose to the stomach. This is used to give milk or medication to infant. This is usually left in place for a number of feeds.

Nasojejunal feeds: A way of feeding babies directly into the small bowel; used to overcome conditions such as severe reflux, vomiting, and aspiration.

Nebulizer: A device for giving medicine by making a fine mist that is inhaled through the nose or mouth; a type of "inhaler."

Necrotizing enterocolitis (NEC): An inflammatory disease of especially the preterm infant's bowel that can cause inflammation and possible destruction of part of the baby's intestines.

Needle aspiration: Removal of trapped air in the pleural space (between the lung and chest wall) by inserting a needle in certain chest wall spaces.

Neonatal abstinence syndrome (NAS): Syndrome constituting symptoms of withdrawal in an infant born to a mother with a history of drug abuse.

Neonatal intensive care unit (NICU): A nursery used to treat sick newborns or neonates. There are four levels: <u>Level I</u>: Basic newborn care; <u>Level II</u>: Advanced newborn care for babies more than thirty-two-weeks gestation; <u>Level III</u>: Care for any baby with severe or life-threatening conditions; <u>Level IV</u>: Regional NICU—higher level of the most acute care providing all medical and surgical subspecialties, transplants, and educational outreach.

Neonatal nurse practitioner (NNP): An advanced practice nurse with specialized training and expertise in neonatal care. NNPs are licensed to diagnose and treat critically ill neonates. In addition, they write orders, interpret results, perform emergency and daily procedures, as well as attend high-risk deliveries.

Neonatologist: A pediatrician with a special training specifically for the care of critically ill newborns for several years; requires a board certification in Neonatal and Perinatal Medicine.

Neurologist (Pediatric): A pediatrician with special training dealing with diseases and care of the brain and nervous system of children; requires board certification in Pediatric Neurology.

NICU: See Neonatal intensive care unit.

Nitric oxide: A gas naturally produced by the body can be given as a medication that is breathed in. This helps to expand the tiny blood vessels in the lung, and is sometimes used in PPHN (persistent pulmonary hypertension of the newborn).

Non nutritive sucking: Sucking on a pacifier or finger (baby's own or caregiver's). This aids in suck development and enhances digestion.

Normal saline: A solution containing 0.9 percent salt or sodium chloride.

NPO: Abbreviation of a Latin term "nil per os" used for nothing per oral; i.e., no feeds to be given orally.

Nutrients: Proteins, carbohydrates, fats, vitamins, and minerals that are needed for proper growth.

Nystatin (Mycostatin): Used as a cream to treat candida or yeast (fungal) infections as in candida diaper dermatitis; also used as oral swab medication for oral candida (thrush).

O

Obstetrician: Physician who specializes in diseases of women during pregnancy and child birth; requires board certification in Obstetrics and Gynecology (women's diseases).

Occupational therapist: A specially trained healthcare provider in the NICU who uses structured activity or stimulation, helping baby learn to coordinate sucking, breathing, and swallowing while remaining comfortable. These techniques are also taught to parents to enhance infant development.

Ophthalmologist: Physician specializing in diagnosing and treating problems of the eyes; requires board certification.

Orogastric tube: A flexible tube inserted through the mouth down the throat and food pipe to the stomach. This is used for providing nutrition and medication as well as to drain gastric secretions if needed.

Oscillator: A ventilator providing high frequency or rapid breaths.

Ostomy: A surgical opening between an internal organ and the body surface; e.g., colostomy, ileostomy.

Oximeter: A device placed on the finger, hand, toe, or ankle (usually right hand) that painlessly measures levels of oxygen in the blood via a sensor.

Oxygen: Gas that is essential to life. Room air has 21 percent oxygen.

Oxygen saturation: The amount of oxygen bound to hemoglobin. This is an indicator of a baby's oxygenation. Maximum saturations are 100 percent in healthy lungs.

Oxygen therapy: Any method of giving supplemental oxygen to the tissues through the lungs using an oxygen mask, nasal cannula, oxyhood, or using a ventilator. Oxygen therapy is measured in liters of flow per minute.

P

Pale: Denotes deficiency of pink skin color; usually caused by reduced blood flow through the skin, or decreased blood or shock.

Palvizumab (Synagis): Protects premature infants from developing RSV or respiratory syncytial virus infection. Injection is given monthly, usually in the thigh muscle, during RSV season (fall to spring).

Patent ductus arteriosus (PDA): Caused by failure of a small blood vessel (ductus arteriosus) to close. Normally this opening between aorta and pulmonary artery closes soon after birth. If it remains open, it may need to be closed by medication or surgery to prevent "flooding" of the lungs.

PDA ligation: A surgical procedure where a small incision is made in the chest and a suture or clips are placed around the patent ductus arteriosus (PDA).

Pediatrician: Physician trained in care and treatment of children; requires board certification in Pediatrics.

Penicillin: Antibiotic used to treat bacterial infections such as Group B Streptococcal (GBS) infections.

Percutaneous central catheter, or Peripherally inserted central catheter (PICC): A long catheter placed in a vein and advanced to a larger vein closer to the heart. A PICC will not need to be replaced as often as a peripheral IV line.

Perinatal asphyxia (peri = around, natal = delivery): Asphyxia or suffocation indicates impaired blood or oxygen supply to the baby around delivery.

Periventricular leukomalacia (PVL): Damages in brain tissue usually around the ventricles, mostly secondary to brain bleed, associated with increased risk of learning or movement issues.

Persistent pulmonary hypertension of the newborn (PPHN): Increased pressure (hypertension) of the lung blood vessels that forces blood away from the lungs, thus decreasing oxygen going to the rest of the body.

Phenobarbital: First-line drug in treatment of neonatal seizures.

Phototherapy: Light treatment used for jaundice in the newborn. This breaks down bilirubin to a soluble form that can be excreted in the urine.

Physical therapist (Physiotherapist): A specially trained health professional who uses exercise, massage, and other forms of treatment to improve recovery.

PLA antigen: Platelet antigen that causes mother's blood to form antibodies that break down fetal platelets.

Placenta: An organ in the uterus that attaches the fetus to the uterus, providing the fetus with nutrition, gas exchange, and waste removal.

Platelets: Blood component associated with clotting.

Pneumatosis: Air bubbles in the bowel wall occurring in necrotizing enterocolitis (NEC).

Pneumomediastinum: Leakage of air into the space in the center of chest containing the heart and major blood vessels.

Pneumonia: Inflammation or infection of lungs.

Pneumothorax: Air leak into the space between the lungs and chest wall.

Poly-Vi-Sol: Oral liquid multivitamin supplement for infants.

Polycythemia: Increased concentration or red blood cells (RBCs) in the blood causing thick blood.

Postnatal: Occurring after birth.

Postpartum: Occurring after delivery.

Pre-ductal oxygen saturation: Oxygen saturation in non-mixed blood before the origin of the ductus arteriosus.

Premature: Babies born at less than thirty-seven-weeks gestation.

Prenatal: Occurring before delivery.

Preterm formulas:
Similac Special Care 20 with Iron / Special Care 24 with Iron / Special Care 30 with Iron provide 20, 24, or 30 calories per ounce (or per 30 cc).
Enfamil Premature 20 with Iron / Enfamil Premature 24 with Iron / Enfamil Premature 30 provide 20, 24, and 30 calories per ounce. (See Nutritionals, page 424.)

Preterm formulas for babies with frequent spitting or reflux: Similac for Spit Up or a similar formula (which has rice starch added). Many other formulas such as Pregestimil, Nutramigen, and Alimentum may be used in varied situations.

Preterm formulas for lactose intolerant babies: Formulas such as Enfamil ProSobee (soy based) or Similac Sensitive (reduced lactose) or Similac Soy Isomil may be used.

Preterm milk fortifiers:

- Prolacta +4, +6, +8, +10 are human milk fortifiers to give extra calories per ounce and other nutrients including protein and calcium.

- Prolacta +4 will provide four extra calories per ounce.
  Similac and Enfamil human milk fortifiers give additional calories and nutrients.

Prolacta: A human milk-based fortifier—see Preterm milk fortifiers.

Prone: Lying on stomach.

Prostaglandin E1: Prostaglandin medication used to keep the PDA open in cyanotic congenital heart disease.

Pulse oximeter: A small device using a light sensor that helps determine oxygen levels. The light sensor is placed, then covered by a wrap (usually on the infant's right hand or wrist) in order to get oxygenation of the pre-ductal or unmixed blood. The device gives a measure of blood oxygen saturation. Saturations above ninety are generally acceptable in babies. In a preterm baby, saturation levels are usually maintained between 88–94%.

R

Radiant warmer: An open bed or a mobile cart that has a heat and light source and connections for other monitoring devices, and provides easy access to the infant.

Radiologist: A trained physician specializing in doing and interpreting x-rays, ultrasounds, and other procedures.

Reglan: See Metoclopramide.

Ranitidine (Zantac): Drug that inhibits stomach acid secretion.

Red blood cells: Cells in blood that carry hemoglobin, which is primarily responsible for carrying oxygen to the tissues.

Resident (Medical): Physician still in training in a specific field of medicine or surgery.

Respirator (or Ventilator): A machine that helps breathing by supplying air and oxygen under pressure via an endotracheal tube (ETT) placed in infant's windpipe or trachea.

Respiratory distress syndrome (RDS): Breathing problem in mostly premature babies with immature lungs and insufficient surfactant (a substance that lines the lung sacs and keeps them open).

Respiratory syncytial virus: A virus that causes infections of respiratory tract, a major cause of bronchiolitis and pneumonia in infants and children.

Respiratory therapist: A trained healthcare professional who assesses breathing and treats with oxygen or via minimally invasive and invasive respiratory support.

Resuscitation bed: An open bed (radiant warmer) on wheels with an overhead heating lamp and a light source, Apgar timer, a plug for recording skin temperature, suctioning equipment, and oxygen terminals that can be connected to wall suction and oxygen source.

Retina: The light-sensitive inner lining of the eye that receives visual images.

Retinopathy of prematurity: A disease affecting the retina of preterm infants. It involves rapid and irregular growth of blood vessels that can lead to bleeding and scarring of retina. This can lead to retinal detachment and blindness.

Rh disease: Blood incompatibility in the mother and baby, causing destruction of red blood cells and jaundice.

Room air resuscitation: Resuscitation with bag and mask without using any supplemental or additional oxygen.

S

Saturation (oxygen): Degree to which oxygen is bound to hemoglobin; measured as percentage with a maximum being 100 percent; over 90 percent generally viewed as acceptable saturations.

Seizures: Abnormal electrical activity of the brain causing involuntary muscle contractions and relaxation (usually of arms and legs). Seizures may be indicative of brain irritation or malformation.

Sepsis: Blood infection.

Shunt: A thin tube that drains fluid from one part of the body to another.

Small for gestational age (SGA): Newborns whose birth weight is less than tenth percentile for their gestation.

Social worker: A professional trained to help families cope with problems and crises. In the NICU, a social worker helps families access community resources and also helps in discharge planning.

Spina bifida: A birth defect involving the spinal cord that requires surgery and may result in varying degrees of paralysis.

Spinal cord: Bundles of nervous tissues that travel from base of brain in a bony canal in the backbone.

Spironolactone (Aldactone): Diuretic—helps rid the body of excess water.

Suctioning: Removal of mucus and secretions from mouth, nose, and throat using a bulb syringe or suction catheter. Suctioning can also be further qualified as "other organ suctioning," e.g., gastric (stomach) suctioning, or laryngeal suctioning (suctioning of the airways).

Sudden infant distress syndrome (SIDS): Death of an infant under one year of age during sleep with unidentifiable causes; also called crib death.

Surfactant: A substance in lungs that helps to keep air sacs open. Surfactant in a liquid form such as Curosurf, Survanta, or Infrasurf is given via the endotracheal tube (ETT) into the airway, and helps to keep the immature lung sacs or alveoli (which lack surfactant) open. Two to three doses may be given eight to twelve hours apart.

Synagis (Palvizumab): Therapy of antibodies given as monthly intramuscular injection used to help prevent a serious lung disease caused by respiratory syncytial virus (RSV) in high risk babies.

Syndrome: A combination of signs and symptoms that are together associated with a certain medical disorder.

T

Tachycardia: Rapid heart rate. Normal heart rate of a newborn is 120 to160 beats per minute.

Tachypnea: Rapid breathing. Normal respiratory rate of a newborn is 40 to 60 breaths per minute.

Teratogen: An agent (drug, chemical toxin) that can cause birth defect if a fetus is exposed to it during development.

Theophylline: Stimulates the respiratory center; used in treatment of apnea of prematurity; also used in treatment of chronic lung disease or BPD to relieve the spasm of muscles in breathing tubes or bronchi, and to dilate them.

Thrombocytopenia: Low platelets.

Thrush: Yeast infection (Candida) in babies seen as white patchy coating on tongue and gums

Topical: Applied to limited area of skin only.

TORCH: Intrauterine congenital infections: Toxoplasmosis, Other viruses, Rubella, Cytomegalovirus, and Herpes simplex virus.

Total parenteral nutrition (TPN): Provision of nutrients, i.e., proteins, carbohydrates, fats, vitamins, and minerals with water through an intravenous line.

Tracheomalacia: Trachea is unusually soft and floppy and collapses during breathing.

Transfusion: Giving blood or blood products directly into a vein or catheter.

Transient tachypnea of the newborn (TTN): Transitory rapid breathing seen in the newborn soon after delivery due to retained lung fluid.

Transillumination: A diagnostic technique for detecting a pneumothorax in an emergency. A bright light source is placed on the infant's chest. The chest area filled with air will "light up all over." This can be compared with the opposite side of the chest. This technique can also be used in other situations.

Trimester: One of the three-month periods of a normal pregnancy. Pregnancy is divided into first, second, and third trimesters.

Trisomy 21 (or Down syndrome): Chromosomal abnormality where there is an extra chromosome or related defect. Trisomy 21 is associated with facial and body dysmorphism (abnormality) and mental retardation.

Trophic feeds: Minute amount of feeds given to preterm infants to stimulate the growth of the immature gut.

Tube feeding: See Gavage feeding.

Twin-to-twin transfusion syndrome: Disease affecting identical twins. The shared placenta may give blood from one twin to the other, causing different sizes of twins.

Tylenol (Acetaminophen): Used for pain and fever reduction.

U

Ultrasound: Using high-frequency sound waves, images are obtained of an internal body structure. No radiation is involved.

Umbilical arterial catheter (UAC): A line placed directly into umbilical artery in the cord; there are two arteries and one vein in the umbilical cord.

Umbilical hernia: A skin-covered protrusion in the navel or umbilicus due to weakness in the abdominal muscles.

Umbilical vein: Vein present during fetal development that carries oxygenated blood from placenta to the fetus. There is one umbilical vein in the umbilicus.

Umbilical venous catheter (UVC): A line is placed directly into the umbilical vein in the cord, which is advanced into the inferior vena cava.

V

Vaccine: A killed or less powerful version of a bacterium or virus, given for production of antibodies, thus giving immunity.

Vancomycin: Antibiotic used to treat infections such as staphylococcal infections. Blood levels are monitored.

Vasoactive: Medications that constrict the systemic blood vessels and increase the heart contractility (the ability of the heart to contract).

Vasodilator: Opens or dilates blood vessels so that there is less resistance to flow.

Vein: Blood vessel leading to the heart.

Ventilator (Respirator): Mechanical breathing machine; types include pressure, volume, and high-frequency ventilators for individual needs.

Ventolin: Opens airways, by relaxing the muscle of the breathing tubes or bronchi.

Ventricles: Small central chambers in the brain; also the two lower chambers of the heart.

Very low birth-weight infant (VLBW): Babies less than 1,500 grams or three pounds five ounces.

Viable: A newborn potentially able to survive.

Vital signs: Temperature, heart rate, respiratory rate, and blood pressure.

Vitamin D: Given as oral drops to supplement the vitamin D in breast milk.

Vitamin K: A routine intramuscular injection of vitamin K given to all newborns to prevent bleeding.

W

Warmer: See Radiant warmer.

Wean: To gradually stop one way and start another as in weaning from a warmer, or weaning from the respirator or oxygen.

White blood cells: Cells in blood that fight infection.

WIC (Women, Infants, and Children) nutrition program: A program that helps pregnant women, new mothers, and children, providing food and nutrition as well as formula for babies.

X

X-ray: Electromagnetic waves producing images of internal body parts.

Y

Yeast infection: Infection with a fungus such as candida.

References, books, and articles of interest

Adcock, Lisa M. "Clinical Manifestations and Diagnosis of Intraventricular Hemorrhage in the Newborn." UptoDate. Wolters Kluwer. December 14, 2015. www.uptodate.com.

American Academy of Pediatrics. *Pediatric Nutrition.* 7th ed. 2014.

———— "Breastfeeding and the use of human milk." *Pediatrics* 129, no. 3 (2012): 598-601.

———— "Healthy Children." Last modified January 5, 2017. www.healthychildren.org.

———— *NICU Journal: A Parent's Journey.* 2010. Spiral-bound edition July 11, 2017.

———— "Screening Examination of Premature Infants for Retinopathy of Prematurity." *Pediatrics* 131, no. 1 (2013): 189-95.

American Academy of Pediatrics and American Heart Association. *Textbook of Neonatal Resuscitation.* 7th ed. 2016.

Avery, Gordon B., Mary Ann Fletcher, and Mhairi G. MacDonald. *Neonatology: Pathophysiology and Management of the Newborn.* 10th ed. Philadelphia: Lippincott, Williams & Wilkins, 2015.

Barr, Frederick E., and Barney S. Graham. "Respiratory Syncytial Virus Infection: Prevention." UptoDate. Wolters Kluwer. March 24, 2016. www.uptodate.com.

Bernbaum, Judy C. *Preterm Infants in Primary Care: A Guide to Office Management.* Columbus, OH: Abbott Laboratories, 2000.

Butte, Nancy F., and Alison Stuebe. "Patient Information: Maternal Health and Nutrition during Breastfeeding (Beyond the Basics)." UptoDate. Wolters Kluwer. July 6, 2016. www.uptodate. com.

Clark, David A., *Atlas of Neonatology—A Companion to Avery's Diseases of the Newborn.* W. B. Saunders Company, 2000.

Drutz, Jan E. "Hepatitis B Virus Immunization in Infants, Children and Adolescents." UptoDate. Wolters Kluwer. February 29, 2016. www.uptodate.com.

Fanaroff, Avroy A., Jonathan M. Fanaroff, and Marshall H. Klaus. *Klaus and Fanaroff's Care of the High-risk Neonate.* 6th ed. Philadelphia: Elsevier/Saunders, 2013.

Gardner, Sandra L., Brian S. Carter, Mary Enzman Hines, and Jacinto A. Hernandez. *Merenstein & Gardner's Handbook of Neonatal Intensive Care.* 8th ed. St. Louis: Elsevier, 2016.

Griffin, Ian J. "Growth Management in Preterm Infants." UptoDate. Wolters Kluwer. April 6, 2016. www.uptodate.com.

Human Milk Banking Association of North America. *2011 Best Practice for Expressing, Storing and Handling Human Milk in Hospitals, Homes, and Child Care Settings.* 3rd ed. 2011.

Kemper, Alex R. "Newborn Screening." UptoDate. Wolters Kluwer. December 16, 2015. www.uptodate.com.

Klein, Alan H., and Jill Alison Ganon. *Caring for Your Premature Baby: A Complete Resource for Parents.* New York: HarperCollins, 1998.

Lactation Education Resources. "Lactation Management Training." www.lactationtraining.com.

Mandy, George T. "Short-term Complications of the Preterm Infant." UpToDate. Wolters Kluwer. November 18, 2015. www.uptodate.com.

McCarty, Read, ed. *You Are Not Alone: 20 Stories of Hope, Heroism, Heartache, and Healing as Told by the Parents of Children Treated in the NICU.* South Weymouth, MA: Children's Medical Ventures, 1998.

Merenstein, Gerald B., and Sandra L. Gardner. *Handbook of Neonatal Intensive Care.* 8th ed. St. Louis: Mosby, 2015.

Mhairi G. MacDonald and Jayashree Ramasethu. *Atlas of Procedures in Neonatology.* 4th ed. 2017.

Paysse, Evelyn A. "Retinopathy of Prematurity." UptoDate. Wolters Kluwer. March 29, 2016. www.uptodate.com.

Prolacta Bioscience. "Give your preemie the best chance to grow strong." 2014. www.prolacta.com/premature-babies-have-increased-nutritional-needs.

Stewart, Jane. "Care of the Neonatal Intensive Care Unit Graduate." UptoDate. Wolters Kluwer. August 27, 2015. www.uptodate.com.

———. "Discharge Planning for High-Risk Newborns." UptoDate. Wolters Kluwer. September 8, 2015. www.uptodate.com.

Wagner, Carol L., and Frank R. Greer. "Prevention of Rickets and Vitamin D Deficiency in Infants, Children and Adolescents." *Pediatrics* 122, no. 5 (2008): 1142-52.

Young, Jeanine. *Developmental Care of the Premature Baby.* London: Ballière Tindall, 1996.

Zaichkin, Jeanette. *Newborn Intensive Care: What Every Parent Needs to Know.* American Academy of Pediatrics, 3rd ed. 2009.

Index

Index

Poems

Dedications to NICU Graduates

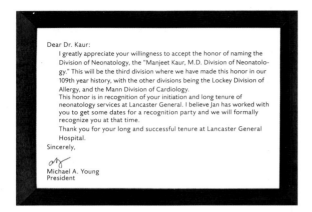

Dear Dr. Kaur:

I greatly appreciate your willingness to accept the honor of naming the Division of Neonatology, the "Manjeet Kaur, M.D. Division of Neonatology." This will be the third division where we have made this honor in our 109th year history, with the other divisions being the Lockey Division of Allergy, and the Mann Division of Cardiology.

This honor is in recognition of your initiation and long tenure of neonatology services at Lancaster General. I believe Jan has worked with you to get some dates for a recognition party and we will formally recognize you at that time.

Thank you for your long and successful tenure at Lancaster General Hospital.

Sincerely,

Michael A. Young
President

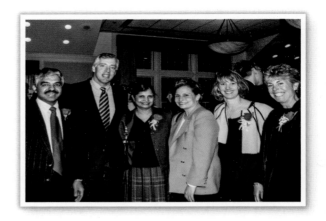

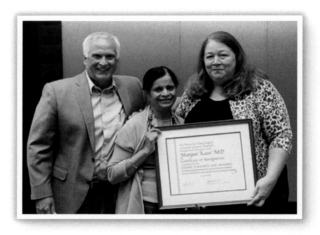

Manjeet Kaur, M.D., (center) receives the Henry S. Wentz, M.D., Award from Drs. Monty Duke and Christine Stabler. The award, named in honor of the former chair of the Department of Family and Community Medicine, is given to a member of the LG Health Medical & Dental Staff who has excelled in medical education, teaching, patient care, and service to the hospital and the community.

In 2016 the Lancaster General Health Foundation initiated the *Dr. Manjeet Kaur NICU Scholarship Fund* to honor the vital contributions that Dr. Kaur has made at Women & Babies Hospital and in our community. The scholarship will provide an annual award to assist with further training and education related to neonatal care.

The inaugural award was made to Jessica Carrier, RN, in September 2017.

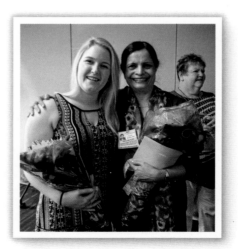